Register Now for Online Access to Your Book!

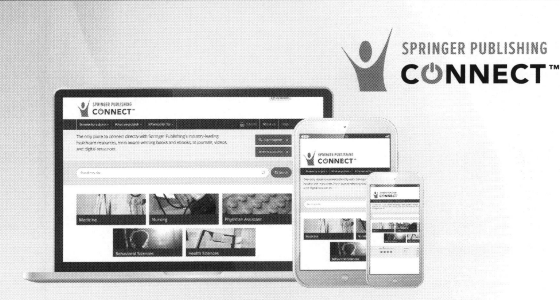

SPRINGER PUBLISHING
CONNECT™

Your print purchase of *Rural Nursing, Sixth Edition,* **includes online access to the contents of your book**—increasing accessibility, portability, and searchability!

Access today at:
http://connect.springerpub.com/content/book/978-0-8261-8364-4
or scan the QR code at the right with your smartphone. Log in or register, then click "Redeem a voucher" and use the code below.

ELRLA6P3

Scan here for quick access.

Having trouble redeeming a voucher code?
Go to https://connect.springerpub.com/redeeming-voucher-code

If you are experiencing problems accessing the digital component of this product, please contact our customer service department at cs@springerpub.com

The online access with your print purchase is available at the publisher's discretion and may be removed at any time without notice.

Publisher's Note: New and used products purchased from third-party sellers are not guaranteed for quality, authenticity, or access to any included digital components.

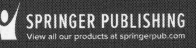

SPRINGER PUBLISHING
View all our products at springerpub.com

Rural Nursing

Charlene A. Winters, PhD, RN, FAAN, is professor emerita in the College of Nursing at Montana State University, Missoula Campus. Dr. Winters taught undergraduate and graduate courses to prepare nurses for practice in rural settings as nurse generalists, nurse leaders, and nurse practitioners. Most recently, Dr. Winters taught courses on searching, appraising, and using evidence to care for rural and vulnerable populations. She is recognized for her research on rural nursing practice, rural nursing theory development, nursing education for rural practice, adaptation to and self-management of chronic illness by rural dwellers, and response to environmental exposures in rural communities. Her research was funded by the National Institutes of Health, the Health Resources and Services Administration, and various foundations and professional organizations. She is editor or coeditor of four previous editions of *Rural Nursing*. Her research is published in numerous peer-reviewed journals. Over the years, Dr. Winters has been an active member of the Western Institute of Nursing, the Council for the Advancement of Nursing Science, the American Academy of Nursing, Sigma Theta Tau International, the American Association of Critical Care Nurses, and the National Association of Clinical Nurse Specialists. She is a charter member of the International Council of Nursing—Rural and Remote Nurses Network and the Montana Association of Clinical Nurse Specialists. Dr. Winters provided leadership as president of the Western Institute of Nursing, member of the Leadership Council for the Council for the Advancement of Nursing Science, member of the editorial boards for *Nursing Research* and *Rural and Remote Health*, contributing editor for *Critical Care Nurse*, and as a chairperson or member of several committees for the American Association of Critical Care Nurses. Dr. Winters is a Fellow in the American Academy of Nursing and the Western Institute of Nursing. She holds a doctorate in nursing from Rush University, College of Nursing, Chicago, Illinois, and baccalaureate and master's degrees in nursing from California State University, Long Beach.

Rural Nursing
Concepts, Theory, and Practice

SIXTH EDITION

Charlene A. Winters, PhD, RN, FAAN
EDITOR

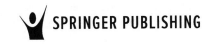 SPRINGER PUBLISHING

Copyright © 2022 Springer Publishing Company, LLC
All rights reserved.
First Springer Publishing edition 2009; subsequent editions 2013, 2018

Springer Publishing Company, LLC
11 West 42nd Street, New York, NY 10036
www.springerpub.com
connect.springerpub.com/

Acquisitions Editor: Joseph Morita
Compositor: diacriTech

ISBN: 978-0-8261-8363-7
ebook ISBN: 978-0-8261-8364-4
DOI: 10.1891/9780826183644

SUPPLEMENTS:
Instructor Materials:
Qualified instructors may request supplements by emailing textbook@springerpub.com
Instructor's Manual ISBN: 978-0-8261-6032-4
Instructor's PowerPoints ISBN: 978-0-8261-8365-1

21 22 23 24 25 / 5 4 3 2 1

Library of Congress Control Number: 2021910008

Charlene A. Winters: orcid.org/0000-0001-8033-9925

Publisher's Note: **New and used products purchased from third-party sellers are not guaranteed for quality, authenticity, or access to any included digital components.**

Cover photo: Island Lake, Beartooth Mountains, Montana. **Photographer:** Megan Hamilton, MSN, RN, CFRN, NRP, Clinical Instructor, Montana State University, College of Nursing.

Printed in the United States of America.

This text is dedicated to my mentor, Dr. Helen J. Lee, whose contributions to the health of rural persons, rural nursing practice and education, and rural nursing theory development are unmatched. Her advice and unwavering support were instrumental to the development of the sixth edition of Rural Nursing. *I am proud to call Helen my friend and colleague.*

Contents

Contributors

Julie H. Alexander-Ruff, EdD, MSN, CPNP-PC, FAAPNP   Assistant Professor, Montana State University College of Nursing, Bozeman Campus, Bozeman, Montana

Darin Bell, MD   Assistant Director of Rural Education, Family Medicine Residency Western Montana, Missoula, Montana

Robin L. Boland, MN, RN, FNP-C   Nurse Practitioner, Endocrinology, Benefis Medical Group, Benefit Health, Great Falls, Montana

Victoria L. S. Britson, PhD, APRN, CNP, FNP-BC, CNE   Family Nurse Practitioner, eSenior Care | Avera eCare, Sioux Falls, South Dakota

Robin J. Brown, PhD, RN   Assistant Professor, South Dakota State University College of Nursing, Brookings, South Dakota

Janice A. Buehler, PhD, RN   Associate Professor (Ret.), Montana State University College of Nursing, Billiings, Montana

Linda Burdette, PhD, RN   Assistant Dean and Associate Professor, South Dakota State University College of Nursing, Aberdeen, South Dakota

Yoshiko Y. Colclough, PhD, RN   Associate Professor, Montana State University College of Nursing, Bozeman Campus, Bozeman, Montana

Kee A. Dunning, MS, MEd, LCPC, LFMT   CEO of Dunning Counseling and Consulting Chief Clinician, The Tumbleweed Program, Billings, Montana.

Pamela Fahs, PhD, RN   Decker College of Nursing and Health Sciences, Decker School of Nursing, Binghamton University, Binghamton, New York

Becka Foerster, MS, RN, CNE   Lecturer, South Dakota State University College of Nursing, Brookings, South Dakota

Nicole Gibson, DNP, RN, FNP-C   Nurse Practitioner-Electrophysiology, Sioux Falls, South Dakota

Lori Hendrickx, EdD, RN, CCRN, CNL   Professor, South Dakota State University College of Nursing, Aberdeen, South Dakota

Tanis Hernandez, MSW, LCSW   Medical Social Worker, Randle, Washington, DC

Barbara B. Hobbs, PhD, RN   Professor Emerita, South Dakota State University, West River Nursing Department, Rapid City, South Dakota

Bette Ide, PhD, RN [Deceased]   Professor, University of North Dakota, College of Nursing, Grand Forks, North Dakota

Mary J. Isaacson, PhD, RN, CHPN   Associate Professor, South Dakota State University College of Nursing, Rapid City, South Dakota

Lynn Jakobs, PhD   Assistant Professor, College of Health and Human Services, School of Nursing, California State University, Fresno, California

Laurie Johansen, PhD, MS, RN, CNE, PHN   Professor and Director of Nursing, Southwest Minnesota State University, Marshall, Minnesota

Sandra W. Kuntz, PhD, RN   Associate Professor Emerita, Montana State University College of Nursing, Kalispell Campus, Helena, Montana

Helen J. Lee, PhD, RN   Professor Emerita, Montana State University College of Nursing, Missoula Campus, Missoula, Montana

Kathleen A Long, PhD, APRN, FAAN   Dean and Professor Emerita, University of Florida, College of Nursing, Gainesville, Florida

D. Dale M. Mayer, PhD, RN   Associate Professor, Montana State University College of Nursing, Missoula Campus, Missoula, Montana

Meg McDonagh, RN, MN, NP   Senior Instructor Emerita, University of Calgary Faculty of Nursing, Cochrane, Canada

Heidi A. Mennenga, PhD, RN, CNE   Associate Professor, South Dakota State University College of Nursing, Brookings, South Dakota

Kailyn Mock, MHA   Assistant Director/Nursing Initiatives, Montana Office of Rural Health and Area Health Education Center, Montana State University College of Nursing, Bozeman, Montana

Sally Moyce, PhD, RN   Assistant Professor, Montana State University College of Nursing, Bozeman Campus, Bozeman, Montana

Elizabeth Nichols, PhD, RN, FAAN   Dean and Professor Emerita, Montana State University College of Nursing, Bozeman Campus, Bozeman, Montana

Mary Kay Nissen, DNP, APRP, CNP, FNP-BC, COHN-S   Nurse Practitioner, Shenandoah Medical Clinic, Shenandoah, Iowa

Chad O'Lynn, PhD, RN, CNE, ANEF   Director of Evaluation, Chamberlain University, Lincoln City, Oregon

Amy Olson, DNP, FNP-BC, BSN   Family Nurse Practitioner, Alaska Native Tribal Health Consortium, Anchorage, Alaska

Judith Pare, PhD, RN   Director of Education Massachusetts Nurses Association, Windham, New Hampshire

Polly Petersen, PhD, RN   Associate Professor (Ret.) (Affiliate), Montana State University College of Nursing, Bozeman, Montana

Susan J. Raph, DNP, RN, NEA-BC   Clinical Professor and Associate Dean for Academic Affairs, Montana State University College of Nursing, Bozeman, Montana

K. M. Reeder, PhD, RN, FAHA   Adjunct Professor, Passan School of Nursing, Wilkes University, Cape Coral, Florida

Marlene Reimer, PhD, RN, CNN(C) [Deceased]   Professor, University of Calgary, Faculty of Nursing, Calgary, Alberta, Canada

Jane A. Schantz, MS, FNP-BC, ACHPN   Decker College of Nursing and Health Sciences, Decker School of Nursing, Binghamton University, Binghamton, New York

Jane Ellis Scharff, MN, RN   Associate Clinical Professor and Campus Director (Ret.), Montana State University College of Nursing Bozeman Campus, Bozeman, Montana

Dayle Sharp, PhD, DNP, McPH, FNP-BC, APRN   Clinical Associate Professor, Director of Family Nurse Practitioner Program, College of Health and Human Services, Department of Nursing, University of New Hampshire, Durham, New Hampshire

Jean Shreffler-Grant, PhD, RN   Professor Emerita, Montana State University College of Nursing, Missoula Campus, Missoula, Montana

Andrea D. Skrocki, MN, APRN, PMHNP-BC   Psychiatric Nurse Practitioner CPG Psychiatry, Missoula, Montana

Stacy M. Stellflug, PhD, APRN, FNP-BC   Assistant Professor and Rural Ready Nurse Practitioner, HRSA Grant Program Director, Montana State University College of Nursing, Billings Campus, Billings, Montana

Marilyn A. Swan, PhD, RN   Associate Professor, College of Allied Health and Nursing, School of Nursing, Minnesota State University, Mankato, Minnesota

Tamara L. Tasseff, PhD, RN, CHPN   Associate Chief Nurse, Veterans Health Administration, VA Black Hills Health Care System, Edgemont, South Dakota

Beth Walstrom, MEd   Research Coordinator, South Dakota State University College of Nursing, Brookings, South Dakota

Clarann Weinert, SC, PhD, RN, FAAN   Professor Emerita, Montana State University College of Nursing, Bozeman, Montana

Charlene A. Winters, PhD, RN, FAAN   Professor Emerita, Montana State University College of Nursing, Missoula Campus, Missoula, Montana

Jana G. Zwilling, PhD, APRN, FNP-C   Clinical Assistant Professor, Director, Family Nurse Practitioner Track, University of North Dakota College of Nursing and Professional Disciplines, Grand Forks, North Dakota

Foreword

Rural healthcare is a complex process where the interface of issues of access with culture, health, and health beliefs provide a challenging practice environment. *Rural Nursing: Concepts, Theory, and Practice, Sixth Edition,* is a valuable textbook and resource for those serving the healthcare needs in rural and frontier areas. Winters' text provides a critical focus on rural populations and continues to be the first-line resource toward understanding rural dwellers, the environment of rural or frontier healthcare, and nursing from multiple perspectives. Whether you are developing and disseminating knowledge about rural health and nursing, learning about rural dwellers, practicing rural nursing, or in an interdisciplinary rural practice, there is much to gain from reading this latest edition of *Rural Nursing: Concepts, Theory, and Practice.* This book highlights the realities of rural nursing from bedside to advanced practice. Theoretical perspectives, as well as new models of practice and research, are found in this edition. Winters supports rural nurses by identifying not only the challenges, but also in highlighting opportunities in rural healthcare and innovative practice.

Rural Nursing: Concepts, Theory and Practice is a critical resource on my bookshelf. This text is a staple in graduate nursing education in the rural nursing doctor of philosophy degree (PhD) and masters degree nurse practitioner programs at Binghamton University. As an editor, I feel confident that this book and the chapters within are some of the most often cited in the rural nursing literature. Winters' *Rural Nursing: Concepts, Theory and Practice, Sixth Edition,* is synonymous with rural nursing.

Pamela Stewart Fahs, PhD, RN
Professor and Dr. G. Clifford and Florence B. Decker Chair in Rural Nursing
Decker School of Nursing; Decker College of Nursing and Health Sciences,
Binghamton University
Editor-in-Chief, *Online Journal of Rural Nursing and Health Care*

Preface

The sixth edition of *Rural Nursing: Concepts, Theory, and Practice*, like the editions before it, focuses on the health of rural dwellers, the provision of healthcare in rural settings, and the skills and knowledge required for effective nursing practice, education, and research within this context. The sixth edition contains 10 new chapters, content on the effect of the coronavirus (COVID-19) on rural populations, seminal chapters on Rural Nursing Theory and rural nursing, and updated chapters retained from previous editions.

The text is divided into five sections. Section I focuses on theory and research and includes an overview of the theory development process, the seminal work on Rural Nursing Theory by Long and Weinert, an update of the theory by Lee and McDonagh, two chapters on rural nursing concepts, and chapters on conducting research in rural and frontier settings. The focus of Section II is rural nursing practice. Included in this section is Scharff's widely quoted seminal chapter on the nature and scope of rural nursing practice and three chapters that expand our understanding of the experiences of rural nurses and nurse practitioners. Section III focuses on healthcare delivery in rural settings and includes chapters on health behavior, suicide, nurses as primary care providers, emergency services, telehealth, palliative care, and complementary and alternative therapy use by rural dwellers. Section IV addresses education and provides insight into learning opportunities in rural clinical settings; interprofessional, collaborative, and transcultural service-learning education; and the skills and competencies nurses and nurse practitioners (NPs) need to care for rural populations. Section V focuses on the care of select vulnerable populations including migrant and seasonal workers, neonates experiencing opiate withdrawal, American Indians requiring palliative and end-of-life care, and the conduct of research with vulnerable populations.

The sixth edition was developed during the worldwide COVID-19 pandemic. Early in the pandemic, COVID-19 incidence was highest among residents of large metropolitan areas (Morbidity and Mortality Weekly Report [MMWR], 2020, para. 2). Largely spared during the early days of the pandemic, rural communities saw an unprecedented spike in infections and hospitalizations in September 2020. In December 2020, the prevalence of COVID-19 cases in nonmetropolitan areas was found to be greater and growing more rapidly than in metropolitan areas (Economic Research Service [ERS], 2021, para. 2); the highest COVID-19 case rates were found in farming-dependent and manufacturing-dependent counties (para 5). When compared to metropolitan residents, rural residents are older, have more underlying health problems, are un- or underinsured, reside in communities with scarce healthcare resources, and long distances to hospitals with specialists and intensive care units (ICUs). For these reasons, rural residents are thought to be more vulnerable to severe illness and death due to COVID-19 (Cromartie et al., 2020; Dobis & McGranahan, 2021). Authors of Chapters 15, 18, 21, 23, 26, and 29 address unique challenges rural communities, providers, and researchers face due to the COVID-19 pandemic.

As with the first five editions of *Rural Nursing: Concepts, Theory, and Practice*, the sixth edition again expands understanding of the rural healthcare environment; previous editions have been used by faculty preparing nurses at the baccalaureate, master, and doctoral levels. Qualified instructors may obtain access to a supplemental Instructor's Manual and PowerPoints from Springer Publishing.

THE NEED FOR RURAL NURSING THEORY AND HISTORY OF THE TEXT

The genesis of this text originated from a vision of Dr. Anna Shannon, dean of the College of Nursing at Montana State University (MSU). The first edition of the rural text was titled *Conceptual Basis for Rural Nursing* (1998). Subsequent editions were retitled, *Rural Nursing: Concepts, Theory, and Practice*. New editions continued to include material written by MSA faculty and students, while expanding to include authors from across the United States, Canada, and Australia.

Dr. Shannon (see Chapter 1) noted that early work on nursing theories placed little emphasis on environment, and when examining the literature, she found an absence of articles on rural nursing. MSU College of Nursing faculty, graduate students, administrators, and consultants committed to develop an integrated, theoretical approach to rural nursing. In 1977, the first year for the rural generalist master's program at MSU, students were required to take a course in rural nursing where a significant amount of research collaboration between students and faculty took place. To learn about rural health and healthcare, students interviewed rural persons regarding their health perceptions, needs, and practices using qualitative research methods. Participants lived in rural areas of less than 2,500 population were chosen by convenience to be interviewed, and primarily worked in the extractive industries—logging, farming, and ranching. Data were generated over several years, creating a rich database. Faculty groups were formed to examine the interview and demographic data and the student papers noting concepts that frequently emerged from the data. This qualitative material, linked with quantitative studies, led to the development of the Rural Nursing Theory first published in 1989 by Dr. Kathleen Long and Dr. Clarann Weinert (see Chapter 2). The early work on the theory conducted by Long and Weinert was built upon four assumptions:

1. Rural was defined as sparsely populated areas.
2. Healthcare needs in rural areas are different than healthcare needs in urban areas.
3. There are healthcare needs common to all rural areas.
4. Models of care that work well in urban centers are not appropriate to rural areas.

The Rural Nursing Theory is a descriptive theory noted as the "most basic type of middle-range theory" (Fawcett, 1999, p. 15). It describes specific characteristics and observations made of rural persons seeking healthcare and their healthcare providers. The published theory contains three theoretical statements and several key concepts (see Chapter 2). What Drs. Long, Weinert, and Shannon knew is that available evidence, that is, research data, an understanding of context and resources, an understanding of healthcare providers' practice and expertise, as well as rural persons' perceptions of health and healthcare, are critical to the provision of evidence-based practice and research in rural settings.

WHY FOCUS ON RURAL?

The number of persons living in rural areas is significant. Rural areas in the United States are home to 14% of the population and occupy 72% of the land mass (Economic Research Service [ERS], 2020). Urban areas (UA) and urban clusters (UC) contain most of the population but occupy only about 3% of the land area in the United States.

Rural areas are important to the economy. Rural industries center around resource-based activities (agriculture, forestry, and mining), recreation, manufacturing, and processing (food, wood, and mining products) industries with known risks to health. The importance of the impact of rural America led President Obama to form the White House Rural Council (White House, 2011).

Rural persons are a vulnerable population. In the opening pages of the first edition of this text (Lee, 1998), Dr. Helen Lee provided a wonderful description of one area of western Montana. The description brought into focus several characteristics thought to describe rural areas . . . wide open spaces, remoteness, distance from large urban settlements, beautiful vistas, sparsely populated areas, farming economies, clean water and air, and healthful living. All over the world, romantic connotations are associated with rural and the rural lifestyle. However, these images do not portray rural accurately. Rural areas, like UAs, are multidimensional and persons living there experience problems.

In the United States, rural persons tend to be older, less educated, and in poorer health when compared to their urban counterparts. They are more likely to earn minimum wage, and lack transportation and access to healthcare providers and other healthcare resources. Rural dwellers experience poorer health and social welfare outcomes than urban dwellers in the areas of mental health, substance abuse, public health, and oral health. The National Advisory Committee on Rural Health and Human Services (Health Resources & Services Administration [HRSA], 2020) was chartered in 1987 to advise the U.S. Secretary of Health and Human Services on the ways to address healthcare problems in rural America. Reports have identified obesity, unhealthy lifestyle, poor access to specialized health and social services, increased healthcare costs, absent telehealth, and suicide, among other significant issues facing rural dwellers. Although rural areas are predominately White, there is ethnic and racial diversity (African American, Hispanic, Asian, and Native American) and vulnerable subpopulations (migrant and seasonal workers and homeless) who generally experience poorer outcomes than rural Whites. Currently, the coronavirus pandemic (COVID-19) has disproportionately affected persons of color in rural and urban communities.

The authors hope readers will find the latest edition thought provoking and useful in their clinical practice, teaching efforts, and research activities.

Charlene A. Winters

REFERENCES

Cromartie, J., Dobis, E. A., Krumel, T. P., McGranahan, D., & Pender, J. (2020). *Rural America at a glance: 2020 edition*. Economic Research Service. U.S. Department of Agriculture. https://www.ers.usda.gov/webdocs/publications/100089/eib-221.pdf?v=4110

Dobis, E. A., & McGranahan, D. (2021). *Rural residents appear to be more vulnerable to serious infection or death from coronavirus COVID-19*. Economic Research Service. https://www.ers.usda.gov/amber-waves/2021/february/rural-residents-appear-to-be-more-vulnerable-to-serious-infection-or-death-from-coronavirus-covid-19/

Economic Research Service, U.S. Department of Agriculture. (2020). *Population & migration: Overview.* https://www.ers.usda.gov/topics/rural-economy-population/population-migration/

Economic Research Service, U.S. Department of Agriculture. (2021). *The COVID-19 pandemic and rural America.* https://www.ers.usda.gov/covid-19/rural-america/

Fawcett, J. (1999). *The relationship of theory and research* (3rd ed.). F. A. Davis.

Health Resources & Services Administration. (2020). *Federal advisory committees. National Advisory Committee on Rural Health & Human Services.* https://www.hrsa.gov/advisory-committees/rural-health/index.html

Lee, H. J. (Ed.). (1998). *Conceptual basis for rural nursing.* Springer Publishing Company.

Morbidity and Mortality Weekly Report. (2020). COVID-19 stats: COVID-19 incidence, by Urban-Rural Classification—United States, January 22–October 31, 2020. *MMWR Morbidity and Mortality Weekly Report, 69*(46), 1753. http://dx.doi.org/10.15585/mmwr.mm6946a6

White House. (2011). *White house rural council.* https://obamawhitehouse.archives.gov/administration/eop/rural-council/executive-order

Qualified instructors may obtain access to a supplementary Instructor's Manual and PowerPoints by emailing textbook@springerpub.com.

Acknowledgments

I want to acknowledge the work of the many colleagues, students, consultants, and research participants whose contributions made this text possible.

SECTION I

Rural Nursing Theory and Research

Section 1 opens with an updated chapter that features the history of the development of the Rural Nursing Theory (RNT). The beginning work at the College of Nursing at Montana State University is featured and followed by a summary of the ongoing work and recommendations for future work. Chapter 2 is the seminal chapter, Rural Nursing: Developing Theory Base (Long and Weinert), which first appeared in the nursing literature in 1989 and has been a part of the previous five editions of this book. An updated Chapter 3 contains the analyzed concepts included in the RNT chapter. Chapter 4 was updated for the sixth edition. The authors examined rural nursing research for the latest findings about concepts contained in the theoretical statements, which led them to recommend changes for two of the three theoretical statements in the original RNT. Lack of anonymity is the topic of Chapter 5, updated for this edition; the authors considered the effect of modern technology on the concept and its related concepts of privacy, familiarity, and confidentially. Chapter 6 is a new chapter that provides insights for conducting research in rural and frontier setting. Chapter 7 was updated for this edition and provides a blueprint for a focused program of research in rural settings. Multiple researchers, distance between the researchers involved, funding from multiple agencies, and the development of an instrument to measure health literacy are considered.

CHAPTER 1

Rural Nursing Theory: Past, Present, and Future

HELEN J. LEE AND CHARLENE A. WINTERS

DISCUSSION TOPICS

- Discuss the strategies you might use to initiate and sustain theory development with your colleagues.
- Identify the areas within rural nursing theory (RNT) that need further development. Identify the specific strategies to address those needs.
- Identify the real-world learning experiences for students, which allow them to explore health needs and perceptions of rural persons from numerous rural groups.

INTRODUCTION

For this sixth edition of *Rural Nursing: Concepts, Theory, and Practice*, we believe it is important to take a step back and detail the history that led to the development of the theory. We also believe it is critical to provide direction to further its development. Therefore, the purpose of this chapter is to provide the (a) history, context, and assumptions; (b) current status and studies; and (c) future directions and needed research of the rural nursing theory (RNT). The historical content is divided into three phases.

HISTORY, CONTEXT, AND ASSUMPTIONS

Within the United States, the average population density is 87.4 persons per square mile (U.S. Census Bureau, 2019) and most persons live in cities. Most states contain rural areas, even New Jersey, where the population density is the highest in the United States at nearly 1,200 individuals per square mile. In contrast, based on 2017 U.S. Census Bureau estimates (Worldatlas, 2017), six states have fewer than 20 persons per square mile (Table 1.1). Montana ranks third in the population density list.

TABLE 1.1 Least Densely Populated States in the United States

Rank	State	Persons/Square Mile
1	Alaska	1.3
2	Wyoming	6.0
3	Montana	6.8–7.1[1]
4	North Dakota	11.0
5	South Dakota	11.3
6	New Mexico	17.2

In 1975, Montana State University (MSU) recruited Anna M. Shannon, a native Montanan, to be the dean of the College of Nursing. Dr. Shannon was convinced that nursing practice in a rural environment was different from that in an urban place. Dr. Shannon also noted paucity in the numbers of articles pertaining to *rural* nursing in the literature base. The articles available were from sociology; the content examined the characteristics of young women entering the nursing profession.

Phase 1 (1977–1998)

Dean Shannon and two faculty members, Drs. Jacqueline Taylor (anthropologist) and Ruth Ludemann (sociologist) wrote federal grant applications to fund the rural generalist master's program beginning in 1977. MSU is a land grant university. The College of Nursing is a state-wide program; the main campus is located in Bozeman and at that time the extended campuses were located in Great Falls, Billings, Butte, and Missoula. Undergraduate students started their nursing courses in Bozeman and then transferred to the extended campuses for clinical courses. A four-quarter master's program was available at the Bozeman campus; students could enroll in adult, family–child, and psychiatric nursing.

Initially, the new graduate rural nursing program rotated around the College of Nursing's campus sites. The length of the program was five quarters. A thesis was required. For two of the rural core nursing courses, students were assigned to select a rural or remote community; in the first course, the community was to be described visually and structurally (population, governance, occupations, and healthcare availability). In the second course, titled *Rural Nursing*, the students interviewed 10 to 12 persons in the chosen community about their perceptions of their health and their healthcare. Course paperwork for both classes was reports of the findings of both activities. Participants were engaged primarily in the extractive industries—farming, ranching, and logging. Procedures for protection of human subjects were followed.[2]

In the spring of 1982, a podium presentation titled *Sparsely Populated Areas: Towards Nursing Theory* was given to the Western Council on Higher Education, a regional nursing research organization now called the Western Institute of Nursing (WIN). Introduced by College of Nursing Dean Shannon, the presentation's purpose was to demonstrate how a nursing school could "maximize its resources, provide opportunities for faculty and student research, and contribute ... to the development of an empirically based theory of nursing" (pp. 70–71). Dr. Taylor (1982) organized the presentation that included

---

1. Estimates may differ based on different data sources.

2. Community and interview data collection were supported in part by U.S. Department of Health and Services, Division of Nursing, Advanced Training Grant to Montana State University Grant (#1816001649AI).

faculty and graduate students' studies about the (a) role of distance in home dialysis, (b) sodium in drinking water and adolescent blood pressure, and (c) beliefs and practices of Crow Indian women, Hmong refugees, and Hutterite colony members. Her concluding remarks included a plan for theory construction and testing using retroduction, a process that includes both inductive and deductive reasoning.

Using the procedures described earlier, the faculty and student groups continued gathering data for the theory base using the student interviews, the community data they collected, and the student papers describing the health beliefs, values, and practices of the rural participants interviewed. Concepts emerging from the data included *health status, health beliefs, isolation, distance, self-reliance, lack of anonymity, familiarity, insider/outsider, old timer/newcomer, and informal healthcare systems.*

In 1983, Dr. Clarann Weinert developed a survey to validate the emerging concepts. Instruments used in the quantitative study and the constructs measured are listed in Table 1.2.

A convenience sample of 62 persons (40 women, 22 men) from 13 sparsely populated counties in Montana responded to the survey. The mean age of the sample was 61.3 years of age; the mean education year was 13.5 years. The survey data were analyzed to inform the qualitative data through the emerging concepts.

Rural Nursing: Developing the Theory Base, by Drs. Kathleen A. Long and Clarann Weinert, was published in 1989 (see a reprint of this paper in Chapter 2 in this text). The assumptions of the emerging theory guided the process: (a) *Rural* was defined as sparsely populated; the entire state of Montana was considered sparsely populated despite the population centers that existed within the state. (b) Healthcare needs of rural environments are different from healthcare needs in urban settings. (c) All rural areas have common needs. (d) Urban models of healthcare are not appropriate or adequate for rural areas.

Three theoretical statements were proposed. The first two statements pertain to rural persons. The first states that rural persons "define health primarily as the ability to work, to be productive and do usual tasks" (Long & Weinert, 1989, p. 120). The second statement indicates that "rural persons are self-reliant and resist seeking help from those seen as 'outsiders' or from agencies seen as national or regional 'welfare' programs" (p. 120). A corollary to the second statement was that healthcare is usually sought through the informal rather than the formal system. The third statement applies to rural healthcare providers (HCPs): they "must deal with a lack of anonymity and much greater role diffusion than providers in urban or suburban settings" (p. 119).

Concepts related to the first statement include *health beliefs, work beliefs,* and *health-seeking behavior. Isolation* and *distance* were the two concepts that assisted in understanding health-seeking behavior of rural individuals. Despite living long distances from healthcare facilities, rural individuals did not view themselves as isolated.

Related to the second theoretical statement are the concepts of *self-reliance* and *independence.* The desire to care for oneself was common among the interviewed rural individuals.

TABLE 1.2 Survey Instruments and Constructs

General Health Perception Scale	Physical health status and health beliefs (Davies & Ware, 1981)
Personal Resource Questionnaire	Informal systems for support and healthcare (Brandt & Weinert, 1981)
Trait Anxiety Scale	Mental health status (Spielberger et al., 1970)
Beck Depression Inventory	Mental health status (Beck, 1967)

Lack of anonymity is a major concept for the providers of nursing and healthcare in a rural environment. Closely associated with practice in a rural area are the related concepts of *old-timer/newcomer* and *insider/outsider*. These interrelated concepts guide rural individuals' interactions and relationships with nurses and other HCPs.

Following the publication of Long and Weinert's (1989) article about the RNT base (see a reprint of this paper in Chapter 2 in this text), several MSU faculty members committed to continue work on the theory. Enrolled graduate nursing students continued choosing and describing rural communities and interviewing their residents regarding their health perceptions. A concurrent activity began during this time; interested graduate students and nursing faculty began analyzing the concepts that emerged during the RNT process. Several students developed their community interviews into theses. These along with concept analyses papers became chapters in *Conceptual Basis for Rural Nursing*, a publication edited by Dr. Helen Lee (1998).[3] The text ultimately became the first of the subsequent editions of *Rural Nursing: Concepts, Theory, and Practice*.

Phase 2 (1999–2006)

MSU College of Nursing faculty, Drs. Helen J. Lee and Charlene A. Winters, continued the theory work through the teaching of the rural nursing course in the graduate nursing curriculum. Presentations about the theory, the concepts, and the faculty–student collaboration were accepted at several Communicating Nursing Research Conferences sponsored by WIN, the Western regional nursing research organization (2001, 2002, and 2004).

During this time, three events led to the formation of a collaborative effort with nurse researchers in Canada. The first was an independent activity project and visit by Meg K. McDonagh from the University of Calgary to explore the emerging RNT work at MSU. The second and third events were the attendance of the core MSU faculty at two conferences, a Canadian Rural Conference in Saskatoon, Saskatchewan, Canada, and the Rural Nursing Research Conference in Binghamton, New York. The collaboration occurred with nurse researchers of the Faculty of Nursing, University of Calgary (Elizabeth H. Tomlinson, Meg K. McDonagh, Dana S. Edge, and Marlene A Reimer). Chad O'Lynn joined the MSU group of researchers. The work, titled North American Study (NAS) Group, led to the appointment of Dr. Winters as a visiting scholar at the University of Calgary Faculty of Nursing and a comparison study conducted across international borders about rural/remote health beliefs between participants in Montana and the Canadian provinces of Alberta and Manitoba. The purposes of NAS were to (a) validate existing RNT concepts, (b) explore new emerging concepts, and (c) determine the areas for further theoretical development and research.

Following the activity of the comparison study group (Winters et al., 2016), the NAS group made these recommendations regarding RNT:

1. Concepts
   a. Add identified new concepts to RNT: *health-seeking behavior* and *choices* (residence, HCP).
   b. Most concept analyses were incomplete and the new concepts identified needed to be developed.
   c. It was noted that validation of all the concepts was needed.

---

3. Funding sources for the publication of *Conceptual Basis for Rural Nursing* was a monetary grant received from the Montana Consortium for Excellence in Healthcare. The Consortium also funded, in part, the content of two chapters within the text. The grant award was facilitated by Jane E. Scharff.

2. These issues arose during the analysis of the data and require further exploration as to their fit with RNT
   a. Economic
   b. Aging communities
   c. Environmental exposure to chemicals, injury from animals, and safety with regard to driving and farm/ranch work injuries.

Dr. Helen Lee and Ms. McDonagh conducted an extensive review of literature that supported or refuted the RNT theoretical statements and concepts. They found that:

> The rural residents' definition of health in the first descriptive statement is changing from that of a functional nature to a more holistic view that includes physical, mental, social, and spiritual aspects. The self-reliance of rural residents in the second relational statement is broadly supported; however, the resistance to seeking help from those seen as 'outsiders' is changing. The third relational statement pertaining to HCPs and their lack of anonymity and role diffusion is supported. The findings for the concept of distance in the original rural theory development work are not supported. This literature appraisal of the rural nursing theory base structure supports a need for change. (Lee & Winters, 2006, p. 24; also see Chapter 4 in this text)

At the end of this phase, Drs. Lee and Winters published the textbook, *Rural Nursing: Concepts, Theory, and Practice* (2006). The Springer Publishers considered it the second edition of *Conceptual Basis for Rural Nursing*. The change in title more accurately reflected the direction of the changing content of the book.

Phase 3 (2007–2012)

The NAS researchers determined that the third relational statement about rural nursing practice would be the next focus of the RNT research group. A study was designed to explore the degree to which nurses and health professionals working in rural and remote settings access and use health research in practice; it was called the Rural Nurse Research Access (RRA) study. The study was initiated with a pilot study in Montana to develop a questionnaire and was conducted in collaboration with graduate nursing students enrolled in the rural nursing course. The qualitative work consisted of a windshield survey of nine rural communities with populations of 3,000 or less and located 50 miles or more from an urban setting. The semistructured interviews were conducted by 29 rural nurses (age range 31–72; years in nursing 3–50; 11 were baccalaureate prepared and eight were associate degree graduates; 21 were employed in critical access hospitals [CAHs]). Verbatim transcripts and field notes were analyzed for common themes. The RRA qualitative findings from the pilot study showed that participants (a) equated the word research with gathering information, an activity that was done two to three times a day to two to three times a month, (b) considered research a workplace activity, (c) stated that their primary sources for health research information were colleagues (managers, staff nurses, and physicians), and (d) used the Internet, if available.

Based on the initial questionnaire findings from the pilot study, a comparative analysis was done with published studies in the literature and revisions were made. Subsequently, the finalized survey instrument was used in Canada to explore practices and attitudes with a mix of healthcare workers including nurses, physicians, and social workers.

Since the U.S. members of the RRA group wanted to focus their study on nurses, the survey was sent to registered nurses working in rural areas in three states—Montana,

Oregon, and South Dakota. Human subject procedures were completed for the institutions involved in all three states. The names of participants were obtained through state boards of nursing files. Nurses working in rural counties (Rural–Urban Continuum Codes 6–9, U.S. Department of Agriculture, 2007) were the targeted recipients of the survey questionnaire. There was a response rate of 61% (Koessl et al., 2010).

The demographics of the RRA quantitative study participants were as follows:

- Their ages ranged from 41 to 60 years.
- Sixty percent had a university degree.
- Sixty percent were employed full time.
- Forty percent were employed in a hospital-based practice.
- More than 50% had been practicing for more than 20 years.
- Less than 50% were practicing in a rural/remote setting.
- Sixty percent did not practice in the same community in which they lived.

The RRA study survey participants indicated that the evidence most frequently used was "a personal experience of caring for patients/clients over time" and "information that I learn about each patient/client as an individual," actions that are consistent with evidence-based practice (EBP; O'Lynn et al., 2009, p. 40; Melnyk et al., 2010). They ranked low-level evidence sources as most commonly used, and were least likely to use a research journal. When compared to Olade (2004), the survey participants were (a) more likely to have used research in the last year, (b) less likely to use more research if they could, and (c) unlikely to use research if it contradicted institutional policy or common sense. Their ability to evaluate research quality was lacking. The perception of practice as evidence-based was higher in younger nurses; 71.5% in nurses less than 30 years of age as compared to 22.2% in those 60 years of age and older (Koessl et al., 2010).

Members of the research team for this study were Helen Lee, Jean Shreffler-Grant, Charlene Winters, and Susan Luparell from MSU; Dana S. Edge, Meg McDonagh, Lianna Barnieh, and Elizabeth "Betty" Tomlinson from University of Calgary; Chad O'Lynn from the University of Portland; and Lori Hendrickx from South Dakota State University.[4]

During this phase, Dr. Lee retired from teaching. The *Rural Nursing: Concepts, Theory, and Practice*, the third edition (2010) by Drs. Winters and Lee was published. This edition contained an update of the RNT from Dr. Lee and Ms. McDonagh to include clearly revised theoretical statements.

1. Rural residents define health as being able to do what they want to do; it is a way of life and a state of mind; there is a goal of maintaining balance in all aspects of their lives.

   Older rural residents and those with ties to extractive industries are more likely to define health in a functional manner—to work, to be productive, and to do the usual tasks.

2. Rural residents are self-reliant and make decisions to seek care for illness, sickness, or injury depending on their self-assessment of the severity of their present health condition and of the resources needed and available. Rural residents with infants and children who experience illness, sickness, or injury will seek care more quickly than for themselves (Lee & McDonagh, 2010, p. 27).

---

4. Funding sources for the phases of the RRA study included MSU College of Nursing grant, Sigma Theta Tau International, Zeta Upsilon Chapter (Montana state wide chapter), Sigma Theta Tau, Omicron Chapter (University of Portland), and South Dakota State University College of Nursing Intramural Funding.

Present Activity (2013–Present)

Dr. Winters continued to teach the rural nursing course as previously described through 2013. After that time, the course was broadened to focus on vulnerable populations; however, rural remained a significant focus within the course. The fourth edition of *Rural Nursing: Concepts, Theory, and Practice* (Winters, 2013) was published with an increased number of international authors. The fourth and fifth editions (Winters & Lee, 2018) expanded to include authors from across the United States. As with the previous editions, the focus was on explicating the concepts and propositions that guide nursing practice, rural healthcare delivery issues, and understanding the characteristics and behaviors of rural persons. Winters stated at a Community Forum for Nursing at South Dakota State University and Sanford USD Medical Center (2012) that:

> *What Drs. Long, Weinert, and Shannon knew is that research data, an understanding of context and resources, as well as rural perceptions of health and healthcare were critical to the provision of EBP. Together, these items constitute the available evidence that should drive rural clinical practice. The rural evidence base is in line with the American Nurses Association (ANA) and other nursing organizations mandate for our EBP interventions.*

The American Nurses Association (ANA) standards of nursing practice and professional performance mandate the use of evidence-based interventions and the integration of research findings into practice (2004). EBP is a problem-solving approach to the delivery of healthcare that integrates the best evidence from well-designed studies and patient care data, and combines it with patient preferences and values, combined with clinical expertise (Melnyk et al., 2010). The Institute of Medicine maintained that EBP is a core competency that every healthcare clinician should have to meet the needs of the 21st-century healthcare system (Greiner & Knebel, 2003). To achieve EBP as a core competency requires improved communication and collaboration, shared responsibility, synchrony of efforts, drawing close clinical research and practice, and an engaged public.

To facilitate rural research and practice (a) there must be an integration of rural experiences in nursing education, (b) nursing students must be recruited from rural settings, and (c) nursing education must be delivered from rural settings (Bushy & Leipert, 2005). Strategies to integrate research and EBP projects require course assignments, collaboration with clinical partners on research applicable to clinical practice, and provision of networking and educational opportunities–academic/clinical partnerships (Miller et al., 2009).

Dr. Winters and her faculty colleagues have worked to increase collaboration efforts in western Montana. Groups, students (high school, undergraduate, and graduate), and faculty collaboration included the following:

- *High school students and faculty collaboration*: MSU researchers collaborated with a Libby Montana high school science teacher and students enrolled in a research elective on a community-based participatory research study conducted in Libby (Kuntz et al., 2009; Winters et al., 2008). The faculty presented a class on research process. Human subjects and research protocol training were provided. In the class, there was discussion and approval of a research proposal. A survey was developed and community-based data collection took place. Students were provided a report of the survey findings. Drs. Winters and Kuntz were the faculty mentors.
- *Undergraduate nursing students and faculty collaboration*: To explore community members' understanding of and interest in research, undergraduate MSU nursing students interviewed residents of Libby, Montana, as part of a community-based

participatory research project (Winters et al., 2008). The interviews informed the research study and also served as an assignment in the students' senior-level community health nursing course. Dr. Kuntz was the faculty mentor.

- *Undergraduate nursing students and faculty collaboration in a clinical course*: To compare body mass index (BMI) of school children in Missoula, Montana, student teams used the compiled data in support of the Coordinated Approach to the Child Health program. Dr. Sandy Kuntz was the faculty mentor.
- *Undergraduate nursing students and faculty collaboration in a research course*: Students in Missoula, Montana, collaborated with hospital nurses and a faculty mentor to test whether hospital procedures for nasogastric tube placement and chest tube dressing changes were evidence based. Dr. Dorothy (Dale) Mayer was the faculty mentor.
- *Graduate nursing students and faculty collaboration*: Students conducted a secondary analysis of previously collected qualitative data to explore the rural context and women's self-management of chronic health conditions. Dr. Winters was the faculty mentor.
- *Graduate nursing students and faculty collaboration*: Students enrolled in a vulnerable population course selected a rural community, vulnerable subpopulation, and health-related issue to explore throughout the semester from the individual, provider, and health system perspective. Students searched and appraised the literature, conducted community and systems assessments, and interviewed individuals as part of the learning experience. Dr. Winters was the faculty mentor.

From each of these experiences, students and faculty learn valuable information about rural communities and rural persons that inform RNT, practice, and research.[5]

FUTURE DIRECTIONS

The collaborative work of MSU faculty in the above-mentioned EBP activities represents brief examples of the total number of activities occurring in the MSU College of Nursing. The examples with undergraduate students originated from one College of Nursing campus in western Montana. Collaboration with faculty members from other campuses in the MSU College of Nursing system would be ideal. Reinstating the RNT work group that existed in earlier years to conduct secondary analyses of qualitative data collected by graduate nursing students enrolled in the vulnerable populations course would provide valuable insight into current rural health issues. MSU is collecting funds to support an endowed research chair within the College of Nursing. When that goal is finally realized, may the rich heritage of this work on RNT be a stepping-stone for future work!

As indicated earlier, toward the conclusion of the comparative analysis across borders study, the NAS investigators identified a blueprint of work that was needed related to RNT development:

- Develop and test instruments to measure the concepts.
- Test the theoretical and relational statements.

5. Funding sources for the phases of the RRA study included MSU College of Nursing grant, Sigma Theta Tau International, Zeta Upsilon Chapter (Montana state wide chapter), Sigma Theta Tau, Omicron Chapter (University of Portland), and South Dakota State University College of Nursing Intramural Funding.

- Compare and contrast the health perceptions and needs of persons living in differing rural cultures and environments:
  - American Indians and Aboriginal peoples.
  - Rural and remote persons in other areas in the United States, Canada, and elsewhere
  - Urban, former urban, and other rural subpopulations
- Compare and contrast the health perceptions and needs of persons of differing circumstances:
  - Ill and well populations
  - Old-timers and newcomers
  - Young and old
  - The urban poor
- Target research on the third relational statement:
  - Effect of technology on generalist role, role diffusion, and professional isolation.
  - Explore gender differences.

The NAS group generated the following research questions:

1. Are the health-seeking behaviors identified unique to rural residents?
2. How do health-seeking behaviors differ from those of health promotion?
3. How do illness variables affect rural persons' health-seeking behaviors? Choice of HCP?
4. What variables affect rural persons' acceptance of "outside" services/HCP?
5. Do various rural groups define health differently?

The above-mentioned needs and questions are still relevant for the RNT work that needs to be done today.

CONCLUSION

More than 40 years have passed since the initial work on RNT began. The RNT base as published is in need of revision. Advances in health service and communication technologies, healthcare practices, along with changes in the perceptions and behaviors of rural residents over the past four decades may account for the emerging concepts identified. The work identified and the generation of additional theoretical statements will increase the potential of generating a middle range theory pertaining to the healthcare of rural persons. Relevance of rural nursing will likely be measured by the ability to evolve and change as new knowledge shapes it.

REFERENCES

American Nurses Association. (2004). *Scope and standards of practice*. Author.

Beck, A. (1967). *Depression: Causes and treatment*. University of Pennsylvania Press.

Brandt, P., & Weinert, C. (1981). The PRQ: A social support measure. *Nursing Research, 30*, 277–280.

Bushy, A., & Leipert, B. (2005). Factors that influence students in choosing rural nursing practice: A pilot study. *Rural and Remote Health, 5*, 387. http://rrh.deakin.edu.au

Davies, A., & Ware, J. (1981). *Measuring health perceptions in the health insurance experiment*. RAND.

Greiner, A. C., & Knebel, E.(Eds.). (2003). *Health professions education: A bridge to quality*. National Academies Press. http://www.nap.edu/catalog/10681.html

Koessl, B. D., Winters, C. A., Lee, H. J., & Hendrickx, L. (2010). Rural nurses' attitudes and beliefs toward evidence-based practice. In C. A. Winters & H. J. Lee (Eds.), *Rural nursing: Concepts, theory, and practice* (3th ed., pp. 327–344). Springer Publishing Company.

Kuntz, S. W., Winters, C. A., Hill, W., Weinert, C., Rowse, K., Hernandez, T., & Black, B. (2009). Rural public health policy models to address an evolving environmental asbestos disaster. *Public Health Nursing, 26*(1), 70–78. https://doi-org.proxybz.lib.montana.edu/10.1111/j.1525-1446.2008.00755.x

Lee, H. J. (Ed.). (1998). *Conceptual basis for rural nursing*. Springer Publishing Company.

Lee, H. J., & McDonagh, M. K. (2010). Updating the rural nursing theory base. In C. A. Winters & H. J. Lee (Eds.), *Rural nursing: Concepts, theory, and practice* (3rd ed., pp. 19–39). Springer Publishing Company.

Lee, H. J., & Winters, C. A. (Eds.). (2006). *Rural nursing: Concepts, theory, and practice* (2nd ed.). Springer Publishing Company.

Long, K. A., & Weinert, C. (1989). Rural nursing: Developing the theory base. *Scholarly Inquiry for Nursing Practice: An International Journal, 3*, 113–127.

Melnyk, B. M., Fineout-Overholt, E., Stillwell, S. B., & Williamson, K. M. (2010). The seven steps of evidence-based practice. *American Journal of Nursing, 110*(1), 51–53. https://doi.org/10.1097/01.NAJ.0000366056.06605.d2

Miller, J., Bryant MacLean, L., Coward, P., & Broemeling, A. M. (2009). Developing strategies to enhance health capacity in a predominantly rural Canadian health authority. *Rural and Remote Health, 9*, 1266. https://doi.org/10.22605/RRH1266

Olade, P. (2004). Evidence-based practice and research utilization activities among rural nurses. *Journal of Nursing Scholarship, 36*(3), 220–225. https://doi-org.proxybz.lib.montana.edu/10.1111/j.1547-5069.2004.04041.x

O'Lynn, C., Luparell, S., Winters, C. A., Shreffler-Grant, J., Lee, H. J., & Hendrickx, L. (2009). Rural nurses' research use. *Online Journal of Rural Nursing and Health Care, 9*(1), 34–45. https://doi.org/10.14574/ojrnhc.v9i1.103

Shannon, A. (1982). Introduction: Nursing in sparsely populated areas. In J. Taylor, Sparsely populated areas: Toward nursing theory. *Western Journal of Nursing Research, 4*(3), 70–71.

Spielberger, C., Gorsuch, R., & Lushene, R. (1970). *STAI manual for the State-Trait Anxiety Questionnaire*. Consulting Psychologist.

Taylor, J. (1982). Sparsely populated areas: Toward nursing theory. *Western Journal of Nursing Research, 4*(3), 69–77.

U.S. Census Bureau. (2019). *Quick facts: Montana*. https://www.census.gov/quickfacts/table/PST045216/30,00

U.S. Department of Agriculture Economic Research Service. (2007). *Rural-urban continuum codes*. https://www.ers.usda.gov/data-products/rural-urban-continuum-codes

Winters, C. A. (2012, April). *Rural nursing theory & nursing research: Developing evidence-based care for rural dwellers*. Presentation at a Community Forum for Nursing, South Dakota State University & Sanford USD Medical Center, Sioux Falls, SD.

Winters, C. A. (Ed.). (2013). *Rural nursing: Concepts, theory, and practice* (4th ed.). Springer Publishing Company.

Winters, C. A., Kuntz, S. W., Weinert, C., & Rowse, K. (2008). *Exploring research communication & engagement in a rural community: The Libby Partnership Initiative*. National Institutes of Health/National Institute of Nursing Research. [1R03NR011242–01].

Winters, C. A., & Lee, H. J. (2018). *Rural nursing: Concepts, theory, and practice* (5th ed.). Springer Publishing Company.

Winters, C. A., & Lee, H. J. (Eds.). (2010). *Rural nursing: Concepts, theory, and practice* (3th ed.). Springer Publishing Company.

Winters, C. A., Thomlinson, E. H., O'Lynn, C., Lee, H. L., McDonagh, M. K., Edge, D. S., & Reimer, M. A. (2006). Exploring rural nursing across borders. In H. J. Lee & C. A. Winters (Eds.), *Rural nursing: Concepts, theory and practice* (2nd ed., pp. 27–39). Springer Publishing Company.

Worldatlas. (2017). *Least densely populated U.S. states*. http://www.worldatlas.com/articles/least-densely-populated-u-s-states.html

CHAPTER 2

Rural Nursing: Developing the Theory Base[1]

KATHLEEN A. LONG AND CLARANN WEINERT

DISCUSSION TOPICS

- Select a rural or frontier community to explore. Conduct a windshield survey of the community, gather epidemiographic data about the community, and interview residents to further define both the common and the locale-specific conditions and characteristics of the rural populations. Compare and contrast the findings with concepts identified by Long and Weinert.
- Design strategies to tailor the formal healthcare system to suit the preferences of rural persons for family and community help during times of illness and injury.
- Identify the opportunities to reduce professional isolation and increase professional networking for advanced practice nurses working in rural and frontier settings.

INTRODUCTION

A logger suffering from "heart lock" does not have a cardiovascular abnormality. He is suffering from a work-related anxiety disorder and can be assisted by an ED nurse who accurately assesses his needs and responds with effective communication and a supportive interpersonal relationship. A farmer who has lost his finger in a grain thresher several hours earlier does not have time during the harvesting season for a discussion of occupational safety. He will cope with his injury assisted by a clinic nurse who can adjust the timing of his antibiotic doses to fit with his work schedule in the fields.

---

1. From Long, K. A., & Weinert, C. (1989). Rural nursing: Developing the theory base. *Scholarly Inquiry for Nursing Practice: An International Journal, 3*, 113–127. Copyright 1989 by Springer Publishing Company. Reprinted with permission.

Many healthcare needs of rural dwellers cannot be adequately addressed by the application of nursing models developed in urban or suburban areas, but require unique approaches emphasizing the special needs of this population. Although nurses are significant, and frequently the sole healthcare providers for people living in rural areas, little has been written to guide the practice of rural nursing. The literature provides vignettes and individual descriptions, but there is a need for an integrated, theoretical approach to rural nursing.

Rural nursing is defined as the provision of healthcare by professional nurses to persons living in sparsely populated areas. Over the last 8 years, graduate students and faculty members at the Montana State University College of Nursing have worked toward developing a theory base for rural nursing. Theory development has used primarily a retroductive approach, and data have been collected and refined using a combination of qualitative and quantitative methods. The experiences of rural residents and rural nurses have guided the identification of key concepts relevant to rural nursing. The goal of the theory-building process has been to identify commonalities and differences in nursing practice across all rural areas and the common and unique elements of rural nursing in relation to nursing overall. The implications of developing a theory of rural nursing for practice have been examined as a part of the ongoing process.

The theory-building process was initiated in the late 1970s. At that time, literature and research related to rural healthcare were limited and focused primarily on the problem of retaining physicians in rural areas and providing assessments of rural healthcare needs and prescriptions for rural healthcare services based on models and experiences from urban and suburban areas (Coward, 1977; Flax et al., 1979). The unique health problems and healthcare needs of extremely sparsely populated states, such as Montana, had not been addressed from the perspective of the rural consumer. No organized theoretical base for guiding rural healthcare practice in general, or rural nursing in particular, existed.

QUALITATIVE DATA

The target population for qualitative data collection was the people of Montana. Montana, the fourth largest state in the United States, is an extremely sparsely populated state, with nearly 800,000 people and an average population density of approximately five persons per square mile. One-half of the counties in Montana have three or fewer persons per square mile, with six of those counties having less than one person per square mile. There is only one metropolitan center in the state; it is a city of nearly 70,000 people, with a surrounding area that constitutes a center of approximately 100,000 (Montana State University Center for Data Systems and Analysis, 1985).

Qualitative data were collected through ethnographic study by Montana State University College of Nursing graduate students. These data provided the initial ideas about health and healthcare in Montana. Since general propositions about rural health and rural healthcare did not exist, gathering of concrete data was the first step toward the subsequent development of more general theoretical propositions.

Graduate students used ethnographic techniques as described by Spradley (1979) to gather information from individuals, families, and healthcare providers. Interview sites were selected by students on the basis of specific interest and convenience. During a 6-year period, data were gathered from approximately 25 locations. In general, each student worked in depth in one community, collecting data from 10 to 20 informants over a period of at least 1 year. Data were gathered primarily from persons in ranching and farming areas and from towns of less than 2,500 persons. In some instances, student interest's led to extensive interviews with specific rural subgroups, such as men in the logging industry or older residents in a rural town (Weinert & Long, 1987). Open-ended interview questions were developed using Spradley's guidelines. The questions emphasized seeking the informants' views without superimposing the cultural biases of the interviewer. The opening question in the interview was, "What is health to you ... from your viewpoint? ... your definition?" Interviewers used standard probes and a standard format of questions regarding health beliefs and healthcare preferences.

Spradley (1979) indicated that the goal of ethnographic study is to "build a systematic understanding of all human cultures from the perspective of those who have learned them" (p. 10). The goal of data collection in Montana was to learn about the culture of rural Montanans from rural Montanans. Emphasis in the cultural learning process was on understanding health beliefs, values, and practices. Rigdon et al. (1987) have noted that understanding the meaning that persons attach to subjective experiences is an important aspect of nursing knowledge. The ethnographic approach captured the meanings that rural dwellers ascribe to the subjective states of health and illness and facilitated the development of a rich database.

As the database developed, the following definitions and assumptions were accepted as a foundation for theory development. "Rural" was defined as meaning sparsely populated. Within this context, states such as Montana, which are sparsely populated overall, are viewed as rural throughout, despite the existence of some population centers within them. Further, based on this definition, rural regions or areas can be identified within otherwise heavily populated states. An assumption is made that, to some degree, healthcare needs are different in rural areas from those of urban areas. Also, all rural areas are viewed as having some common healthcare needs. Finally, another assumption is made that urban models are not appropriate to, or adequate for, meeting healthcare needs in rural areas.

RETRODUCTIVE THEORY GENERATION

Faculty work groups were developed to examine and organize the qualitative data. The work groups involved three to five nursing faculty members, each with rural nursing experience, but with varied backgrounds and expertise. Thus, a work group included experts from various clinical areas, as well as persons with direct experience either in small rural hospitals or in larger metropolitan centers within rural states. Standard ethnographic content analysis (Spradley, 1979) was used to sort and categorize the ethnographic data. Groups worked toward consensus about the meaning and organization of specific data. Recurring themes were identified and viewed as having relevance and importance for the rural informants in relation to their views of health.

A retroductive approach, as originally described by Hanson (1958), was used for examining the initial ethnographic data and to build the theory base. Specific concepts and relational statements were derived from the data, and more general propositions were induced from these statements. The new propositions were then used for developing additional specific statements that could be supported by existing data or were categorized for later testing. The retroductive approach was literally a "back-and-forth" process that permitted persons familiar with the data to move between the data and beginning-level theoretical propositions. The process was orderly and consistent, and required group consensus about data interpretation and the relevance of derived propositions. The retroductive process continued in work groups over several years as additional ethnographic data were gathered. Consultants participated at key points in the process, to raise questions, add insights, and critically evaluate the group's theory-building approach. Walker and Avant (1983) have noted that the retroductive process "adds considerably to the body of theoretical knowledge. It is, in fact, the way theory develops in the 'real world'" (p. 176).

QUANTITATIVE DATA

Following several years of ethnographic study, the faculty members involved in theory development wished to enrich the qualitative database by collecting relevant quantitative data. Kleinman (1983) stated, "Qualitative description, taken together with various quantitative measures, can be a standardized research method for assessing validity. It is especially valuable in studying social and cultural significance, for example, illness beliefs interaction norms, social gain, ethnic help seeking, and treatment responses" (p. 543). Hinds and Young (1987) noted, "The combination of different methodologies within a single study promotes the likelihood of uncovering multiple dimensions of a phenomenon's empirical reality" (p. 195).

A survey developed by Weinert in 1983 attempted to validate some of the rural health concepts that had emerged from the ethnographic data. These concepts were health status and health beliefs, isolation and distance, self-reliance, and informal healthcare systems. Survey instruments with established psychometric properties were selected to measure the specific concepts of interest. A mail questionnaire completed by the respondents included the Beck Depression Inventory (Beck, 1967) and the Trait Anxiety Scale (Spielberger et al., 1970) to tap mental health status, and the General Health Perception Scale (Davies & Ware, 1981) to measure physical health status and health beliefs. A background information form assessed demographic variables, including the period of residence and geographic locale. The Personal Resource Questionnaire (Brandt & Weinert, 1981) assessed the use of informal systems for support and healthcare.

The convenience sample of survey participants was located through the agricultural extension service, social groups, and informal networks. All the participants lived in Montana completed the questionnaires in their homes, and returned them by mail to the researcher. The 62 survey participants were middle-class Whites, with an average of 13.5 years of education and a mean age of 61.3 years, who had lived in Montana for an average period of 45.6 years. The survey sample consisted of 40 women and 22 men residing in one of the 13 sparsely populated Montana counties. The most populated county has a population density of 5.9 persons per square mile, and one town of nearly 6,000 people. In the most sparsely populated county, there is one town with 600 people and an average population density of 0.5 persons per square mile.

Findings from the quantitative study were used throughout the theory development process to support or refute concept descriptions and relational statements derived from the ethnographic data. Survey findings are discussed in the following section as they relate to key concepts and relational statements.

REFINING THE BUILDING BLOCKS OF THEORY

To order the data and foster the formation of relational statements, an organizational scheme for theory development was adopted. Using the paradigm first described by Yura and Torres (1975) and later by Fawcett (1984), ethnographic data were categorized under the four major dimensions of nursing theory: person, health, environment, and nursing. The data were then ordered from the more general to the more specific. This process led to the identification of constructs, concepts, variables, and indicators.

An example helps in illustrating this process. Ethnographic data had been gathered from "gypo" loggers. These men are independent logging contractors from northwestern Montana who work in rugged isolated areas, usually living in trailers or tents while working. Examples of quotes from these loggers and their associates as found in the data: A logger states, "We worry about the here and now;" a local physician says, "Loggers enter the healthcare system during times of crisis only;" and the public health nurse in the area says, "Loggers don't want to hear about healthcare problems; they don't return until the next accident." Table 2.1 shows the scheme used for organizing these data.

The concepts "present time" orientation and crisis orientation to health are identified. These are placed under the person dimension. In this example, the constructs are not fully developed, but are viewed as either psychological or sociocultural, or both. The important variables identified thus far are definitions of time and of crisis. Possible indicators are measures of time, such as hours or seasons, and measures of crisis, such as numbers of illnesses or injuries.

Key Concepts

In the process of data organization, it was noted that some concepts appeared repeatedly in ethnographic data collected in several different areas of the state. In addition, aspects of several of these concepts were supported by the quantitative survey data (Weinert, 1983). Using Walker and Avant's (1983) model of concept synthesis, these concepts were identified as key concepts in relation to understanding rural health needs and rural nursing practice. These key concepts are as follows: work beliefs and health beliefs, isolation and distance, self-reliance, lack of anonymity, outsider/insider, and old-timer/newcomer.

As key concepts in this theory, work beliefs and health beliefs are viewed differently in rural dwellers as contrasted with urban or suburban residents. These two sets of beliefs appear to be closely interrelated among rural persons. Work or fulfilling one's usual functions is of primary importance. Health is assessed by rural people in relation to work role and work activities, and health needs are usually secondary to work needs.

The related concepts of isolation and distance are identified as important in understanding rural health and nursing. Specifically, they help in understanding healthcare-seeking behavior. Quantitative survey data indicated that rural informants who lived outside towns traveled a distance of almost 23 miles, on an average, for emergency healthcare, and over 50 miles for routine healthcare. Despite these distances, ethnographic data indicated that rural dwellers tended to see health services as accessible and did not view themselves as isolated.

TABLE 2.1. Data Ordering Scheme

Dimension	Psychological/sociocultural
Concept	"Present time" orientation
	Crisis orientation to health
Variable	Definitions of time
	Definitions of crisis
Indicator	Hours, minutes, days
	Seasons, work seasons
	Number of injuries
	Number of illnesses

Self-reliance and independence of rural persons are also seen as key concepts. The desire to do for oneself and care for oneself was strong among the rural persons interviewed; this has important ramifications in relation to the provision of healthcare.

Two key concept areas, lack of anonymity and outsider/insider, have particular relevance to the practice of rural nursing. Lack of anonymity, a hallmark of small towns and surrounding sparsely populated areas, implies a limited ability for rural persons to have private areas of their lives. Rural nurses almost always reported being known to their patients as neighbors, as part of a given family, as members of a certain church, and so on. Similarly, these nurses usually know their patients in several different social and personal relationships beyond the nurse–patient relationship. The old-timer/newcomer concept, or the related concept of outsider/insider, is relevant in terms of the acceptance of nurses and of all healthcare providers in rural communities. The ethnographic data indicated that these concepts were used by rural dwellers in organizing their view of the social environment and in guiding their interactions and relationships. Survey data revealed that those who had lived in Montana for over 10 years, but less than 20 years, still considered themselves to be "newcomers" and expected to be viewed as such by those in their community (Weinert & Long, 1987).

Relational Statements

In an effort to move from a purely descriptive theory to a beginning-level explanatory one, some initial relational statements were generated from the qualitative data and were supported by the quantitative data that had been collected thus far. The statements are in the early stages of testing.

The first statement is that rural dwellers define health primarily as the ability to work, to be productive, and to do usual tasks. The ethnographic data indicate that rural persons place little emphasis on the comfort, cosmetic, and life-prolonging aspects of health. One is viewed as healthy when he or she is able to function and is productive in one's work role. Specifically, rural residents indicated that pain was tolerated, often for extended periods, so long as it did not interfere with the ability to function. The General Health Perception Scale indicated that rural survey participants reported experiencing less pain than an age-comparable urban sample (Weinert & Long, 1987). Further, scores on the Beck Depression Inventory and the Trait Anxiety Scale (Weinert, 1983) revealed that they experienced less anxiety and less depression.

The second statement is that rural dwellers are self-reliant and resist accepting help or services from those seen as "outsiders" or from agencies seen as national or regional "welfare" programs. A corollary to this statement is that help, including needed healthcare, is usually sought through an informal rather than a formal system. Ethnographic data supported both the second statement and its corollary. Numerous references were found to show, for example, a preference for "the 'old doc' who knows us" over the new specialist who was unfamiliar. Data from the Personal Resource Questionnaire (Weinert, 1983) indicated that rural dwellers relied primarily on family, relatives, and close friends for help and support. Further, the rural survey respondents reported using healthcare professionals and formal human service agencies much less frequently than did comparable urban respondents in previous studies.

A third statement is that healthcare providers in rural areas must deal with a lack of anonymity and a much greater role diffusion than providers in urban or suburban settings. This statement has a marked significance for rural nursing practice. Although limited ethnographic and survey data have been collected from rural nurses thus far, some emerging themes have been identified. In addition to identifying a sense of isolation from professional peers, rural nurses emphasize their lack of anonymity and a sense of role diffusion. There is an inability to keep separate the activities and the behaviors of the individual nurse's various roles. In a small town, for example, the nurse's behavior as a wife, a mother, and a church attendee are all significantly related to her effectiveness as a healthcare professional in that community. Further, in their professional role, nurses reported experiencing role diffusion. Nurses are expected to perform a variety of diverse and unrelated tasks. During a single shift, a nurse may work in obstetrics delivering a baby, care for a dying patient on the medical–surgical unit, and initiate care of a trauma patient in the ED. Likewise, during an evening shift or on weekends, a nurse may be required to carry out tasks reserved for the pharmacist or dietitian on the day shift.

RELATIONSHIP OF CONCEPTS AND STATEMENTS TO THE LARGER BODY OF NURSING KNOWLEDGE

How people define health and illness has a direct impact on how they seek and use healthcare services and is a key concept in understanding client behavior and in planning intervention.

Definition of Health

The rural Montana dwellers defined health primarily as the ability to work and to be productive. The work of other researchers supports the finding that residents of sparsely populated areas view health in terms of ability to work and to remain productive. Ross (1982), a nurse anthropologist, studied the health perceptions of women living in the Lake District along the coast of Nova Scotia. She conducted in-depth interviews with 60 women of both British and French backgrounds in small coastal fishing communities. Similar to the rural dwellers in Montana, these women described good health as being "able to do what you want to do" and to be "able to work." Lee's (1991) recent work in Montana supports earlier findings on which the rural nursing theory was built. She found that work and health practices were closely related among farmers and ranchers; health is viewed as a functional state in relation to work. Scharff's (1987) interviews with nurses practicing in small rural hospitals in eastern Washington, northern Idaho, and western Montana indicated that they viewed the health needs of rural people as overlapping those of people living in urban situations in many instances. The nurse informants, however, noted that rural people equate health with the ability to work or function in their daily activities. Rural people were viewed as delaying healthcare until they were very ill, thus often needing hospitalization at the point of seeking care.

Self-Reliance

The statement derived from the Montana data that "rural dwellers resist accepting help from outsiders or strangers" has been supported by data from research in rural Maryland (Salisbury State College, 1986). People living in the rural eastern shore area were described as highly resistant to care from persons viewed as outsiders, and rural shore residents often refused to go "across the bridge" to Baltimore to seek healthcare, even though this was a trip of less than 100 miles and would allow access to sophisticated, specialized treatment. Like the rural people in Montana, these Maryland residents sought healthcare information and assistance from local, and often informal, sources.

The self-reliance of rural persons and their resistance to outside help were also reported by Counts and Boyle (1987) in relation to the residents of the Appalachian area. Self-reliance was noted as a major feature that must be considered in planning nursing care services for this population.

The rural Nova Scotia women studied by Ross (1982) indicated informal personal networks of family, friends, and neighbors as important sources of health information who also provided the physical, financial, emotional, and social support that contributed to well-being. When these women were asked what connection there was between health and the availability of hospitals, doctors, and other medical care, 42% indicated that health knowledge and care was the individual's responsibility; 25% thought professionals were useful to a certain point in providing advice and services such as routine physical exams; 19% indicated that these services were for sick persons, not healthy persons; and 9% felt the formal healthcare system had no relationship to health (Ross, 1982, p. 311). One woman commented, "Health is not a topic to discuss with doctors and nurses" (Ross, 1982, p. 309).

Rural Nursing

The Montana data and the theory derived from it indicate that nurses and other health-care providers in rural areas must deal with a lack of anonymity. Nurses are known in a variety of roles to their patients, and in turn, know their patients in a variety of roles. Most of the nurses interviewed by Scharff (1987) felt that by knowing their patients personally they could give better care. Other nurses, however, noted that providing professional care for family or friends can be a frightening experience. Nurses indicated that there was no anonymity for them in the rural community, which at times was reassuring and at other times, constricting (Scharff, 1987).

The concept of role diffusion in the rural hospital setting was very apparent in Scharff's (1987) work. She reported that a rural hospital nurse must be a jack-of-all-trades who often practices within the realm of numerous other healthcare disciplines, including respiratory therapy, laboratory technology, dietetics, pharmacy, social work, psychology, and medicine. Examples of the intersections between rural nursing and other disciplines include doing EKGs, performing arterial punctures, running blood gas machines, drawing blood, setting up cultures, going to the pharmacy to pour drugs, going to the local drugstore to get medications for patients, ordering x-rays and medications, delivering babies, directing the actions of physicians, and cooking meals when the cook gets snowed in. As Scharff noted, some of these functions are carried out by urban nurses practicing in particular settings such as a trauma center or an ICU. Rural nurses, however, are usually not circumscribed by assignment to a particular unit or department and are expected to function in multiple roles, even during one work shift.

This generalist work role and the lack of anonymity of rural nurses are substantiated by findings and descriptions from several other rural areas of the United States (Biegel, 1983; St. Clair et al., 1986). A study of nurses in rural Texas noted, "Nurses play roles as nurse, friend, neighbor, citizen, and family member" within a community; further, rural nurses in their work roles were described as needing to be "all things to all people" (St. Clair et al., 1986, p. 28).

Generalizability

The issue of a situation or locale-specific theory and its relationship to the larger body of nursing knowledge needs serious consideration. The work of Scharff (1987) indicated that the core of rural nursing is not different from that of urban nursing. The intersections, however, those "meeting points at which nursing extends its practice into the domains of other professions"; the dimensions, that is, the "philosophy, responsibilities, functions, roles, and skills"; and the boundaries that "respond to new and growing needs and demands from society" (American Nurses Association, 1980) appear to be very distinct for rural nursing practice.

Questions still remain as to how generalizable findings from Montana residents are to other rural populations. Clearly, there is a need for more organized and rigorous data collection in relation to rural nursing before these questions can be answered. A sound theory base for rural practice requires a continued research, conducted across diverse rural settings.

IMPLICATIONS FOR NURSING PRACTICE

The findings from the Montana research about people living in sparsely populated areas have implications for nursing practice in rural areas. Since work is of major importance to rural people, healthcare must fit within work schedules. Healthcare programs or clinics that conflict with the rural economic cycle, such as haying or calving, will not be used. Since health is defined as the ability to work, health promotion must address the work issue. For example, health education related to cardiovascular disease should highlight the strategies for preventing conditions that involve long-term disability such as stroke. These aspects will be more meaningful to rural dwellers than preventive aspects that emphasize a longer, more comfortable life.

The self-reliance of rural dwellers has specific nursing implications. Rural people often delay seeking healthcare until they are gravely ill or incapacitated. Nursing approaches need to address two distinct aspects: nonjudgmental intervention for those who undergo a delayed treatment and a strong emphasis on imparting knowledge of preventive health. If the nurse can provide adequate information regarding health, the rural dwellers' desire for self-reliance may lead to health-promotion behaviors. With a good information base, rural people can make appropriate decisions regarding self-care versus the need for professional intervention.

Healthcare services must be tailored to suit the preferences of rural persons for family and community help during periods of illness. Nurses can provide instruction, support, and relief to family members and neighbors, who are often the primary care providers for sick and disabled persons.

The formal healthcare system needs to fit into the informal helping system in rural areas. A long-term community resident, such as the drugstore proprietor, can be assisted in providing accurate advice to residents through the provision of reference materials and a telephone backup system. One can anticipate greater acceptance and use by rural residents of an updated but old and trusted healthcare resource, rather than a new professional but "outsider" service (Weinert & Long, 1987).

Nurses who enter rural communities must allow for extended periods prior to acceptance. Involvement in diverse community activities, such as civic organizations and recreational clubs, may assist the nurse in being known and accepted as a person. In rural communities, acceptance as a healthcare professional is often tied to personal acceptance. Thus, it appears that rural communities are not appropriate practice settings for nurses who prefer to maintain entirely separate professional and personal lives.

The stresses that appear to affect nurses in rural practice settings have particular importance. Rural nurses see themselves as cutoff from the professional mainstream. They are often in situations where there is no collegial support to assist in defining an appropriate practice role and its boundaries. The educational preparation of those who wish to practice in rural settings needs to emphasize not only generalist skills, but also a strong base in change theory and leadership techniques. Nurses in rural practice need a sound orientation to techniques for accessing diverse sources of current information. If the closest library is several hundred miles away, for example, can all arrangements for interlibrary loan and access to material via telephone, bus, or mail be arranged? Networks that link together nurses practicing in distant rural sites are particularly useful, both for information exchange and for mutual support.

CONCLUSION

It is becoming increasingly clear that rural dwellers have distinct definitions of health. Their healthcare needs require approaches that differ significantly from urban and suburban populations. Subcultural values, norms, and beliefs play key roles in how rural people define health and from whom they seek advice and care. These values and beliefs, combined with the realities of rural living— such as weather, distance, and isolation— markedly affect the practice of nursing in rural settings. Additional ethnographic and quantitative data are needed to further define both the common and the locale-specific conditions and characteristics of rural populations. Continued research can provide a more solid base for the nursing theory that is required to guide the practice and the delivery of healthcare to rural populations.

ACKNOWLEDGMENTS

Qualitative data collected and analyzed by the Montana State University College of Nursing graduate students and faculty form the basis for a substantial portion of this chapter. Ethnographic data collection and analysis were supported, in part, by a U.S. Department of Health and Human Services, Division of Nursing, and Advanced Training Grant to the Montana State University College of Nursing (#1816001649AI). The project that provided the survey data was funded by a Montana State University Faculty Research/Creativity Grant. This chapter is based partially on a paper presented at the Western Society for Research in Nursing Conference, Tempe, Arizona, on May 1987.

REFERENCES

American Nurses Association. (1980). *Nursing. A social policy statement* (No. NP-6320M9/82R). Author.
Beck, A. (1967). *Depression: Causes and treatment*. University of Pennsylvania Press.
Biegel, A. (1983). Toward a definition of rural nursing. *Home Health Care Nursing, 1*, 45–46. https://doi.org/10.1097/00004045-198309000-00012
Brandt, P., & Weinert, C. (1981). The PRQ: A social support measure. *Nursing Research, 30*, 277–280. https://doi.org/10.1097/00006199-198109000-00007
Counts, M., & Boyle, J. (1987). Nursing, health and policy within a community context. *Advances in Nursing Science, 9*, 12–23. https://doi.org/10.1097/00012272-198704000-00009
Coward, R. (1977). Delivering social services in small towns and rural communities. In R. Coward (Ed.), *Rural families across the life span: Implications for community programming* (pp. 1–17). Indiana Cooperative Extension Services.
Davies, A., & Ware, J. (1981). *Measuring health perceptions in the health insurance experiment*. RAND.

Fawcett, J. (1984). *Analysis and evaluation of conceptual models of nursing*. F. A. Davis.

Flax, J., Wagenfeld, M., Ivens, R., & Weiss, R. (1979). *Mental health and rural America: An overview, and annotated bibliography*. U.S. Government Printing Office.

Hanson, N. (1958). *Patterns of discovery*. Cambridge University Press.

Hinds, P., & Young, K. (1987). A triangulation of methods and paradigms to study nurse-given wellness care. *Nursing Research, 36*, 195–198. https://doi.org/10.1097/00006199-198705000-00025

Kleinman, A. (1983). The cultural meanings and social uses of illness: A role for medical anthropology and clinically oriented social science in the development of primary care theory and research. *Journal of Family Practice, 16*, 539–545.

Lee, H. J. (1991). Relationship of hardiness and current life events to perceived health and rural adults. *Research in Nursing and Health. 14*(5), 351–359. https://doi.org/10.1002/nur.4770140506

Montana State University Center for Data Systems and Analysis. (1985). *Population profiles of Montana counties: 1980*. Author.

Rigdon, I., Clayton, B., & Diamond, M. (1987). Toward a theory of helpfulness for the elderly bereaved: An invitation to a new life. *Advances in Nursing Science, 9*, 32–43. https://doi.org/10.1097/00012272-198701000-00007

Ross, H. (1982). *Women and wellness: Defining, attaining, and maintaining health in Eastern Canada*. [Doctoral dissertation, University of Washington]. Dissertation Abstracts International, 42, DEO 82–12624.

Salisbury State College. (1986, June). *Discussion of Salisbury State College rural health findings*. Proceedings from Contemporary Issues in Rural Health Conference, Salisbury, Maryland.

Scharff, J. (1987). *The nature and scope of rural nursing: Distinctive characteristics*. Unpublished master's thesis, Montana State University, Bozeman, Montana.

Spielberger, C., Gorsuch, R., & Lushene, R. (1970). *STAI manual for the State-Trait anxiety questionnaire*. Consulting Psychologist.

Spradley, J. (1979). *The ethnographic interview*. Holt, Rinehart, & Winston.

St. Clair, C., Pickard, M., & Harlow, K. (1986). Continuing education for self-actualization: Building a plan for rural nurses. *Journal of Continuing Education in Nursing, 17*, 27–31.

Walker, L., & Avant, K. (1983). *Strategies for theory construction in nursing*. Appleton-Century-Crofts.

Weinert, C. (1983). *Social support: Rural people in their new middle years*. Unpublished raw data. College of Nursing. Montana State University, Bozeman, MT.

Weinert, C., & Long, K. (1987). Understanding the health care needs of rural families. *Journal of Family Relations, 36*, 450–455. https://doi.org/10.2307/584499

Yura, H., & Torres, G. (1975). *Today's conceptual frameworks with the baccalaureate nursing programs* (NLN Pub. No. 15–1558, pp. 17–75). National League for Nursing.

CHAPTER 3

Concept Analysis

HELEN J. LEE, CHARLENE A. WINTERS, ROBIN L. BOLAND,
SUSAN J. RAPH, AND JANICE A. BUEHLER

DISCUSSION TOPICS

- In the Swan and Hobbs (2017) concept analysis of lack of anonymity, the consequences of the concept include familiarity, privacy, and anonymity. Select another concept and determine the linkages between it and other identified rural nursing concepts.
- Select a concept, look at the attributes listed, and list potential empirical referents that might be used to measure the concept.
- The concept of work beliefs has yet to be analyzed. What search terms would you select to begin your search?

INTRODUCTION

Long and Weinert (1989) stated that during the initial "process of data organization … some concepts appeared repeatedly in the ethnographic data collected in several different areas of the state" (p. 118; also see Chapter 2). Following the initial publication of their article in 1989, faculty in the Rural Nursing Theory Special Committee within the Montana State University (MSU)-Bozeman College of Nursing embarked on a plan to analyze identified concepts. The committee's efforts were enhanced through coursework involvement of graduate nursing students enrolled in the MSU College of Nursing's rural generalist program. The purpose of this chapter is to summarize the analyzed concepts contained in *Conceptual Basis of Rural Nursing* (Lee, 1998), other conducted relevant research (Boland & Lee, 2006; Raph & Buehler, 2006), and the concept analysis work on lack of anonymity (Swan & Hobbs, 2017). The summary provides a quick reference of the analyzed concepts and allows for easy identification of areas needing further work.

THE CONCEPTS AND THEORETICAL STATEMENTS

The concepts are organized according to the framework provided in the rural nursing theory base. Following each theoretical statement are concept summaries pertinent to that statement. Each concept summary is presented using the analysis framework selected by the chapter authors from *Conceptual Basis of Rural Nursing* (Lee, 1998). Elements of the framework, whether explicit or implicit, contained in the chapters are presented; elements not evident are indicated by statements such as "none given" or "not identified."

First Statement: How Rural Dwellers Define Health

The first statement is that

> ... *rural dwellers define health primarily as the ability to work, to be productive, to do usual tasks" (Long & Weinert, 1989, p. 120).*

Work beliefs and health beliefs were key concepts; isolation and distance were identified as related concepts. Health beliefs, isolation, and distance were three of the four concepts analyzed.

HEALTH BELIEFS (LONG, 1993)

Method of analysis: Smith's (1983) four models of health—clinical, role performance, adaptive, and eudaemonistic.

Definition: Rural dwellers often conceptualize health within the role performance model (Long, 1993).

Defining attributes:

1. "Ability to work ... [and] perform one's daily activities" (p. 124)
2. "Determine health needs primarily in relation to work activities" (p. 124)
3. "As a result of their environment, rural dwellers are more frequently called upon to be independent and self-reliant" (p. 124)

Antecedents: Beliefs held will affect "health-promotion behaviors, healthcare seeking, and acceptance of preventive and treatment interventions" (p. 123).

Consequences: Knowledge of client's concept of health is important for the development of relevant and acceptable assessment approaches and intervention strategies (p. 123).

Empirical referents: Not identified.

ISOLATION (LEE ET AL., 1998)

Method of analysis: Wilson's method (Walker & Avant, 1995)

Definition: None given.

Essential attributes:

1. Separation—"Being divided from the rest" (Lee et al., 1998, p. 69)
2. Relativeness—"Something dependent on external conditions for its specific nature ... existing or having its specific nature only by relation to something else; not absolute or independent" (p. 69)
3. Perception—"Consciousness or awareness" (p. 69)

Antecedents: "Presence of an indicator directing attention to the condition of isolation (geographical terrain, distance, changes imposed by weather, economic costs, time, or personal preference)" (p. 69).

Consequences: "Decreased communication or interaction with other individuals that results in social or professional isolation" (p. 70).

Empirical referents: Not identified.

DISTANCE (HENSON ET AL., 1998)

Method of analysis: Wilson's method (Walker & Avant, 1988)

Definition: "Implies a degree of separation between two or more entities. ... The nature of separation may be in space, time or behavior" (Henson et al., 1998, p. 51).

Essential attributes:

1. Mileage—"Total number of miles traveled" (p. 56)
2. Time—"Measurement in minutes it takes to travel from one place to another" (p. 56)
3. Perception—"Variation in awareness of data that is different from others' awareness" (p. 56)

Antecedent: "Access to healthcare" (p. 58)

Consequence: "Potential for compromised healthcare" (p. 58)

Empirical referents:

1. Objective
   a. "Distance" (miles, kilometers; p. 58)
   b. "Travel time" (p. 58)
   c. MSU Rurality Index (county of residence population, distance to emergency care; Weinert & Boik, 1995)
2. Subjective
   a. "Perception" (Henson et al., 1998, p. 58)

Second Statement: Self-Reliance

The second statement is that

> ... rural dwellers are self-reliant and resist accepting help or services from those seen as "outsiders" or from agencies seen as national or regional "welfare" programs. A corollary to this statement is that help, including needed healthcare, is usually sought through an informal rather than a formal system. (Long & Weinert, 1989, p. 120)

Key concepts analyzed were self-reliance, outsider, insider, old-timer, newcomer, resources, informal networks, and lay care network.

SELF-RELIANCE (CHAFEY ET AL., 1998)

Method of analysis: Qualitative research inquiry (Morse, 1995)

Definition:

1. "The capacity to provide for one's own needs" (Agich, 1993, as cited in Chafey et al., 1998, p. 158)
2. "The desire to do for oneself and care for oneself" (Long & Weinert, 1989, p. 119)

Sample: Cohort of nine women between 70 and 85 years of age, living in small rural towns.

Data collection: Interview using structured guide developed to elicit participants' perceptions of self-reliance (Chafey et al., 1998, p. 160).

Characteristics:

1. Primary
   a. Learned—"A skill emanating from previous learning events that started in their youth (family chores and assumption of responsibilities), continued into adulthood, and was reinforced by later life events (retirement, death of a parent or spouse)" (p. 162)
   b. Decisional choice—"Making one's own decisions and choices" (p. 164)
   c. Independence—"Independence or dependence on self, dependence on others, self-assertion or freedom of action, and self-identity" (p. 166)
2. Secondary—Embodied an aspect of their self-reliance experience.
   a. Self-confidence (p. 170)
   b. Self-competence (pp. 170–171)

OUTSIDER (BAILEY, 1998)
Method of analysis: Wilson's method (Walker & Avant, 1988)

Definition: "Being exterior to the group, matter, or boundary in question" (Bailey, 1998, p. 140)

Defining attributes:

1. Differentness—"In terms of cultural orientation, standards, lifestyle, education, religion, occupation, social status, worldview, interests, or experience"; "the quality or state of being different" (pp. 143–144)
2. Unfamiliarity—With the matter in question (p. 144)
3. Unconnectedness—"Having no family or personal ties" (p. 144)

Antecedents: "Lacking understanding or knowledge of the social context, beliefs, rituals, customs, and history of the community" (p. 144).

Consequences: "One may be excluded from access to knowledge and information, not be accepted, not be recognized, be isolated, and be distrusted" (p. 144).

Empirical referents: Not identified.

INSIDER (MYERS, 1998)
Method of analysis: Wilson's method (Walker & Avant, 1995)

Definition: "Someone who is a member of a group and has access to special or privileged information" (Myers, 1998, p. 127).

Defining attributes:

1. "Member of a group" (p. 132)
2. "Having access to privileged information" (p. 132)
3. "An awareness of implicit assumptions and social context" (p. 132)
4. "A long-time occupant" (p. 132)

Antecedents: "Acceptance by the group" (p. 135)

Consequences:

1. "Power ... because of having information that others lack" (p. 135)
2. "Reserved social position ... that is unavailable to others" (p. 135)
3. "Lack of objectivity" (p. 135)
4. "Committed to the group" (p. 135)

Empirical referents: Not identified.

OLD-TIMER (CANIPAROLI, 1998)

Method of analysis: Wilson's method (Walker & Avant, 1995)

Definition:

1. "One who is long established in a place or position" (Caniparoli, 1998, p. 103)
2. "A man who has lived in the county a long time" (American slang, 1968, as cited in Caniparoli, 1998, p. 103)

Defining attributes:

1. "Age" (p. 108)
2. "Length of time spent in a community" (p. 108)
3. "Establishment of a relationship within the community" (p. 108)

Antecedents: "Identification as an old-timer" (p. 110)

Consequences: "Establishes a relationship within the community ... [that] can be viewed as positive or negative depending on the role of the viewer" (p. 110).

Empirical referents: Not identified.

Concept Verification Research: Boland conducted a qualitative study with a convenience sample of nine participants living in small rural communities in central Montana (Boland & Lee, 2006). The study findings confirmed the three defining attributes for old-timer and identified land ownership as the key element of the third attribute. The old-timers spoke of their functions within the community as working together for survival, holding social events to accomplish work and play, to share traditions, and act as historians.

Most participants identified themselves as "old-timers" despite earlier historical literature describing "old-timers" as persons who were "mysterious, unusual and fiercely independent" (Caniparoli, 1998, p. 106). These study participants expressed doubt about their level of influence within the communities, originally attributed to them in the earlier rural nursing theory development. Loss of influence was attributed to changing times (fewer farms and ranches, increased identification with the nearby larger towns and cities) and "the loss of respect for elderly people in today's society" (Boland & Lee, 2006, p. 50).

NEWCOMER (SUTERMASTER, 1998)

Method of analysis: Wilson's method (Walker & Avant, 1995)

Definition: "One that has recently arrived" (Sutermaster, 1998, p. 113)

Defining attributes:

1. "Newly arrived" (p. 120)
2. "Unaware of the history of the area/institution" (p. 120)
3. "Their existence may result in change" (p. 120)

Antecedents: "Individuals or families would have had a need or desire to move" (p. 121).

Consequences: "There is a new individual or family living in the community" (p. 121).

Empirical referents: Not identified.

RESOURCES (BALLANTYNE, 1998)
Method of analysis: Wilson's method (Walker & Avant, 1995)

Definition:

> *Resources are properties, resorts, or assets that are finite by nature and are made available for use by populations through an allocation process. Resources are accessed and used in response to a population's or individual's motivation for need satisfaction. ... Furthermore, these three elements can be visualized in a circle with the flow of energy between the allocated resource, accessibility of the resource, and use of the resource. (Ballantyne, 1998, p. 181)*

Defining attributes:

1. Property—"Resource is a property or an asset that has value for consumption by populations in need of that property" (p. 181)
2. Expedient—"Continuance or plan for solution of a particular problem" (p. 181)
3. Resort—"Turning inward to one's resources" (p. 181)

Antecedents: Knowledge of "local, regional, and national availability" (p. 187)

Consequences: "Allocation, accessibility, and use" (p. 187)

Empirical referents: Not identified.

INFORMAL NETWORKS (GROSSMAN & McNERNEY, 1998)
Method of analysis: Wilson's method (Walker & Avant, 1995)

Definition: "Networks are interconnected relationships, durable patterns of interactions, and interpersonal threads that comprise a social fabric" (Grossman & McNerney, 1998, pp. 201–202).

Defining attributes:

1. Volunteer—includes family members, coworkers, and neighbors who offer assistance free of charge (p. 204)
2. Information exchange (p. 204)
3. Support—has two components: emotional (being a friend, listening) and physical (assistance with daily living, health promotion, and maintenance activities; p. 204)
4. Guidance—"May be given as advice, consultation (availability of resources, referral to healthcare providers, sources of alternative treatments), and information" (p. 204)

Antecedents:

1. "A bond ... the tie that exists among ... the core of the informal network (family, friends, neighbors, and coworkers)" (p. 206)
2. "Are generated in response to a perceived need" (p. 206)
3. Consequences: "The perceived need is met or not met" (p. 206)

Empirical referents: Not identified.

LAY CARE NETWORK (TURNBULL, 1998)
Method of analysis: Wilson's method (Walker & Avant, 1988)

Definition: None given.

Defining attributes:

1. Interconnection or net—"An interconnection is the means by which one thing connects with another, whereas a net consists of fibers woven together for catching something" (Turnbull, 1998, p. 195).
2. Of the people—"Belonging to, concerned with, or performed by the 'people' in a nonprofessional capacity" (p. 195).
3. Sense of concern—"The idea that one develops or maintains an interest in the well-being of a person or object, to oversee with the intent to protect" (Oxford, 1989 as cited in Turnbull, 1998, p. 195).

Antecedents: Not identified.

Consequences: Not identified.

Empirical referents: Not identified.

Conclusion: Turnbull (1998) recommended "further refinement of the concept, 'lay care provider,' and suggests a change in the wording of the concept itself" (p. 198). The literature review clearly delineates between lay providers and informal care providers, whereas the wording "lay care providers" combines two different concepts.

Third Statement: Lack of Anonymity and Role Diffusion

The third statement is that "Health care providers in rural areas must deal with a lack of anonymity and much greater role diffusion than providers in urban or suburban settings" (Long & Weinert, 1989, p. 120). The key concepts are lack of anonymity and role diffusion. Related concepts are familiarity and professional isolation. Analyzed were lack of anonymity, familiarity, and professional isolation.

LACK OF ANONYMITY (LEE, 1998; SWAN & HOBBS, 2017)
In the rural nursing theory literature base, this concept was first analyzed by Lee (1998). More recently, Swan and Hobbs (2017) have completed extensive work updating the concept of lack of anonymity; content of their analysis is included with this summary. A second article on the lack of anonymity is included in this edition of *Rural Nursing: Concepts, Theory, and Practice* (see Chapter 5).

Method of analysis: Wilson's method (Walker & Avant, 2011)

Definition: "A condition in which one cannot remain nameless or unknown" (Lee, 1998, p. 77)

Defining attributes: (Swan & Hobbs, 2017, p. 1078)

1. "Identifiable"
2. "Establishing boundaries for public and private self"
3. "Interconnectedness in a community"

Antecedents: Swan and Hobbs's antecedent update includes "(a) environmental context, (b) opportunities to become visible, (c) developing relationships, and (d) unconscious or limited awareness of public or personal privacy" (p. 1080).

Consequences: Swan and Hobbs consequence update includes "(a) familiarity, (b) visibility, (c) collective responsibility, (d) awareness of privacy, and (e) manage/balance lack of anonymity" (p. 1080).

Empirical referents: Using the material evolving from their in-depth concept analysis work, Swan and Hobbs (2017) identified empirical referents for use in the development of an instrument: Lack of Anonymity Measure-24 (LOAN-24). Swan and Hobbs (2018) tested the instrument by using the expertise of rural content experts located 25 to 1,500 miles away from their offices.

Concept Verification Research: Raph conducted a pilot study focusing on the phenomenon "lack of anonymity" with four informants employed in a western rural "frontier" county health department (Raph & Buehler, 2006). Using grounded theory technique, four differing interactive categories emerged through the data analysis: (a) personally affirming interactions were defined as "friendly encounters that did not place the informant in a professional role" (p. 199); (b) professional affirming interactions were those seeking clarification on "general information about vaccines, appointments, or needed after-hour services ... usually (taking place in) public places in the community" (pp. 199–200); (c) professionally threatening interactions "placed healthcare providers in a position of potentially doing harm if not handled correctly" (p. 200); and (d) personally threatening encounters were those that "provoked fear and anger" (p. 201). The four categories, placed in a continuum from positive to negative, extend the second and third defining attributes of the lack of anonymity (Lee, 1998, p. 84) and verify the consequences of the "greater difficulty in maintaining personal and professional privacy."

FAMILIARITY (McNeely & Shreffler, 1998)
Method of analysis: Wilson's method (Walker & Avant, 1988)

Definition:

> ... an antithetical concept that includes the positive ideas of thorough knowledge of or an acquaintance with and closeness and intimacy, such as one would find in a family or deep friendship, and the contrasting perspective of offensive, unwarranted, intimate conduct that might include behaviors such as flirting, sexual harassment, domestic violence, abusive relationships, or incest. (McNeely & Shreffler, 1998, p. 91)

Defining attributes:

1. "Friendly relationship or close acquaintance" (p. 98)
2. "Intimacy" (p. 98)

3. "Informality" (p. 98)
4. "The exhibited familiarity is welcome or unwelcome depending on the perceptions of the receiver" (p. 98)

Antecedents: Not identified.

Consequences: Not identified.

Empirical referents: Not identified.

PROFESSIONAL ISOLATION (SHREFFLER, 1998)

Method of analysis: Wilson's method (Walker & Avant, 1988)

Definition: None given.

Defining attributes:

1. "an actual separation from or a deficiency in a resource needed to fulfill one's professional responsibilities or needs (objective component)" (Shreffler, 1998, p. 426)
2. "professional need is perceived as partially or wholly unmet (subjective component)" (p. 426)
3. "the actual separation or deficiency is on a continuum" (p. 426)
4. "the individual is not voluntarily separating herself/himself from an available professional resource" (p. 426)
5. "the objective component is more likely to be present in rural areas" (p. 426)

Antecedents: The individuals

1. experience "separation from or deficiency in resources needed to fulfill professional responsibilities" (p. 429)
2. have "needs for resources to fulfill their professional responsibilities" (p. 429)
3. "can make choices about the use of available resources" (p. 429)
4. "are able to perceive whether professional needs are met" (p. 429)

Consequences: They "are specific to the need that is unmet and the vulnerabilities of the individual in the occupation or job position" (p. 429).

Empirical referents

1. "The availability of the needed resource is measured and found deficient" (p. 429)
2. "Individuals. ... express awareness of an unmet need or exhibit signs of the consequence of the unmet need" (pp. 429–430)

CONCLUSION

The concepts contained in *Conceptual Basis of Rural Nursing* (Lee, 1998) and updated content about lack of anonymity published by Swan and Hobbs (2017) have been explicated in this chapter. Most analyses were conducted using the Wilson method (Walker & Avant, 1988, 1995, 2011). However, some of the elements (e.g., definitions, antecedents, consequences, and empirical referents) were not addressed. Furthermore, some key concepts were not analyzed (e.g., work beliefs, role diffusion). Further development of the concepts is needed. Paramount is the need for validation of concepts with rural dwellers from multiple settings and varying races and ethnicities.

REFERENCES

Agich, G. J. (1983). *Autonomy and long term care.* Oxford University Press.

Bailey, M. C. (1998). Outsider. In H. J. Lee (Ed.), *Conceptual basis for rural nursing* (pp. 139–148). Springer Publishing Company.

Ballantyne, J. (1998). Health resources and the rural client. In H. J. Lee (Ed.), *Conceptual basis for rural nursing* (pp. 178–198). Springer Publishing Company.

Boland, R., & Lee, H. (2006). Old-timers. In H. J. Lee & C. A. Winters (Eds.), *Rural nursing: Concepts, theory, and practice* (2nd ed., pp. 43–52). Springer Publishing Company.

Caniparoli, C. D. (1998). Old-timer. In H. J. Lee (Ed.), *Conceptual basis for rural nursing* (pp. 102–112). Springer Publishing Company.

Chafey, K., Sullivan, T., & Shannon, A. (1998). Self-reliance: Characteristics of their own autonomy by elderly rural women. In H. J. Lee (Ed.), *Conceptual basis for rural nursing* (pp. 156–177). Springer Publishing Company.

Grossman, L. L., & McNerney, S. (1998). Informal networks. In H. J. Lee (Ed.), *Conceptual basis for rural nursing* (pp. 200–208). Springer Publishing Company.

Henson, D., Sadler, T., & Walton, S. (1998). Distance. In H. J. Lee (Ed.), *Conceptual basis for rural nursing* (pp. 51–60). Springer Publishing Company.

Lee, H. J. (1998). Lack of anonymity. In H. J. Lee (Ed.), *Conceptual basis for rural nursing* (pp. 76–88). Springer Publishing Company.

Lee, H. J., Hollis, B. R., & McClain, K. A. (1998). Isolation. In H. J. Lee (Ed.), *Conceptual basis for rural nursing* (pp. 139–148). Springer Publishing Company.

Long, K. A. (1993). The concept of health: Rural perspectives. *Nursing Clinics of North America, 28,* 123–130.

Long, K. A., & Weinert, C. (1989). Rural nursing: Developing the theory base. *Scholarly Inquiry for Nursing Practice: An International Journal, 3*(2), 113–132.

McNeely, A. G., & Shreffler, M. J. (1998). Familiarity. In H. J. Lee (Ed.), *Conceptual basis for rural nursing* (pp. 89–101). Springer Publishing Company.

Morse, M. J. (1995). Exploring the theoretical basis of nursing using advanced techniques of concept analysis. *Advances in Nursing Science, 17*(3), 31–46. https://doi.org/10.1097/00012272-199503000-00005

Myers, D. D. (1998). Insider. In H. J. Lee (Ed.), *Conceptual basis for rural nursing* (pp. 125–138). Springer Publishing Company.

Raph, S., & Buehler, J. A. (2006). Rural health professionals' perceptions of lack of anonymity. In H. J. Lee, & C. A. Winters (Eds.), *Rural nursing: Concepts, theory, and practice* (2nd ed., pp. 197–204). Springer Publishing Company.

Shreffler, M. J. (1998). Professional isolation: A concept analysis. In H. J. Lee (Ed.), *Conceptual basis for rural nursing* (pp. 420–432). Springer Publishing Company.

Smith, J. A. (1983). *The idea of health: Implications for the nursing profession.* Teachers College Press.

Sutermaster, D. J. (1998). Newcomer. In H. J. Lee (Ed.), *Conceptual basis for rural nursing* (pp. 113–124). Springer Publishing Company.

Swan, M. A., & Hobbs, B. B. (2017). Concept analysis: Lack of anonymity. *Journal of Advanced Nursing, 73*(5), 1075–1084. https://doi.org/10.1111/jan.13236

Swan, M. A., & Hobbs, B. B. (2018). Querying rural content experts using an online questionnaire. *Online Journal of Rural Nursing and Health Care, 18*(2), 189–208. http://dx.doi.org/10.14574/ojrnhc.v18i2.533

Turnbull, T. S. (1998). Lay care network. In H. J. Lee (Ed.), *Conceptual basis for rural nursing* (pp. 189–199). Springer Publishing Company.

Walker, L., & Avant, K. (1988). *Strategies for theory construction in nursing* (2nd ed.). Appleton-Century-Crofts.

Walker, L., & Avant, K. (1995). *Strategies for theory construction in nursing* (3th ed.). Appleton-Century-Crofts.

Walker, L., & Avant, K. (2011). *Strategies for theory construction in nursing* (5th ed.). Prentice Hall.

Weinert, C., & Boik, R. (1995). MSU rurality index: Development and evaluation. *Research in Nursing and Health, 18,* 453–464. https://doi-org.proxybz.lib.montana.edu/10.1002/nur.4770180510

CHAPTER 4

Updating the Rural Nursing Theory Base

HELEN J. LEE AND MEG McDONAGH

DISCUSSION TOPICS

- Select one of the relational statements from the Rural Nursing Theory statements and diagram it. Include additional concepts that might be related to the statement.
- Lack of anonymity has changed over the years since it was first identified as a concept in Rural Nursing Theory. Identify whether there are other concepts that have changed over time. In what way?
- Identify a concept and select the fields of study from which you could analyze it.

Many disciplines exist to generate, test, and apply theories that will improve the quality of people's lives.

—Fawcett, 1999, p. 1

INTRODUCTION

"Sparsely Populated Areas: Toward Nursing Theory" was the title of a symposium presented by Montana State University (MSU) College of Nursing at the Western Council on Higher Education for Nursing (now Western Institute of Nursing). The symposium would demonstrate how the college could leverage opportunities for faculty and student research and contribute to the development of a theory of rural nursing (Shannon, 1982). This chapter includes a summary of the Rural Nursing Theory structure subsequently published in 1989 by Long and Weinert. It is followed by a review of the literature supporting or refuting the viability of the theoretical statements and concepts. Based on the review, we propose a revised Rural Nursing Theory structure and make suggestions for future work.

THE ORIGINAL RURAL NURSING THEORY STRUCTURE

The quality of the lives of rural persons and the lack of empirical studies about their healthcare was of concern to MSU College of Nursing researchers. A middle-range theory emerged from a recognized need for a framework that acknowledges the unique perceptions of rural persons and the generalist experience of nurses who practice in rural settings. Prior to the development of the theory, it was assumed that nursing care of rural persons was similar to the care of persons living in urban environments.

The resulting descriptive theory is the "most basic type of middle-range theory" (Fawcett, 1999, p. 15). Middle-range theory focuses "on a limited dimension of the reality of nursing" and grows at the "intersection of practice and research to provide guidance for everyday practice and scholarly research rooted in the discipline of nursing" (Smith & Liehr, 2003, p. xi). The theory emerged from observations gathered through qualitative and quantitative descriptive studies conducted in the sparsely populated rural setting of Montana. It describes specific characteristics and observations made of rural persons seeking healthcare and their healthcare providers. The published theory contains three theoretical statements and several key concepts (Long & Weinert, 1989; also see Chapter 2).

The first statement is descriptive and states that *"rural dwellers define health primarily as the ability to work, to be productive, to do usual tasks"* (Long & Weinert, 1989, p. 120). Key concepts associated with this statement are work beliefs and health beliefs. The second statement is relational and proposes that *"rural dwellers are self-reliant and resist accepting help or services from those seen as 'outsiders' or from agencies seen as national or regional 'welfare' programs"* (Long & Weinert, 1989, p. 120). Rural persons preferred to seek healthcare from insiders, persons with whom they were familiar. Additional key concepts pertaining to this statement are old-timer and newcomer. A corollary to the second statement is that "help, including needed medical care, is usually sought through an informal rather than a formal system" (p. 120). The third statement is relational and focuses on healthcare providers; it indicates that *lack of anonymity and role diffusion are experienced more acutely among rural providers than among providers in urban or suburban settings.* Lack of anonymity also applies to the recipients of healthcare in rural areas, as all persons in that environment have a "limited ability ... to have private areas of their lives" (Long & Weinert, 1989, p. 119).

In addition to the above-mentioned three statements, an understanding of the concepts isolation and distance is important in the healthcare-seeking behavior of rural residents. Isolation refers to separation from or being placed alone (Lee et al., 1998). Distance is measurable time, physical space between places, and personal perception of that space (Henson et al., 1998). Qualitative data upon which the theoretical work was based indicated that rural residents did not feel isolated, despite the fact that they averaged 23 miles of travel to their nearest ED and over 50 miles to their primary healthcare source (Long & Weinert, 1989, p. 119).

RELATED NURSING LITERATURE

The content of Long and Weinert's (1989) Rural Nursing Theory article was and is widely quoted in nursing literature, including community health and rural nursing texts, and in presentations given about rural nursing. However, periodic rural nursing literature reviews contain few citations specifically focusing on health perceptions and needs of rural persons. We located three qualitative studies through conference proceedings, the contents of which were subsequently published (Bales et al., 2006; Lee & Winters, 2004; Thomlinson et al., 2004). Other sources included two nursing master's theses (Bales, 2006; Moran, 2005); a study that focused on the healthcare meanings, values, and practices of Anglo-American male population in the rural American midwest (Sellers et al., 1999); a study exploring rurality and health in midlife women (Thurston & Meadows, 2003); and a study examining the health-information-seeking experiences of rural women in Ontario, Canada (Wathen & Harris, 2006, 2007). We also located several journal articles, mostly qualitative rural research, that included rural concepts found in Long and Weinert's article. A book titled *Rural Nursing: Aspects of Practice* (Ross, 2008) contains research evidence of studies that Ross and her colleagues conducted in New Zealand. Ross (2008, p. xviii) stated that the groundwork for her work was shaped by edited texts of Bushy (1991a, 1991b, 2000), Lee (1998) and Lee & Winters (2006).

In the following sections, each theoretical statement is followed by findings from the literature supporting or refuting the statement.

Theoretical Statement 1 (Descriptive)

"... [R]ural dwellers define health primarily as the ability to work, to be productive, to do usual tasks" (Long & Weinert, 1989, p. 120).

Four qualitative studies conducted in the United States examined health perceptions; one with rural men aged 25 to 49, one with rural men and women aged 28 to 63, and two with older rural persons aged 60 to 85. Three provided support for the above-mentioned descriptive statement that defines health as the ability to carry out important functions (Niemoller et al., 2000; Pierce, 2001; Sellers et al., 1999). In the fourth study, Averill (2002) found that definitions of health varied across her southwest U.S. sample that included older retirees, more recent retirees, and Hispanic elders. The older retirees from mining and ranching communities viewed health in a similar manner to the original qualitative theory development samples, whereas more recent retirees focused on strategies to remain healthy—proper diet, regular exercise, and regular health exams. The Hispanic elders in Averill's sample frequently mentioned incorporating home remedies and herbal preparations into their health maintenance practices.

Participants in the several health perceptions and needs studies (Bales, 2006; Bales et al., 2006; Lee & Winters, 2004; Moran, 2005; Thomlinson et al., 2004; Winters, Thomlinson, et al., 2006) conducted in the United States and Canada were more likely to define health holistically. Lee and Winters (2004) found that for rural persons working in service occupations, being able to function included being physically, mentally, and emotionally fit. Participants in a study conducted by Bales et al. (2006) thought that being healthy meant being mentally and physically active, eating well, and having an overall sense of well-being. Thomlinson et al. (2004) interpreted their participants' responses by saying that health was a "holistic relationship between the physical, mental, social and spiritual aspects of their lives" (p. 261). This same view of health was echoed by Canadian middle-aged women in Thurston and Meadows's (2003) study and by the older adults residing in Appalachia who completed surveys and participated in focus groups (Goins et al., 2011).

Australian women in de la Rue and Coulson's (2003) study, aged 73 to 87, equated health with not being ill. They knew maintenance of their health was influenced by their geographical location and their desire to remain living on the land.

SUMMARY

The literature both supports and refutes the first theoretical statement. Support appears in studies of rural male adults and of older persons and retirees from the extractive industries (mining and farming). Lack of support for the functional definition of health emerges from a variety of settings and from differing rural samples. It may be that age, the rural environmental setting, the influence of the work ethic, and the culture are factors in defining health (de la Rue & Coulson, 2003). Potentially, younger rural participants may be influenced by increased media exposure and its emphasis on health promotion and the use of preventive health practices. In addition, healthcare providers may be expanding their view of health beyond the illness care model and may be sharing this with their clients.

Theoretical Statement 2 (Relational)

"... [R]ural dwellers are self-reliant and resist accepting help or services from those seen as 'outsiders' or from agencies seen as national or regional welfare programs" (Long & Weinert, 1989, p. 120).

The attribute of self-reliance dominates the literature about rural persons and their health-seeking behaviors (Davis & Magilvy, 2000; Jirojwong & MacLennan, 2002; Lee & Winters, 2004; Niemoller et al., 2000; Ross, 2008; Sellers et al., 1999; Thomlinson et al., 2004; Wathen & Harris, 2006, 2007; Winters, Thomlinson, et al., 2006). Care was sought by rural residents after first "consulting books" (Jirojwong & MacLennan, 2002, p. 251) and trying "to deal with an illness themselves" (Thomlinson et al., 2004, p. 10). Because of the presence of chronic illnesses, older adults were knowledgeable about nearby medical care resources, including physicians, physician's assistants, and nurse practitioners (Niemoller et al., 2000; Pierce, 2001; Roberto & Reynolds, 2001), and if available, would use them "to achieve their desired level of independence" (Niemoller et al., 2000, p. 39). However, if the desired resources were not available, these same older adults stated they would "manage" (Niemoller et al., 2000, p. 39).

Canadian women (aged 20–82) in the study conducted by Wathen and Harris (2006) shared differing strategies when faced with an urgent health situation. Some would visit a hospital ED, whereas others would self-medicate and wait until the next morning to contact their family doctor. Decision-making was influenced by the perception of the knowledge and skills of available professional practitioners and, in some situations, by the results of previous interactions about managing their chronic illnesses. In addition, decisions were affected by the distances they needed to travel, particularly in winter.

COROLLARY TO RELATIONAL STATEMENT 2 (DESCRIPTIVE)

"... [H]elp, including needed healthcare, is usually sought through an informal rather than a formal system" (Long & Weinert, 1989, p. 120).

The literature revealed a variety of findings related to the relational statement corollary. Bales (2006) found that mothers with children living in U.S. frontier settings would seek advice from family, friends, and neighbors and would initiate self-care activities if healthcare situations were not considered serious. However, if the illness or injury was gauged as serious, professional healthcare was immediately accessed no matter the distance involved. Bypassing the informal for the formal system because of the seriousness of the illness or injury also was found in studies conducted by Buehler et al. (1998) and Thomlinson et al. (2004).

Participants in two Canadian studies (Thomlinson et al., 2004; Wathen & Harris, 2006, 2007) indicated that family, friends, and neighbors were cited as a major source of support, particularly during the information-gathering phase (Wathen & Harris, 2006). Those particularly valued were persons who held a healthcare professional role or had experienced a disease or illness firsthand (Wathen & Harris, 2006). Although older rural women in the U.S. study conducted by Pierce (2001) stated that they were eager to help neighbors and the less fortunate, they also shared their reluctance to tell family and neighbors about their own needs unless really necessary.

Help gained through accessing informal knowledge via the media, popular magazines, books, libraries, and the Internet was cited in three studies (Roberto & Reynolds, 2001; Thomlinson et al., 2004; Wathen & Harris, 2007). A sample of older women living in the United States actively sought information about living with their osteoporosis (Roberto & Reynolds, 2001): Members of a Canadian sample stated that they frequently made use of formal information sources through libraries, books, and computers (Thomlinson et al., 2004; Wathen & Harris, 2007).

SUMMARY

The second theoretical statement and its corollary are both sustained and refuted by the findings in the literature. Self-reliance continues to be a characteristic attribute of rural persons and influences the way they respond to illness or injury and their subsequent care-seeking behaviors. The informal system (family, friends, and neighbors) is still frequently used as a resource. However, the rural cultural barrier to accessing care through formal resources appears to be changing. The increased knowledge and the need to have information about health and the chronic illnesses they are experiencing may be removing the cultural barrier of approaching "outsiders" for health and medical care. In part, this may be occurring because desired health information can now be obtained through the use of the Internet while maintaining anonymity. Prior to the current age of information technology, maintaining anonymity while seeking health information was not an option.

Theoretical Statement 3 (Relational)

"... [H]ealth care providers in rural areas must deal with a lack of anonymity and much greater role diffusion than providers in urban or suburban settings" (Long & Weinert, 1989, p. 120).

The findings for the two concepts forming this relational statement—lack of anonymity and role diffusion—are sustained in the literature about healthcare providers from Australia, New Zealand, and the United States. In relation to the lack of anonymity, authors stated that "in close knit communities ... news travels fast" (Lau et al., 2002, Results and Discussion, paragraph 7) and that "social life realities in small communities frequently blur professional boundaries" (Blue & Fitzgerald, 2002, pp. 319–320). Social factors pertaining to practice in rural communities include privacy issues for both the professional and the clients for whom they give care (Lau et al., 2002). Healthcare practitioners in rural environments who are known by their clients may find that older women prefer receiving professional care from a familiar person (Courtney et al., 2000; Pierce, 2001), whereas middle-aged women prefer to go elsewhere for care because of that familiarity (Brown et al., 1999; Lee & Winters, 2004). Lee and Winters found this is particularly true for women's healthcare and mental health.

According to the work by Swan and Hobbs (2017), the meaning of the concept, "lack of anonymity," has also undergone change since the earlier work of Long and Weinert (1989). With the advent of widespread access to the Internet and the use of social media, maintaining any sense of anonymity has become increasingly difficult for everyone, including rural nurses. And while Lee et al. (1998) found that personal and professional boundaries may be diminished, Swan and Hobbs (2017) and Chipp et al. (2011) found that the issue may be related to how one establishes boundaries for one's personal and professional self. Another key factor related to the current meaning of lack of anonymity is the environmental context of those involved, specifically rural nurses. Previously this was thought to be a physical, geographic, and relational context and now it would seem that environment also includes digital and temporal.

Role diffusion was found in studies conducted with psychiatrists and nurses in Australia (Lau et al., 2002) and by Rosenthal (1996) in her study of rural nursing in America. Hegney (1997) described role diffusion in both generalist and extended roles in her study of Australian rural nursing practice. Role diffusion was evident in the practice of hospice nurses in New Zealand (McConigley et al., 2000). The reality in sparsely populated areas is that with fewer persons available to perform multiple tasks, more tasks must be undertaken by the individuals who practice in these areas.

SUMMARY

The third theoretical statement about lack of anonymity and role diffusion is well supported in the literature. Familiarity, the opposite of anonymity, can be a facilitator or a barrier to seeking health and illness care from local healthcare practitioners. Familiarity is a distinguishing feature of rural nursing that allows rural nurses a special knowledge of those for whom they provide care within their communities (Hegney, 1997).

The lack of anonymity that healthcare providers experience in rural communities is a paradox. On the one hand, it is often the familiarity and knowing of community members and the lack of anonymity that draws healthcare professionals to rural areas. Yet, it is often these same attributes that can later drive them away.

CONCLUSION

The review of the literature up to early 2017 pertaining to the descriptive middle-range Rural Nursing Theory base revealed a variety of findings. The rural residents' definition of health in the first descriptive statement is changing from that of a functional nature to a more holistic view that includes physical, mental, social, and spiritual aspects. The self-reliance of rural residents in the second relational statement is broadly supported; however, the resistance to seeking help from those seen as outsiders is changing. The third relational statement pertaining to healthcare providers and their lack of anonymity and role diffusion is supported. The findings for the concept of distance in the original rural theory development work are not supported. This literature appraisal of the Rural Nursing Theory base structure supports a need for change.

THE REVISED RURAL NURSING THEORY

Based on a review of the literature up through early 2017, we recommended the following revisions to the first two theoretical statements originally proposed by Long and Weinert in 1989.

Theoretical Statement 1 (Descriptive)

"Rural residents define health as being able to do what they want to do; it is a way of life and a state of mind; there is a goal of maintaining balance in all aspects of their lives" (Lee & McDonagh, 2006, p. 314).

"Older rural residents and those with ties to extractive industries are more likely to define health in a functional manner—to work, to be productive, and to do usual tasks" (Lee & McDonagh, 2006, p. 314).

Essential to understanding rural persons' motivation for illness treatment, health maintenance, and health promotion is knowledge of their health perceptions (Long, 1993). The earlier replacement statements provide a broader view of the health perceptions that have been found with more recent research among rural individuals, families, and communities. They reflect both the earlier emphasis on role performance evident among older residents and among those employed in extractive industries and the expanded view of health perception definitions elicited from other individuals living in rural communities.

Theoretical Statement 2 (Relational)

"Rural residents are self-reliant and make decisions to seek care for illness, sickness, or injury depending on their self-assessment of the severity of their present health condition and of the resources needed and available" (Lee & McDonagh, 2006, p. 315).

"Rural residents with infants and children experiencing illness, sickness, or injury will seek care more quickly than for themselves" (Lee & McDonagh, 2006, p. 315).

These theoretical statements refer to the health-seeking behaviors of rural residents. Key concepts from the 1989 model included self-reliance, seeking care from insiders, and the use of the informal system. Research findings continue to assert that self-reliance is a key characteristic identified in the management of healthcare situations by rural persons. However, changes were seen in the health-seeking behaviors of these residents as they seek advice and care from insiders and outsiders and make use of both informal and formal systems of care.

Additional concepts emerged from the comparative research about rural persons' health behaviors: health-seeking behaviors and choice (Winters, Thomlinson, et al., 2006). *Health-seeking behaviors*, defined as "conscious behaviors designed to promote healthy relationships among physical, mental, social and spiritual aspects of one's life so that life balance is maintained" (Winters, Thomlinson, et al., 2006), include three subthemes: symptom–action–timeline (SATL) process (Buehler et al., 1998), resources, and self-reliance.

Conscious *choice* is made in at least two domains of rural persons' lives. The first is the choice to live in a rural environment; the second is in accessing healthcare resources. Choosing to live in a rural environment is closely associated with the concept of place (see discussion later in this chapter).

Theoretical Statement 3 (Relational)

Healthcare providers in rural areas continue to experience lack of anonymity and role diffusion. Although the literature review demonstrates that the meaning of lack of anonymity has been expanded, the concept is still well supported. Therefore, the original statement was well supported in the literature review; no changes are recommended.

Updated Literature Review

From the latter half of 2017 to March 2020, 33 articles were found between PubMed and Cumulative Index to Nursing and Allied Health Literature (CINAHL) that related to either Rural Nursing Theory or one or more of the key concepts previously identified. Of these articles, two were duplicates and approximately six corroborated our previous work on Rural Nursing Theory. No new research was found that offered knowledge to the development of Rural Nursing Theory.

FUTURE DIRECTIONS

Exploration of the literature regarding rural health perceptions and needs reveal many new avenues for future exploration. Themes of *distance* and *resources* were identified repeatedly in the literature reviewed. Newly proposed concepts emerging from the literature review included *health-seeking behaviors*, *choice*, *environmental context*, and *social capital*. Each of these concepts is addressed in the following sections.

Distance

Although *distance* was not part of the three theoretical statements making up the Rural Nursing Theory base, the content of the rural literature accessed for this review frequently touched on the concept. In the seminal article by Long and Weinert (1989), the participants included in the multiple studies tended to see health services as accessible and did not view themselves as isolated. Canadian authors MacLeod et al. (1998) stated that distance may not be a problem but said the concept exerts a strong influence in providing healthcare in rural areas. This view affirms the assertion of Johnson et al. (1995) that one's geographic location may influence or even determine the form of health-seeking behaviors rural residents demonstrate. Pierce (2001) found that the older women described distance and geographical barriers with concern; yet, they seemed to take problems with accessibility "in stride" (p. 52). In addition, the study participants did express concern about the quality of nearby health services.

The remainder of the research all refuted the initial findings about distance and access to healthcare in Long and Weinert's (1989) theory-based article. Fitzgerald et al. (2001), Moran (2005), Pieh-Holder et al. (2012), and Racher and Vollman (2002) stated that access to healthcare services is a major concern for rural and remote residents and for the health professionals serving them in Australia, Canada, and the United States. In a quantitative study examining the relationship between distance and the nearest mammography facilities in Kentucky, researchers found a significant relationship between the presence of advanced diagnoses and longer average travel distances (Huang et al., 2009).

Australian rural healthcare experts were asked how rural and remote areas are different; Wakerman et al. (2017) found "geographic distance" and "access to healthcare" to be the chief characteristic of that difference.

Access to care is particularly a concern for rural individuals with chronic illness; an expressed problem was finding the "best" doctor (Fitzgerald et al., 2001). Distance to emergency care was an expressed concern of service providers in rural areas (Lee & Winters, 2004) and of mothers of children living in frontier areas (Bales, 2006; Pieh-Holder et al., 2012). Wong and Regan's (2009) study participants averaged at least two chronic illnesses each; they made trade-offs between their safety because of poor winter driving conditions and meeting their health needs. In a survey of middle-aged women, Brown et al. (1999) concluded that experiencing difficulties with accessing healthcare results in greater reliance on self-treatment and self-care, thereby leading to the development of "attitudes of independence and self-reliance [sic]" (p. 151).

Resources

In addition to distance, the concept of *resources* directly impacts access to healthcare services. Gulzar (1999) and Racher and Vollman (2002) discuss the complexity of accessing health services. The rurality or remoteness of a given place affects the access to health services. Within the rural environment, factors such as geography, politics, and economics, as well as the acceptability and the education of healthcare providers, all influence the residents' access to and choice of health resources. Studying patterns of healthcare use and feedback loops among residents may add to the understanding of the complexity of accessing healthcare services in rural and remote areas (Racher & Vollman, 2002). Delivery of health services across sparsely populated areas presents unique challenges because of the vast distances involved and the scarcity of health professionals. For example, the greater the nurse-to-patient or physician-to-patient ratio and the more rural or remote the community, the more limited the health resources are for rural and remote community members.

Health-Seeking Behaviors

Health-seeking behaviors were defined as "conscious behaviors designed to promote healthy relationships among physical, mental, social and spiritual aspects of one's life so that life balance in maintained" (Winters, Thomlinson, et al., 2006, p. 34). The authors included three subthemes, SATL process, resources, and self-reliance, as part of health-seeking behaviors. The SATL process (Buehler et al., 1998) is used to describe the social process and to identify symptoms of sickness, illness, or injury and then seek the appropriate level of requisite care. The level of care sought may be self, lay, or professional, depending upon the perceived seriousness and type of symptom. Accessing resources is a part of the SATL process (see Chapter 16). Self-reliance, defined as behaviors to promote or maintain health without seeking assistance from others, was prevalent in the data from Montana and the Canadian provinces of Alberta and Manitoba. Winters, Thomlinson, et al. (2006, p. 35) considered self-reliance a subtheme of health-seeking behavior because of its paramount influence on a person seeking healthcare in sparsely populated rural areas.

Choice

Choice, the making of conscious decisions to live in a rural environment and access healthcare resources, was a new theme that emerged from a comparison study (Winters, Thomlinson, et al., 2006). Explicitly evident in the Montana data and implicitly identified in the Canadian study through the participants' expressions of the benefits of living in rural environments, the theme of choice is associated with the concept of "place." Although we think of place in a geographical context, it is a broader entity that shapes one's political, economic, spatial, geographic, and cultural views of the world (Kelly, 2003). De la Rue and Colson (2003) found that rural participants' well-being and health were influenced by the "geographical location of living on the land" (p. 5). "Place" provided these rural residents with a kind of emotional or spiritual connectedness that affected the outcomes of their health experiences.

Wathen and Harris (2007) stated that rural living affected the choice of resources that members of their Canadian study would consult about a chronic health concern or an acute medical problem. If the available rural doctor "might not be the best or too up-to date" (p. 643), they preferred their informal system (colleagues, friends, and family), medical books, pharmacists, and/or the veterinarian.

Choice in making decisions related to accessing healthcare can be affected by several factors. Questions often asked to aid in determining a course of action are the following: Where is the closest facility that will provide the healthcare needed? What are the qualifications of the persons who staff that facility? What level of confidence is there in the local facility's healthcare providers? Does familiarity with the professionals who staff the facility make a difference in making the choice of where to go? Is anonymity an important factor in this situation? Does the healthcare facility accept the insurance (true in the U.S. healthcare system) carried by the individual or family seeking care (Moran, 2005)? What hours does the facility stay open? What are the weather conditions? During stormy conditions, what roads are better maintained (freezing rain, snow, and ice; summer rain, wind, and flooding). In an acute emergency, can a helicopter or a fixed-wing land nearby? These represent only a fraction of the factors and questions that play a role in the decision-making for accessing healthcare.

Environmental Context

Appearing repeatedly throughout the literature reviewed were terms like *place, geographical location, context,* or *environmental context.* According to Jones and Ross (2003, p. 16), nursing practice is "shaped by its situatedness" (p. 16). Authors speak of the context of a place and the resources needed that are particular to a context or place (Andrews, 2002, 2003; Andrews & Moon, 2005; MacLeod et al., 2008; Poland et al., 2005; Thurston & Meadows, 2004; Winters, Cudney et al., 2006). According to Lauder et al. (2006), "'Context' is an important unit of analysis ... A rural heath context is both physical and relational and aspects of rural environments ... may enhance or impede health" (p. 75). According to Swan and Hobbs's (2017) work on the lack of anonymity, with the prevalence of Internet use and social media, "environmental context" should now also include the cyber or digital realm.

Health perceptions, needs, and actions of rural persons are also influenced by the environmental context. This was particularly evident in the research reported by de la Rue and Coulson (2003), Thomlinson et al. (2004), and Winters, Cudney, et al. (2006). In their intervention study of rural women with chronic illnesses, Winters and her colleagues found that four themes emerged through the "overarching theme of distance: (a) physical setting, (b) social/cultural/-economic environment, (c) nature of women's work, and (d) accessibility/-quality of health care" (pp. 284–285).

Social Capital

Social capital is a concept that comes from sociology and has come into increasing importance over the last 25 years (Shooker et al., 2008). Rankin (2002, as cited in Lauder et al., 2006) defines social capital as "forms of association that express trust and norms of reciprocity" (p. 75). The Policy Research Initiative for the government of Canada (PRI; 2005 as cited in Shooker et al., 2008) further clarifies social capital as the "networks of social relations that may provide individuals and groups with access to resources and supports" (p. 87). "Creating supportive environments is about building social capital" (p. 87) and is similar to the notion of building "rural health services research capacity" (Hartley, 2005, p. 12).

Nurses practicing in rural settings tend to be more actively engaged professionally and personally in the rural communities in which they live and work (Bushy, 2000; Petersen et al., 2017; Scharff, 1998). However, the present role of nurses in creating supportive healthcare environments is not well understood; recognition, conceptualization, and measurement are needed "to more fully appreciate the impact nurses have on rural health access and services" (Lauder et al., 2006, p. 74).

Three qualitative studies about nurses spoke to the necessity of developing social capital within rural communities (Conger & Plager, 2008; Gibb et al., 2003; MacKinnon, 2008). APRN graduates realized the importance of "rural connectedness" through the development of support networks with other healthcare providers, relationships with urban healthcare centers, connections with local communities, and support through electronic means (Conger & Plager, 2008; Petersen et al., 2017). Nurses providing maternity care realized that they needed to know "their community—who lives in their community, what their skills are, and whether they are available to address local health needs or respond to emergency situations" (MacKinnon, 2008, p. 6). Nurses in solo mental health practice recognized the necessity of assisting rural and remote clients "to achieve a level of social functioning to integrate the person back into their community network" (Gibb, 2003, p. 248). To do this, they found that they needed to work more closely with the potential support structures identified within the clients' community. This was best achieved by fostering a caring home environment, trying to keep people with their families and in their place of employment (Gibb et al., 2003). By having such a support structure, rural mental practitioners can avoid sending the mental health client to a psychiatric institution when a crisis occurs. However, in a recent study from Ontario, Canada (Buck-McFadyen et al., 2018), it was found that although rural residents had higher social capital scores there was no difference in self-reported health between rural and urban populations.

Summary

Theories are developed for the purposes of describing, explaining, and predicting phenomena (Fawcett, 2000). The intent of the early theory development work at the College of Nursing at MSU was to use the descriptive research data collected in sparsely populated rural areas to develop a middle-range theory, one that would provide a framework for nurses providing care to rural dwellers (Shannon, 1982). What evolved was a descriptive theory, the most basic type of middle-range theory (Fawcett, 1999).

Although controversy exists about the placement and abstraction level of middle-range theories within the hierarchical structure of nursing theories (Peterson & Bredow, 2004), the basic theory structure, regardless of level, is similar—theoretical statements that describe or link key concepts (Fawcett, 1999). The interweaving of those concepts and statements provides a pattern of ideas, which provide a new perspective on phenomena (Smith & Liehr, 2003). The pattern, once published and subjected to testing, should remain open to scrutiny, debate, and, if necessary, to change and to incorporate new ideas.

By subjecting the middle-range Rural Nursing Theory to testing in several studies (Bales, 2006; Bales et al., 2006; Lee & Winters, 2004; Moran, 2005; Thomlinson et al., 2004; Winters, Thomlinson et al., 2006) and in the findings from several related studies, it was evident that change had occurred over the past 30 years that had altered the applicability of the original published Rural Nursing Theory base by Weinert and Long (1989). This change is demonstrated by the revisions to theoretical statements and the new emerging concepts.

VISION FOR THE FUTURE

Because of the descriptive nature of the middle-range Rural Nursing Theory, additional descriptive research is needed (Fawcett, 1999). Concept analysis methods can take several approaches, including the Wilson method (Walker & Avant, 1995), the evolutionary method (Rogers, 1993), the empirical or inductive approach (Morse, 1995), or a combination thereof. Testing of the proposed changes to the Rural Nursing Theory relational statements through qualitative studies (ethnography, grounded theory, phenomenology, narrative inquiry, historical inquiry, and photovoice) and participatory action research needs to take place in other sparsely populated areas. Development and testing of instruments to measure the concepts are also needed. Conducting surveys to measure the attributes, attitudes, knowledge, and opinions using open-ended and semistructured interviews and questionnaires is required (Fawcett, 1999). With a compilation of these focused research efforts can emerge a model, a schema, or a list of logically ordered statements that, when present, will provide guidance for the care of rural dwellers (Smith & Liehr, 2003).

Moving the Work Forward

In the early 2000s, a core group of nurse researchers from Montana and Alberta periodically met to review and critique theoretical material and models. Members of this North American Study (NAS) group discussed and planned projects to further Rural Nursing Theory development while offering research and educational opportunities to graduate students within their courses or independent studies. In 2005, a rural nursing and theory listserv group was initiated, which provided a mechanism for online discussion for furthering rural nursing research and theory development. This listserv has now been dormant for some time.

The NAS and listserv members did identify the following questions for continued exploration of rural healthcare behaviors: (a) Are these health-seeking behaviors unique to rural residents? (b) Will health-seeking behavior activities of the Health–Needs–Action Process (HNAP; see Chapter 13) fit under the same middle-range theory framework as those for health promotion? (c) How do illness variables affect rural persons' health-seeking behaviors? (d) How do illness variables affect rural people's choices of healthcare providers? (e) Are rural dwellers more accepting of "outsiders" if they are healthcare professionals working in partnerships with the rural community and local health professionals?

CONCLUSION

The *revised statements* for the middle-range Rural Nursing Theory as published by Lee and McDonagh (2010) have been ready for testing for 10 years. The emerging concepts identified in the review of the rural nursing literature are also ready for exploration, testing, and tool development. In order for this middle-range theory to become more robust it is crucial that nurse researchers with an interest in rural nursing conduct further research to enhance the development of Rural Nursing Theory. These efforts can provide the structure to increase the potential for the development of acceptable, adaptable, and evidence-based nursing care interventions for rural persons.

REFERENCES

Andrews, G. J. (2002). Towards a more place-sensitive nursing: An invitation to medical and health sensitive health geography. *Nursing Inquiry*, 9(4), 221–238. https://doi.org/10.1046/j.1440-1800 .2002.00157.x

Andrews, G. J. (2003). Locating a geography of nursing: Space, place, and the progress of geographical thought. *Nursing Philosophy*, 4, 231–248. https://doi.org/10.1046/j.1466-769X.2003.00140.x

Andrews, G. J., & Moon, G. (2005). Space, place, and the evidence base: Part I—An introduction to health geography. *Worldviews on Evidence Based Nursing*, 2, 55–62. https://doi.org/ 10.1111/j.1741-6787.2005.05004.x

Averill, J. B. (2002). Voices from the Gila: Health care issues for rural elders in south-western New Mexico. *Journal of Advanced Nursing*, 40, 654–662. https://doi.org/10.1046/j.1365-2648.2002.02425.x

Bales, R. L. (2006). Health perceptions, needs, and behaviours of remote rural women of childbearing and childrearing age. In H. J. Lee & C. A. Winters (Eds.), *Rural nursing: Concepts, theory and practice* (2nd ed., pp. 66–78). Springer Publishing Company.

Bales, R. L., Winters, C. A., & Lee, H. J. (2006). Health needs and perceptions of rural persons. In H. J. Lee & C. A. Winters (Eds.), *Rural nursing: Concepts, theory, and practice* (2nd ed., pp. 53–65). Springer Publishing Company.

Blue, I., & Fitzgerald, M. (2002). Interprofessional relations: Care studies of working relationships between registered nurses and general practitioners in rural Australia. *Journal of Clinical Nursing*, 11, 314–321. https://doi.org/10.1046/j.1365-2702.2002.00591.x

Brown, W. J., Young, A. F., & Byles, J. E. (1999). Tyranny of distance? The health of mid-age women living in five geographical areas of Australia. *Australian Journal of Rural Health*, 7, 148–154. https:// doi.org/10.1046/j.1440-1584.1999.00236.x

Buck-McFadyen, E., Akhtar-Danesh, N., Isaacs, S., Leipert, B., Strachan, P., & Valaitis, R. (2019). Social capital and self-rated health: A cross-sectional study of the general social survey data comparing rural and urban adults in Ontario. *Health and Social Care in the Community*, 27, 424–436. https://doi .org/10.1111/hsc.12662

Buehler, J. A., Malone, M., & Majerus, J. M. (1998). Patterns of responses to symptoms in rural residents: The symptom-action-time-line process. In H. J. Lee (Ed.), *Conceptual basis for rural nursing* (pp. 318–328). Springer Publishing Company.

Bushy, A. (Ed.) (1991a). *Rural nursing* (Volume 1). Sage.

Bushy, A. (Ed.) (1991b). *Rural nursing* (Volume 2). Sage.

Bushy, A. (2000). *Orientation to nursing in the rural community*. Sage.

Chipp, C., Dewane, S., Brems, C., Johnson, M. E., Warnwe, T. D., & Roberts, L. W. (2011). "If only someone had told me …": Lessons from rural providers. *The Journal of Rural Health*, 27(1), 122–130. https://doi.org/101111/j.1748-0361.2010.00314.x

Conger, M. M., & Plager, K. A. (2008). Advanced practice nursing practice in rural areas: Connectedness versus disconnectedness. *Online Journal of Rural Nursing and Health Care*, 8(1), 24–38. http://rno-journal.Binghamton.edu/index.php/RNO/article /view/127

Courtney, M., Tong, S., & Walsh, A. (2000). Older patients in the acute care setting: Rural and metropolitan nurses' knowledge, attitudes and practices. *Australian Journal of Rural Health*, 8, 94–102. https://doi.org/10.1046/j.1440-1584.2000.00256.x

Davis, R., & Magilvy, J. K. (2000). Quiet pride: The experience of chronic illness by rural older adults. *Journal of Nursing Scholarship*, 32, 385–390. https://doi.org/10.1111/j.1547-5069.2000.00385.x

de la Rue, M., & Coulson, I. (2003). The meaning of health and well-being: Voices from older rural women. *Rural and Remote Health*, 3(192), 1–10. www.rrh.org.au/journal/article/192

Fawcett, J. (1999). *The relationship of theory and research* (3rd ed.). F. A. Davis.

Fawcett, J. (2000). *Analysis and evaluation of contemporary nursing knowledge: Nursing models and theories.* F. A. Davis.

Fitzgerald, M., Pearson, A., & McCutcheon, H. (2001). Impact of rural living on the experience of chronic illness. *Australian Journal of Rural Health, 9,* 235–240. https://doi.org/10.1046/j.1440-584.2001.00398.x

Gibb, H. (2003). Rural community mental health nursing: A grounded theory account of sole practice. *International Journal of Mental Health Nursing, 12,* 243–250. https://doi.org/10.1046/j.1447-0349.2003.t01-2-.x

Gibb, H., Livesey, L., & Zyla, W. (2003). At 3 am who the hell do you call? Case management issues in sole practice as a rural community mental health nurse. *Australasian Psychiatry, 11*(Suppl. 1), S127–S130. https://doi.org/10.1046/j.1038-5282.2003.02005.x

Goins, R. T., Spencer, S. M., & Williams, K. (2011). Lay meanings of health among rural older adults in Appalachia. *The Journal of Rural Health, 27*(1), 13–20. https://doi.org/10.1111/j.1748-0361.2010.00315.x

Gulzar, L. (1999). Access to health care. *Journal of Nursing Scholarship, 31,* 13–19. https://doi.org/10.1111/j.1547-5069.1999.tb00414.x

Hartley, D. (2005). Rural health research: Building capacity and influencing policy in the United States and Canada. *Canadian Journal of Nursing Research, 37*(1), 7–13. https://cjnr.archive.mcgill.ca/article/viewFile/1923/1917

Hegney, D. (1997). Rural nursing practice. In L. Siegloff (Ed.), *Rural nursing in the Australian context* (pp. 25–43). Royal College of Nursing.

Henson, D., Sadler, T. & Walton, D. (1998). Distance. In H. J. Lee (Ed.) *Conceptual basis for rural nursing* (pp. 51–60). Springer Publishing Company.

Huang, B., Dignan, M., Han, D., & Johnson, O. (2009). Does distance matter? Distance to mammography facilities and stage at diagnosis of breast cancer in Kentucky. *Journal of Rural Health, 25*(4), 366–371. https://doi.org/10.1111/j.1748-0361.2009.00245.x

Jirojwong, S., & MacLennan, R. (2002). Management of episodes of incapacity by families in rural and remote Queensland. *Australian Journal of Rural Health, 10,* 249–255. https://doi.org/10.1111/j.1440-1584.2002.tb00040.x

Johnson, J. L., Ratner, P. A., & Bottorff, J. L. (1995). Urban–rural differences in the health-promoting behaviors of Albertans. *Canadian Journal of Public Health, 86,* 103–108. https://www.jstor.org/stable/41991258

Jones, S., & Ross, J. (2003). *Describing your scope of practice: A resource for rural nurses.* Centre for Rural Health. http://www.moh.govt.nz

Kelly, S. E. (2003). Bioethics and rural health: Theorizing place, space, and subjects. *Social Science & Medicine, 56,* 2277–2288. https://doi.org/10.1016/S0277-9536(02)00227-7

Lau, T., Kumar, S., & Thomas, D. (2002). Practicing psychiatry in New Zealand's rural areas: Incentives, problems and solutions. *Australasian Psychiatry, 10*(1), 33–38. https://doi.org/10.1046/j.1440-1665.2002.0389a.x

Lauder, W., Reel, S., Farmer, J., & Griggs, H. (2006). Social capital, rural nursing and rural nursing theory. *Nursing Inquiry, 13*(1), 73–79. https://doi.org/10.1111/j.1440-1800.2006.00297.x

Lee, H. J. (Ed.). (1998). *Conceptual basis for rural nursing.* Springer Publishing Company.

Lee, H. J., Hollis, B. R., & McClain, K. A. (1998). Isolation. In H. J. Lee (Ed.), *Conceptual basis for rural nursing* (pp. 61–75). Springer Publishing Company.

Lee, H. J., & McDonagh, M. K. (2006). Examining the rural nursing theory base. In H. J. Lee, & C. A. Winters (Eds.), *Rural nursing: Concepts, theory, and practice* (2nd ed., pp. 17–26). Springer Publishing Company.

Lee, H. J., & McDonagh, M. K. (2010). Updating the rural nursing theory base. In C. A. Winters & H. J. Lee (Eds.), *Rural nursing: Concepts, theory, and practice* (3rd ed., pp. 19–39). Springer Publishing Company.

Lee, H. J., & Winters, C. A. (2004). Testing rural nursing theory: Perceptions and needs of service providers. *Online Journal of Rural Nursing and Health Care, 4*(1), 51–63. http://www.rno.org/journal/issues/vol-4/issue.1/Lee_article.htm

Lee, H. J., & Winters, C. A. (Eds.). (2006). *Rural nursing: Concepts, theory and practice* (2nd ed.). Springer Publishing Company.

Long, K. A. (1993). The concept of health: Rural perspectives. *The Nursing Clinics of North America*, *28*(1), 123–130.

Long, K. A., & Weinert, C. (1989). Rural nursing: Developing the theory base. *Scholarly Inquiry for Nursing Practice: An International Journal*, *3*, 113–127. https://doi.org/10.1891/0889-7182.3.2.113

MacKinnon, K. A. (2008). Labouring to nurse: The work of rural nurses who provide maternity care. *Rural and Remove Health Care*, *8*, 1–15. https://www.rrh.org.au/journal/article/1047

MacLeod, M., Browne, A. J., & Leipert, B. (1998). International perspective: Issues for nurses in rural and remote Canada. *Australian Journal of Rural Health*, *6*, 72–78. https://doi.org/10.1111/j.1440-1584.1998.tb00287.x

MacLeod, M. L. P., Misener, R. M., Banks, K., Morton, A. M., Vogt, C., & Bentham, D. (2008). "I'm a different kind of nurse": Advice from nurses in rural and remote Canada. *Canadian Journal of Nursing Leadership*, *21*(3), 40–53. https://doi.org/10.1891/0889-7182.3.2.113

McConigley, R., Kristjanson, L., & Morgan, A. (2000). Palliative care nursing in rural Western Australia. *International Journal of Palliative Nursing*, *6*(2), 80–90. https://doi.org/10.12968/ijpn.2000.6.2.8948

Moran, C. A. (2005). *Replication study of rural nursing theory: A Missouri perspective.* Unpublished thesis, University of Central Missouri, Warrensburg, Missouri.

Morse, M. J. (1995). Exploring the theoretical basis of nursing using advanced techniques of concept analysis. *Advances in Nursing Science*, *17*(3), 31–46. https://doi.org/10.1097/00012272-199503000-00005

Niemoller, J. K., Ide, B. A., & Nichols, E. G. (2000). Issues in studying health-related hardiness and use of services among older rural adults. *Texas Journal of Rural Health*, *18*, 35–43.

Petersen, P., Sharp, D. & Paré, J. (2017). A story of emergent leadership: Understanding the lived experiences of nurses working in a rural hospital setting. *Online Journal of Rural Nursing and Health Care*, *17*(2), 103–125. https://dx.doi.org/10.14574/ojrnhc.v17i2.454

Peterson, S. J., & Bredow, T. S. (2004). *Middle range theories: Application to nursing research.* Lippincott Williams & Wilkins.

Pieh-Holder, Callahan, C., & Young, P. (2012). Qualitative needs assessment: Healthcare experiences of underserved populations in Montgomery County, Virginia, USA. *Rural and Remote Health*, *12*, 2045. https://www.rrh.org.au/journal/article/1816

Pierce, C. (2001). The impact of culture of rural women's descriptions of health. *The Journal of Multicultural Nursing and Health*, *7*, 50–53, 56. https://search.proquest.com/openview/e69f62bfbcd6247e354be6d573bbac75/1?pq-origsite=gscholar&cbl=32370

Poland, B., Lehoux, P., Holmes, D., & Andrews, G. J. (2005). How place matters: Unpacking technology and power in health and social care. *Health & Social Care in the Community*, *13*, 170–180. https://doi.org/10.1111/j.1365-2524.2005.00545.x

Racher, F. E., & Vollman, A. R. (2002). Exploring the dimensions of access to health services: Implications for nursing research and practice. *Research and Theory for Nursing Practice: An International Journal*, *16*, 77–90. https://doi.org/10.1891/rtnp.16.2.77.53003

Roberto, K. A., & Reynolds, S. G. (2001). The meaning of osteoporosis in the lives of rural women. *Health Care for Women International*, *22*, 599–611. https://doi.org/10.1080/07399330127198

Rogers, B. L. (1993). Concept analysis: An evolutionary view. In B. L. Rogers & K. A. Kraft (Eds.), *Concept development in nursing: Foundations, techniques and application* (pp. 73–92). Saunders.

Rosenthal, K. A. (1996). *Rural nursing: An exploratory narrative description.* Unpublished dissertation, University of Colorado, Denver.

Ross, Jean. (Ed.). (2008). *Rural nursing: Aspects of practice.* Rural Health Opportunities, Ministry of Health.

Scharff, J. (1998). The distinctive nature and scope of rural nursing practice: Philosophical bases. In H. Lee (Ed.), *Conceptual basis for rural nursing* (pp. 19–38). Springer Publishing Company.

Sellers, S. C., Poduska, M. D., Propp, L. H., & White, S. E. (1999). The health care meanings, values, and practices of Anglo-American males in the rural Midwest. *Journal of Transcultural Nursing*, *10(4)*, 320–330. https://doi.org/10.1177/104365969901000410

Shannon, A. (1982). Introduction: Nursing in sparsely populated areas. In J. Taylor (Ed.), Sparsely populated areas: Toward nursing theory. *Western Journal of Nursing Research, 4*(Suppl. 3), 70–71. https://doi.org/10.1177/019394598200400316

Shooker, M., Scott, C. M., & Vollman, A. R. (2008). Creating supportive environments for health: Social network analysis. In A. R. Vollman, E. T. Anderson, & J. McFarlane (Eds.), *Canadian community as partner: Theory & multidisciplinary practice* (2nd ed.). Lippincott Williams & Wilkins.

Smith, M. K., & Liehr, P. R. (Eds.). (2003). *Middle range theory of nursing*. Springer Publishing Company.

Swan, M. A., & Hobbs, B. B. (2017). Concept analysis: Lack of anonymity. *Journal of Advanced Nursing,* *73*(5), 1075–1084. https://doi.org/10.1111/jan.13236

Thomlinson, E. H., McDonagh, M. K., Reimer, M., Crooks, K., & Lees, M. (2004). Health beliefs of rural Canadians: Implications for practice. *Australian Journal of Rural Health, 12,* 258–263. https://doi .org/10.1111/j.1440-1854.2004.00627.x

Thurston, W. E., & Meadows, L. M. (2003). Rurality and health: Perspectives from mid-life women. *Rural and Remote Health, 3*(219), 1–12. https://www.rrh.org.au/journal/article/219

Wakerman, L., Bourke, L., Humphreys, J. S., & Taylor, J. (2017). Is remote health different to rural health? *Rural and Remote Health, 17,* 3832. https://www.rrh.org.au/journal/article/3832

Walker, L., & Avant, K. (1995). *Strategies for theory construction in nursing* (3rd ed.). Appleton-Century-Crofts.

Wathen, C. N., & Harris, R. M. (2006). An examination of the health information seeking of women in rural Ontario, Canada experience. *Journal of the American Society for Information Science & Technology, 11*(4)/paper 267. https:eric.ed.gov/?id=EJ1104643

Wathen, C. N., & Harris, R. M. (2007). "I try to take care of it myself." How rural women search for health information. *Qualitative Health Research, 17*(5), 639–651. https://doi.org/10.1177/1049732307301236

Winters, C. A., Cudney, S. A., Sullivan, T., & Thuesen, A. (2006). The rural context and women's self-management of chronic health conditions. *Chronic Illness, 2,* 273–289. https://doi.org/10.1177/17423953060020040801

Winters, C. A., Thomlinson, E. H., O'Lynn, C., Lee, H. J., McDonagh, M. K., Edge, D. S., & Reimer, M. A. (2006). Exploring rural nursing theory across borders. In H. J. Lee & C. A. Winters (Eds.), *Rural nursing: Concepts, theory, and practice* (2nd ed., pp. 27–39). Springer Publishing Company.

Wong, S., & Regan, S. (2009). Patient perspectives on primary health care in rural communities: Effects of geography on access, continuity, and efficiency. *Rural and Remote Health, 9,* 1142. https://www .rrh.org.au/journal/article/1142

CHAPTER 5

Lack of Anonymity: Changes for the 21st Century

Marilyn A. Swan and Barbara B. Hobbs

DISCUSSION TOPICS

- Lack of anonymity involves being known and connected to others. According to the text, lack of anonymity is greater in rural settings and can influence nurses' care. However, the Internet and the use of social media are creating new relationships that can affect patients' healthcare knowledge and access. As a rural nurse, what factors might influence a patient to use the local healthcare services rather than distant providers (Internet or place-bound)?
- Lack of anonymity and privacy issues can arise with Internet use and social media. How has social media use affected your anonymity and privacy? How has your need for privacy and anonymity affected your social media use?
- Confidentiality is an ethical principle for nursing. Regardless of the setting, nurses are expected to maintain confidentiality; however, lack of anonymity found in the rural setting can add to the challenge. How would you, or have you, addressed a breach in confidentiality?
- In the rural setting, nurses may find it difficult setting work and family boundaries for their privacy. What strategies could be used to set boundaries?
- Understanding the challenges nurses encounter in rural settings, what factors, traits, behaviors, and beliefs do you think make an effective rural nurse? What factors, traits, behaviors, and beliefs might limit one's effectiveness?
- Have you ever been faced with caring for a patient you know on a personal basis? What was your experience and how has that experience informed your practice?
- If you are a rural nurse, what measures do you use to foster and support professional and personal privacy for yourself and others?

INTRODUCTION

Strike up a conversation in any rural diner and it will not take long to learn from the locals how everybody knows everybody else. Being known and named, that is, lack of anonymity, is an ever-present reality of daily life in rural communities and commonly

described in rural literature (Lee, 1998). Rural nursing investigators identify lack of anonymity as an aspect of rural life and experienced by rural nurses in their personal and
professional lives (Hegney, 1996; Long & Weinert, 1989). As a concept, lack of anonymity
is firmly established in rural life; however, lack of anonymity is often described in literature alongside privacy, confidentiality, and familiarity. Being closely related concepts, it
makes sense that they are discussed together. However, these four concepts are not synonymous, and there is benefit in examining each to gain understanding about how the
concepts differ from each other, and how they influence rural nursing practice.

Rural dwellers, people who live in rural and remote areas, are interconnected to each
other and their community. Rural nurses, like rural dwellers, experience this interconnectedness in their personal and professional lives. Being known as a rural nurse has
been described as "life in a fishbowl," where you are recognized and observed in and
out of work (Rosenthal, 2010). By being known and connected within a rural community, rural nurses gain social capital (Lauder et al., 2006). Social capital is described as
social connection within a community that bridges people and builds trust (Whitley &
McKenzie, 2005). Trust is necessary in relationships that involve privacy and confidentiality. In rural areas, trusting relationships develop and grow even in the presence of lack
of anonymity. Through the experience of lack of anonymity, rural nurses are uniquely
placed to impact health and well-being of rural dwellers and their communities.

The purpose of this chapter is to take a 21st-century view by beginning to reconsider
our thinking on lack of anonymity. We begin by defining and describing the related concepts and explore a model of how the concepts may be associated with lack of anonymity.
Gaining an understanding of the concepts is necessary as we explore how the concepts
affect rural nursing practice. We end with case studies and questions that highlight the
different concepts in hypothetical situations experienced by a rural nurse.

LACK OF ANONYMITY AND RELATED CONCEPTS

The focus of this section is to provide a summative overview of four concepts that are
foundational to the discussion on lack of anonymity. We begin with concepts, as the relationship between concepts and knowledge development helps us to better understand
nursing practice (Rodgers, 2000). The more insight we have into a concept related to rural
practice environments, the better prepared we can be for rural nursing practice.

Lack of Anonymity and Anonymity

It is beneficial to understand anonymity when discussing lack of anonymity; understanding what a concept is not can aid in understanding the concept. Lee defines lack
of anonymity as "a condition in which one cannot remain nameless or unknown" (Lee,
1998, p. 77). In contrast, Marx (1999) defines anonymity as "a person cannot be identified" (p. 100) which is like Zimbardo's (1969) description of anonymity as the loss of
individual uniqueness or characteristics. Essentially, anonymity means a person is not
known. In rural health literature, discussion on anonymity is often limited. The ability
to be anonymous, or unknown, is to be alone and without relationship with others. And
here is where we need to begin our rethinking. Anonymity means an individual is not
known, whereas lack of anonymity requires being known, suggesting that there is a relational quality to lack of anonymity. In essence, we cannot be anonymous by ourselves;
we need the presence of another person.

The relational quality of lack of anonymity is described in literature. Stewart Fahs (2017) described leaders in rural healthcare as embedded within a community. Rolland (2016) captured the lack of anonymity experienced by rural ED nurses as they provided care to people known to them. Kozica et al. (2015) identified lack of anonymity as a barrier rural woman face when considering whether to participate in a healthy lifestyle class. Swan and Hobbs (2017) maintain that individuals are identifiable and interconnected to communities. These examples support the contention that lack of anonymity, in its variation and contexts, is about being relational.

Anonymity has significant societal implications. Bodle (2013) suggested that anonymity is fundamental to freedom of expression and privacy rights. Anonymity can allow individuals to speak freely in opposition to an idea, policy, or government without retaliation, social exclusion, or loss of personal privacy (McIntyre vs. Ohio Elections Commission, 1995). For example, the influential Federalist Papers were written anonymously to encourage support for the ratification of the U.S. Constitution by New York citizens (Congress.gov, n.d.). The U.S. Supreme Court has ruled on several cases that involve anonymity and afford protections under the U.S. Constitution for those who may take unpopular stances in society (McIntyre vs. Ohio Elections Commission, 1995). Significant discussions are occurring regarding the practice and ethics of anonymity versus no anonymity, particularly in online environments (Bodle, 2013). Being anonymous frees an individual of the accountability, reputation, and responsibility associated with lack of anonymity (Swan & Hobbs, 2017). This contributes to the positive side of anonymity, including free expression of ideas, truth-telling, and self-disclosure of private information not normally shared (Bodle, 2013; Novak, 2014). For example, an anonymous informant, or participant, may share information that might not otherwise be known, such as in a research study or journalistic inquiry. The benefits of anonymity, as previously described, are compelling and worth protecting; however, anonymity has drawbacks.

Contemporary discussions on anonymity focus on digital technology and online environments. A debate persists between those seeking online anonymity, including the use of pseudonyms, versus a growing online culture that requires user identification, such as Facebook and Google+ (Bodle, 2013). There is ample documentation that anonymous online environments provide opportunity for criminals to conceal their identities from an unsuspecting public, and have depersonalization effects resulting in aggressive, hateful speech (Bodle, 2013; Novak, 2014). When someone believes that they are protected by anonymity, they may act in more aggressive ways, or in ways that they would not act if they were known. The relational quality of lack of anonymity implies some level of trust; trust is common in rural communities. Insider status and trusting relationships found in many rural communities may insulate rural dwellers from the negatives of anonymity. Because rural dwellers have trusting relationships with people they know, they may be at greater risk for being preyed upon through the Internet. Taking time to consider the role of anonymity in society is an important exercise as we reflect on the lack of anonymity experienced in rural communities.

So, what does this have to do with rethinking lack of anonymity and anonymity? Lack of anonymity is inherent in a rural environment and occurs without an individual's consent. This means that the rural nurse and the rural dweller both experience lack of anonymity in healthcare encounters. The relational quality of lack of anonymity places rural nurses in practice environments where trusting relationships are commonplace. Anonymity is one way to protect privacy rights, but anonymity is not interchangeable with privacy.

Privacy

Privacy issues are commonly reported with lack of anonymity (Novak, 2014). Although closely related, the concepts are distinctly different; by definition, privacy involves concealment, individuals attempting to keep something to themselves. Individuals manage privacy by not sharing personal information with another, or, by self-disclosing private information to another with the expectation that the information will not be shared. In the latter, a trusting relationship is an essential component of privacy (Townsend, 2009). Privacy is largely personal, with an acceptable level of disclosure varying from person to person.

Since privacy is personal, there is a misperception that privacy is fully under an individual's control. For example, a simple "like" in Facebook shares posted information with friends of a friend, and so forth. Once personal information is shared in a public forum, individual control may be lost. Complicating this further is that an individual may not know, or have control over, what is shared about him or herself on social media websites. Privacy issues are a reality in rural healthcare and research. Noone and Young (2009) identified breaks in privacy for adolescent females seeking contraceptives at a rural clinic by being seen and identified by people in the waiting room. Stein's (2010) ethnographic research into gay and lesbian civil rights in a rural community is upended when journalists reveal the name of the town used during the study. With the promised anonymity and confidentiality compromised, Stein was surprised to learn that the study participants were upset, not by being identified, but that their privacy was compromised (2010). These are examples of private information being disclosed without consent.

Like anonymity, privacy has societal implications. The U.S. Supreme Court established a *right to privacy* as implied in the Constitution in *Griswold vs. Connecticut* in 1965 (Garrow, 2011). Following this decision, the right to privacy was further supported in *Katz vs. U.S.* and *Roe vs. Wade* (Fradella et al., 2011; Rausch, 2012). Privacy, particularly as it pertains to digital and online communication, remains in the public and political forum. As of this writing, the Email Privacy Act passed by the U.S. House of Representatives is awaiting action by the Senate (Congress.gov, 2017). In 2017, the Trump administration reversed the Internet privacy protections implemented under the Obama administration; telecommunication companies can now track people's personal Internet information without consent (Lohr, 2017). Privacy and individual rights to privacy will continue to be the topics of national conversation. The ongoing debate of what is private, or not, may lie in the variability between individuals on what is acceptable to disclose to others.

As we consider how to rethink lack of anonymity, we need to recognize that the concepts of lack of anonymity and privacy are not synonymous. Privacy issues can arise with or without the presence of lack of anonymity. Lack of anonymity may be experienced without loss of privacy. Privacy appears to be connected to how rural dwellers manage boundaries of the personal and public self (Long & Weinert, 1989; Swan & Hobbs, 2017).

Confidentiality

Confidentiality is often linked to privacy and anonymity. The linkage to anonymity is commonly related to journalistic protection of sources, or the use of anonymity in research to ensure confidentiality of study participants (Novak, 2014). In research, confidentiality is maintained by de-identifying, or making study participants, or situations, anonymous. In the strictest sense, study participants are never truly anonymous, as the researcher knows who participated (Novak, 2014). Confidentiality is relational and requires trust in, or with, another individual (Novak, 2014; Townsend, 2009). In healthcare, confidentiality is a central belief of ethical care; nurses have a duty to protect information known about or disclosed by a patient or family during the provision of care (American Nurses Association, 2015). For example, using social media to disclose information about a patient or family breaches confidentiality.

Townsend (2009) suggests that confidentiality works differently within the intimate nature of rural communities. The close relationships and contact at social and community events may place the rural nurse in situations where patients are encountered outside of the healthcare setting. Therefore, rural nurses must be hypervigilant in maintaining confidentiality. In contrast, nurses working in urban settings are less likely to meet patients in social settings; thus, reducing the opportunity to violate confidentiality.

Familiarity

It may be surprising to learn that familiarity is a physiologic process. There is ample evidence that the brain has neural systems for memories that can identify objects, individuals, situations, words, environments, and more, as familiar (Graves et al., 2007; Stone & Valentine, 2005). The familiar stimulates memories stored in the brain and can occur unconsciously (Viswanathan et al., 2016). Yet how the neural systems of memory function are not well understood (Voss et al., 2012). Repetition, or repeated exposure, appears to lead to familiarity (Dahl et al., 2001) and there is evidence that people tend to be more familiar with what they deem to be "good" (Stone & Valentine, 2005). This explains why people are drawn to what they know and may experience a *feeling of knowing* when recognizing the familiar (Jurjanz et al., 2011). Similarly, people become familiar with a location, or environment, and specific elements located within a space (Hayfield & Schug, 2019).

Familiarity also has both cognitive (thinking) and behavioral (emotional) dimensions. The pull toward what is familiar can limit creativity, ideas, and exploration into new ways of thinking (Viswanathan et al., 2016). As such, the cognitive dimension requires that an individual be aware of what they find familiar and be intentional about looking at circumstances in a new way. The behavioral dimension can be directly observed in how an individual interacts with others and within a specific environment or location (Asencio, 2011). For example, a rural nurse may interact more intimately with a patient or family with whom they have a close relationship than a patient or family whom they know from the community. The difference between lack of anonymity and familiarity appears related to the depth of the relationship (Gale et al., 1990).

Further analysis reveals that familiarity is much broader and deeper than originally described. As we look at familiarity, the rural environment and relationships need consideration. In their concept analysis on familiarity, McNeely and Shreffler (1998) defined familiarity within the rural context as a "friendly relationship or close acquaintance, intimacy, informality, and the exhibited familiarity is welcome or unwelcome" (p. 98). Familiarity is complex and encompasses the relationships between person and/or things with which they are well acquainted. Familiarity develops from historical knowledge, geographic/environmental location, close social proximity, and through relationships and interactions with people (Asencio, 2011; Hayfield & Schug, 2019; Jurjanz et al., 2011). Familiar relationships can be friendly to intimate and may be welcome or unwelcome. Familiarity, unlike privacy and confidentiality, does not necessarily include trust. It is possible to be familiar with someone and not trust them; the *unwelcome* element of familiarity may intersect with personal privacy and boundaries.

Support for the familiarity definition is found in literature. Ryan and McKenna (2013) studied the factors that rural family caregivers considered before placing an older adult in a nursing home. The study identified that familiarity with the nursing home staff, residents, and the rural community was a factor in making the decision about nursing home placement. This finding supports that familiarity is a feeling of belonging. Belonging is composed of affective (attachment) and personal (emotional) feelings that make an individual feel they are *at home* (Hayfield & Schug, 2019). Social connections and networks, such as the personal relationship with the nursing home staff, can activate this sense of belonging.

Familiarity appears to exist on a continuum. Imagine being at the local rural diner when someone new to the community enters. The newcomer is familiar in their strangeness within that location and place (Hayfield & Schug, 2019). Over time, their familiarity increases. Through repeated interactions with people in the rural community, the newcomer becomes familiar as they build social relationships, participate in the community life, and assimilate into the culture. They are no longer a stranger. In this case, both familiarity and lack of anonymity increase. Conversely, newcomers who do not interact and build rural relationships may remain less familiar, however, may still experience lack of anonymity in the rural community.

What does this have to do with rethinking lack of anonymity? Lack of anonymity and familiarity are often discussed together, and the difference between the two concepts is not always clear. Both concepts are relational and center on knowing about another person or entity. Swan and Hobbs's (2017) analysis identified familiarity as a consequence of lack of anonymity. Thus, experiencing lack of anonymity contributes to the development of familiarity.

MODEL OF LACK OF ANONYMITY

The purpose of examining concepts is to gain insight into how the concepts affect nursing practice. The previous review defines, describes, and provides a high-level overview of each concept from current literature. To explain the linkages between lack of anonymity with the concepts of privacy, confidentiality, and familiarity, a model of lack of anonymity has been developed (see Figure 5.1).

Lack of anonymity and familiarity are both relational and occur through individual interactions with others in rural communities. Previous research supports that Familiarity is an outcome of Lack of Anonymity (Swan & Hobbs, 2017). Once a person is known or recognized, but are not familiar, they are no longer anonymous and

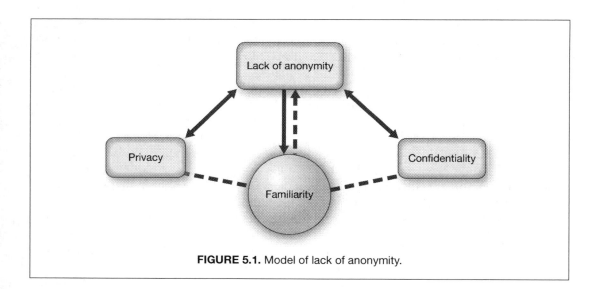

FIGURE 5.1. Model of lack of anonymity.

therefore experience lack of anonymity. Thus, the arrow connecting Lack of Anonymity to Familiarity indicates that an individual will experience lack of anonymity before experiencing familiarity. However, as Familiarity exists on a continuum, as a person becomes more familiar in a rural community it influences the amount of Lack of Anonymity experienced. The dashed unidirectional arrow reflects the feedback effect of Familiarity on Lack of Anonymity.

Based on evidence in the literature, the bidirectional arrows from Lack of Anonymity to Privacy and Confidentiality suggest that there is a relationship and influence between the concepts. For example, a rural nurse who experiences high lack of anonymity may encounter more issues with privacy and confidentiality in his or her personal and professional life. A dash line from Familiarity to Privacy and Confidentiality indicates that the evidence is not clear on the relationship of the concepts to each other; however, since familiarity is a consequence of lack of anonymity, this suggests that there may be a relationship. The model is evolving and requires further research be done to fully understand the relationship between the concepts; additionally, there may be other concepts not considered in this review that require inclusion.

IMPLICATIONS

Rural Nursing Practice

Lack of anonymity is a reality in rural environments, affecting the rural nurse and the rural dweller. Rural dwellers experience relationships with others in a community; familiarity provides opportunity to make friends and have meaningful relationships. People can call others by name and can identify each other's unique qualities and characteristics. Experiencing lack of anonymity by being identifiable and known can be challenging for rural nurses. Rural nurses report issues with personal privacy that may require navigating professional issues and relationships in a community setting. Establishing personal and professional boundaries will help rural nurses with maintaining personal privacy.

Accountability and responsibility are characteristics of rural dwellers; rural dwellers generally engage in honest communication that promotes trusting relationships. Rural nurses provide care to people whom they know and with whom they may have significant relationships. Thus, rural nurses may know medical and personal information about a patient that an urban nurse may not know. Similarly, this knowledge may afford rural nurses the opportunity to establish a trusting relationship prior to a health encounter. A preexisting trust relationship may prompt the sharing of confidential information with a rural nurse. Rural nurses have reported challenges in maintaining confidentiality while maintaining personal and professional boundaries (Swan & Hobbs, 2017). Establishing these boundaries may well be one of the most difficult challenges for rural nurses who experience lack of anonymity in their everyday lives. Future research into how rural nurses manage confidentiality in rural and remote communities may reveal strategies that could be taught or implemented across disciplines in rural healthcare facilities. Gaining knowledge on confidentiality supports ethical nursing practice for rural nurses.

Rural dwellers may also know their nurse, a situation that may or may not be comforting. Noone and Young (2009) describe the paradoxical nature of lack of anonymity; some rural dwellers find comfort in knowing their healthcare providers on a personal level, whereas others do not. There is ample evidence in the literature that rural dwellers find comfort in knowing their nurse, but rural nurses should not assume that all rural dwellers are comfortable *being known* by their nurse. Some rural dwellers may have concern that private health information may be made public. This paradoxical nature may explain some of the variation in privacy expectations among individuals. Rural nurses need to consider how being known to their patient may potentially affect the information disclosed by the patient. Extra care and attention to privacy and confidentiality may be warranted as reassurance to rural dwellers.

The Internet, communication technology, and telemedicine increase access to health information and healthcare providers outside of a rural community. Researchers at the Pew Research Center (2019) report that 86% of U.S. citizens are using the Internet at least occasionally. Greater connectivity and access to health information may act to bridge rural dwellers to outside healthcare resources and information, thus affecting the social capital of rural nurses. Additionally, recognizing that care may be obtained outside of the rural community, specific health history questions should be asked to verify patients' knowledge and ensure their understanding is consistent with the best evidence and current health information.

This review supports that familiarity is integrated in the life of rural dwellers and is more complex than originally believed. Lack of anonymity is often portrayed as a negative of rural communities; however, there is growing evidence that lack of anonymity plays a positive role in relationships and the development of familiarity. Understanding these positive aspects of lack of anonymity and familiarity will provide greater insight into how the concepts affect care provided in rural practice settings. Equally, more research is needed to understand how familiarity may limit thinking and exploration of ideas. The tendency to stay with what is familiar may provide comfort, but during a health challenge, rural nurses should take extra care to ensure that thinking is not limited to what is familiar.

Privacy is a personal issue that may be experienced in rural environments. Lack of anonymity, or being known, can limit privacy. For example, rural dwellers may opt out of mental health services to prevent being recognized by their car parked in the clinic lot (Graber, 2011; Kitchen Andren et al., 2013). In this case, the health and well-being of the patient is being affected out of concern for personal privacy. Rural nurses may need to ask specific questions regarding patients' concerns and seek to understand how privacy issues may affect healthcare choices.

Nursing Research

The concepts described are closely related but are not synonymous or interchangeable. Clearly defining concepts is essential to ensure that the right concept is being studied and measured; without clear definitions, findings may be inconsistent, and conceptual clarity may be diminished. For example, a rural nurse may experience lack of anonymity but have issue with a lack of privacy. Since lack of anonymity, to some degree, is present in a rural environment, the central issue may be the rural nurse's expectation of personal privacy. Thus, privacy is the concept of interest, not necessarily lack of anonymity. Care must be taken to prevent lack of anonymity from being a catchall term; rethinking lack of anonymity and how it influences a rural environment may well reveal new concepts requiring exploration. The state of rural nursing science will advance with the use of common definitions of rural concepts.

In addition, further research on privacy and lack of anonymity is needed to help to identify and delineate the personal issues of privacy from the relational components of lack of anonymity. This delineation is critical to ensure that we are asking research questions appropriate to the concept. Future studies exploring the rural dwellers' expectations of personal privacy would add greater depth to our understanding. Further, it is unknown whether the expectation of personal privacy in rural environments is different than the expectation of those living in urban environments.

CASE STUDIES

The following case studies have been developed to demonstrate how the concepts of lack of anonymity, privacy, confidentiality, and familiarity are encountered in the daily work of a rural nurse.

Karen is a registered nurse in a small rural community. She grew up on a farm outside of town and is related to or knows most of the people in the community. Karen, her husband, and their two school-aged children live in town. Karen and her family are active in youth sports and church activities.

Karen met Leah in the sixth grade, after Leah and her family moved to town. Karen and Leah were friends and used to hang out together. That changed in high school, when Leah began to "party" and experiment with alcohol, marijuana, and other drugs. Karen was not interested in partying with Leah, and the two drifted apart. Today, Leah is a part-time waitress at the local diner. Leah is divorced, mother to three school-aged children, and rents an apartment in town.

CASE STUDY 1

Karen provided nursing care to Leah's child during a recent hospitalization that provided time for Leah and Karen to visit and catch up on their life activities. A couple of weeks after the child was discharged, Karen stopped at the grocery store after work to pick up a few groceries. The store was busy, and Karen was pressed for time. While shopping, Karen ran into Leah, who stopped her and started to ask detailed questions related to her child's condition and medical care received during the hospital stay.

How should Karen respond?

What concept is best represented in the case study? How do you recognize the concept?

CASE STUDY 2

Karen was walking down the hallway that connects the hospital and clinic and found Leah in the hallway holding one child and trying to entertain the other two. Karen greeted Leah and asked whether she needed any help. Leah declined help and said that she did not want to sit in the waiting room and be seen by others. Leah expressed concern that people would determine that she was here to see a visiting specialist, who came to the clinic once a month, and guess at why she needed care. Leah stated, "I don't want people knowing anything about me."

How should Karen respond?

What concept is best represented in the case study? How do you recognize the concept?

(continued)

(continued)

Case Study 3

Karen cared for Leah's child a third time in the ED. During the encounter, Karen learned that Leah's child had a serious, chronic health condition. Leah wept as she shared the diagnosis; she shared the challenges of being the sole parent responsible for the care needs of her family and the financial hardship of paying the medical bills along with living expenses. Karen felt compassion for Leah and connected Leah to the local social service and volunteer agencies for additional support. Leah was appreciative and gave Karen a hug and thanked her for providing great care. A few days later, Karen received a friend request from Leah on a social network. Karen thought this might be a good way to support Leah and accepted the friend request. In reviewing the social network postings, Karen learned that Leah's child was responding well to a medicine listed in the post that Karen knew had been prescribed on discharge from the ED. Karen was excited for Leah and posted a comment that she was glad that the medicine from the ED visit was helping. The next day, Karen was pulled into her manager's office and was told that she violated patient confidentiality.

How should Karen respond?

What concept is best represented in the case study? How do you recognize the concept?

Case Study 4

Leah's child has had a series of recent hospitalizations and Karen has been involved in providing nursing care. Leah is always pleased to see Karen and initiates conversations about their children and mutual interests. During the most recent hospitalization, Leah was struggling with making a treatment decision for her child. Over several shifts, Karen was assigned to Leah's child and had many conversations with Leah about treatment options. Leah told Karen that she appreciated her thoughts and education on different treatment options and shared how the information Karen provided helped her to decide on the best treatment option for her child.

How should Karen respond?

What concept is best represented in the case study? How do you recognize the concept?

CONCLUSION

Lack of anonymity is relational and a reality of rural life. Rural dwellers are identifiable and will become known to others in the community. Likewise, as a rural nurse, being known and recognizable is expected. As a result, rural nurses may need to manage aspects of their personal and professional lives to control their privacy. Trusting relationships exist in rural communities and extend into rural practice settings. As such, rural nurses need to recognize how breaking a trusting relationship will influence the ability to ensure patient privacy and confidentiality. Likewise, sharing confidential or private information about another can also affect the patient–nurse trusting relationship.

The analysis prompts us to rethink how we view lack of anonymity, and consider how lack of anonymity influences, both positively and negatively, rural nursing practice. The relational quality of lack of anonymity, confidentiality, and familiarity reflect the interconnectedness found in rural communities. These stand in contrast to the personal nature of privacy. These four concepts help us to understand rural nursing practice. The model of lack of anonymity suggests that more research is needed to fully understand how the concepts, and possibly others, are related.

Rural nurses are uniquely positioned to influence health and well-being in rural communities. Rethinking lack of anonymity for the 21st century requires us to look deeply into rural concepts in order to open up new possibilities for research and to further our understanding and advance rural nursing science.

REFERENCES

American Nurses Association. (2015). *Code of ethics for nurses with interpretive statements*. American Nurses Publishing.

Asencio, E. K. (2011). Familiarity, legitimation, and frequency: The influence of others on the criminal self-view. *Sociological Inquiry*, *81*(1), 34–52. https://doi.org/10.1111/j.1475-682x.2010.00352.x

Bodle, R. (2013). The ethics of online anonymity or Zuckerberg vs. "Moot." *Computers and Society*, *43*(1), 22–35. https://doi.org/10.1145/2505414.2505417

Congress.gov. (n.d.). *About the federalist papers*. https://www.congress.gov/resources/display/content/About+the+Federalist+Papers

Congress.gov. (2017, February 6). *H. R. 387-Email Privacy Act*. https://www.congress.gov/bill/115th-congress/house-bill/387

Dahl, D. W., Manchanda, R. V., & Argo, J. J. (2001). Embarrassment in consumer purchase: The roles of social presence and purchase familiarity. *Journal of Consumer Research*, *28*(3), 473–481. https://doi.org/10.1086/323734

Fradella, H. F., Morrow, W. J., Fischer, R. G., & Ireland, C. (2011). Quantifying Katz: Empirically measuring "reasonable expectations of privacy" in the fourth amendment context. *American Journal of Criminal Law*, *38*(3), 289–373.

Gale, N., Golledge, R., Halperin, W. C., & Coudelis, H. (1990). Exploring spatial familiarity. *Professional Geographer*, *42*(3), 299–313. https://doi.org/10.1111/j.0033-0124.1990.00299.x.

Garrow, D. J. (2011). The legal legacy of Griswold v. Connecticut. *Human Rights*, *38*(2), 24–25.

Graber, M. A. (2011). The overlapping roles of the rural doctor. *American Medical Association Journal of Ethics*, *13*(5), 273–277. https://doi.org/%2010.1001/virtualmentor.2011.13.5.ccas1-1105

Graves, W. W., Grabowski, T. J., Mehta, S., & Gordon, J. K. (2007). A neural signature of phonological access: Distinguishing the effects of word frequency from familiarity and length in overt picture naming. *Journal of Cognitive Neuroscience*, *19*(4), 617–631. https://doi.org./10.1162/jocn.2007.19.4.617

Hayfield, E. A., & Schug, M. (2019). 'It's like they have a cognitive map of relations': Feeling strange in a small island community. *Journal of Intercultural Studies*, *40*(4), 383–398. https://doi.org/10.1080/07256868.2019.1628719

Hegney, D. (1996). The status of rural nursing in Australia: A review. *Australian Journal of Rural Health*, *4*, 1–10. https://doi.org/10.1111/j.1440-1584.1996.tb00180.x

Jurjanz, L., Donix, M., Amanatidis, E. C., Meyer, S., Poettrich, K., Huebner, T., Baeumler, D., Smolka, M. N., & Holthoff, V. A. (2011). Visual personal familiarity in amnestic mild cognitive impairment. *PLOS ONE*, *6*(5), 1–7. https://doi.org/10.1371/journal.pone.0020030

Kitchen Andren, K. A., McKibbin, C. L., Wykes, T. L., Lee, A. A., Carrico, C. P., & Bourassa, K. A. (2013). Depression treatment among rural older adults: Preferences and factors influencing future service use. *Clinical Gerontologist*, *36*(3), 241–259. https://doi.org/10.1080/07317115.2013.767872

Kozica, S. L., Harrison, C. L., Teede, H. J., Ng, S., Moran, L. J., & Lombard, C. B. (2015). Engaging rural women in healthy lifestyle programs: Insights from a randomized controlled trial. *Trials*, *16*, 413. https://doi.org/10.1186/s13063-015-0860-5

Lauder, W., Reel, S., Farmer, J., & Griggs, H. (2006). Social capital, rural nursing and rural nursing theory. *Nursing Inquiry*, *13*(1), 73–79. https://doi.org/10.1111/j.1440-1800.2006.00297.x

Lee, H. J. (1998). Lack of anonymity. In H. J. Lee (Ed.), *Conceptual basis for rural nursing* (1st ed., pp. 76–88). Springer Publishing Company.

Lohr, S. (2017, April 3). *Trump completes repeal of online privacy protections from Obama era*. https://www
.nytimes.com/2017/04/03/technology/trump-repeal-online-privacy-protections.html?_r=0

Long, K. A., & Weinert, S. C. (1989). Rural nursing: Developing the theory base. *Scholarly Inquiry for Nursing Practice: An International Journal*, 3(2), 113–127.

Marx, G. T. (1999). What's in a name? Some reflections on the sociology of anonymity. *The Information Society*, 15, 99–112. https://doi.org/10.1080/019722499128565

McIntyre v. Ohio Elections Commission, 514 U.S. 334 U.S. (1995). https://www.law.cornell.edu/supct/html/93-986.ZO.html

McNeely, A. G., & Shreffler, M. J. (1998). Familiarity. In H. Lee (Ed.), *Conceptual basis for rural nursing* (1st ed., pp. 89–101). Springer Publishing Company.

Noone, J., & Young, H. M. (2009). Preparing daughters: The context of rurality on mothers' role in contraception. *The Journal of Rural Health*, 25(3), 282–288. https://doi.org/10.1111/j.1748-0361.2009.00231.x

Novak, A. (2014). Anonymity, confidentiality, privacy, and identity: The ties that bind and break in communication research. *Review of Communication*, 14(1), 36–48. https://doi.org/10.1080/15358593.2014.942351

Pew Research Center. (2019, July 25). *About three-in-ten U.S. adults say they are 'almost constantly' online*. https://www.pewresearch.org/fact-tank/2019/07/25/americans-going-online-almost-constantly/

Rausch, R. L. (2012). Reframing Roe: Property over privacy. *Berkley Journal of Gender, Law & Justice*, 27(1), 28–63.

Rodgers, B. L. (2000). Philosophical foundations of concept development. In B. L. Rodgers & K. A. Knafl (Eds.), *Concept development in nursing* (2nd ed., pp. 7–37). Saunders.

Rolland, R. A. (2016). Emergency room nurses transitioning from curative to end-of-life care: The rural influence. *Online Journal of Rural Nursing and Health Care*, 16(2), 58–85. https://doi.org/10.14574/ojrnhc.v16i2.396

Rosenthal, K. A. (2010). The rural nursing generalist in the acute care setting: Flowing like a river. In C. A. Winters & H. J. Lee (Eds.), *Rural nursing concepts: Theory and practice* (3rd ed., pp. 269–283). Springer Publishing Company.

Ryan, A., & McKenna, H. (2013). 'Familiarity' as a key factor influencing rural family carers' experience of the nursing home placement of an older relative: A qualitative study. *BMC Health Services Research*, 13, 252. https://doi.org/10.1186/1472-6963-13-252

Stein, A. (2010). Sex, truths, and audiotape: Anonymity and the ethics of exposure in public ethnography. *Journal of Contemporary Ethnography*, 39(5), 554–568. https://doi.org/10.1177/0891241610375955

Stewart Fahs, P. (2017). Leading-following in the context of rural nursing. *Nursing Science Quarterly*, 30(2), 176–178. https://doi.org/10.1177/0894318417693317

Stone, A., & Valentine, T. (2005). Accuracy of familiarity decisions to famous faces perceived without awareness depends on attitude to the target person and on response latency. *Consciousness & Cognition*, 14(2), 351–376. https://doi.org/10.1016/j.concog.2004.09.002

Swan, M. A., & Hobbs, B. B. (2017). Concept analysis: Lack of anonymity. *Journal of Advanced Nursing*, 73(5), 1075–1084. https://doi.org/10.1111/jan.13236

Townsend, T. (2009). Ethics conflicts in rural communities: Privacy and confidentiality. In W. A. Nelson (Ed.), *Handbook for rural health care ethics: A practical guide for professionals* (1st ed., pp. 128–141). University Press of New England.

Viswanathan, V., Tomko, M., & Linsey, J. (2016). A study on the effects of example familiarity and modality on design fixation. *AI EDAM*, 30(2), 171–184. https://doi.org/10.1017/S0890060416000056

Voss, J., Lucas, H., & Paller, K. (2012). More than a feeling: Pervasive influences of memory without awareness of retrieval. *Cognitive Neuroscience*, 3(3/4), 193–226. https://doi.org/10.1080/17588928.2012.674935

Whitley, R., & McKenzie, K. (2005). Social capital and psychiatry: Review of the literature. *Harvard Review of Psychiatry*, 13(2), 71–84. https://doi.org/10.1080/10673220590956474

Zimbardo, P. G. (1969). The human choice: Individuation, reason and order versus deindividuation, impulse and chaos. In W. Arnold & D. Levine (Eds.), *Nebraska Symposium on Motivation* (1st ed., Vol. XVII, pp. 237–307). University of Nebraska Press.

CHAPTER 6

Rural Nursing Theory and Research on the Frontier

LYNN JAKOBS

DISCUSSION TOPICS

- Use the frontier counties maps on the National Center for Frontier Communities (NCFC) website, frontierus.org/resources/, to evaluate the relationship of frontier county populations compared to total U.S. counties in regard to age and racial distribution, as well as poverty levels. Discuss how *place* affects these sociodemographic indices.
- Based on the information gathered in the first activity, develop a list of research topics appropriate to the frontier setting.
- Besides the methods of recruitment mentioned in this chapter, discuss other recruitment methods appropriate for frontier settings.
- Discuss the possible uses for Rural Nursing Theory when planning, conducting, or analyzing frontier research.

INTRODUCTION

Rural life may entail residing in a county with a population of 100,000, access to a small hospital, several grocery stores, multiple options for primary medical care, a paid ambulance service, and a local ED. Contrast this to life in the frontier, which may entail living in a county with a population of 3,000, one gas station/grocery store, possibly a rural medical clinic, a volunteer ambulance service, and access to an ED at least an hour away. Studies involving access to medical care or access to healthy food in each of these settings would likely yield vastly different results, although both settings fall under the umbrella designation of *rural*. This example demonstrates the importance of properly describing the research setting. This chapter provides an overview of these and other issues when conducting research in the frontier, including the use of Rural Nursing Theory as a conceptual framework.

RURAL CULTURE AND RESEARCHER AUTHENTICITY

Prior to a discussion of rural taxonomies, it is important to briefly discuss rural culture and rural authenticity. Studies have demonstrated that rural dwellers have common characteristics that can be considered integral to a *rural culture*. These characteristics include a distrust of outsiders, a strong sense of independence and self-reliance, and a preference for interacting with other local residents as opposed to someone from outside the community (Long & Weinert, 1989). Researchers who have a rural background and understand both the cultural and healthcare nuances of rural and remote areas may find it easier to build trust and gain entrance into these areas (Farmer et al., 2012).

Cultural characteristics have implications for researchers who want to study healthcare issues in rural/frontier areas. This concept was exemplified by Sharp (2010), when he conducted research with rural nurse practitioners (NPs). Sharp wrote that truth, value, or credibility was achieved because of the time he spent practicing as an NP in a rural area (p. 41). Sharp's practice experience allowed for an understanding of both rural culture and the typical experiences of rural NPs, which allowed him to connect with his participants. Furthermore, researchers with rural backgrounds may have a greater understanding of the types of problems related to this geographic setting. Authenticity may be even more vital in frontier settings where communities are more isolated.

TAXONOMIES FOR RURAL AND FRONTIER RESEARCH

The Rural Designation

It is important for researchers to accurately describe their research setting or population; this entails choosing the appropriate taxonomy to determine the rurality of the setting. The use of specific geographic designations ensures others that a standardized method was utilized, particularly if other researchers want to either duplicate the study, or repeat the study in a different geographic setting.

Government agencies use different taxonomies to determine rurality. A community's standing on the lists of rural or frontier counties may change every 10 years as new census data are reported (Hart, 2012). The more common taxonomies are listed in Table 6.1. The Office of Management and Budget's (OMB) taxonomy divides the United States into three categories: (a) metropolitan, (b) nonmetropolitan, and (c) micropolitan; the nonmetropolitan areas are further subdivided into 10 categories. The most frontier-like of these categories, number 12, could be considered a frontier area (Hart, 2012).

Taxonomies were created by agencies to fit their own purposes; hence, there may be some overlap between the taxonomies for some rural areas. For example, one region may have four different rural configurations depending on the taxonomy chosen to determine rurality (Smith et al., 2013). Therefore, it is important to utilize the taxonomy that best fits the rural research question or purpose.

The Frontier Designation

To avoid comparing heterogeneous populations, frontier researchers should utilize a standard designation. In the mid-1980s, Congress decided that for the purposes of healthcare policy they would define frontier as a county with less than seven persons per square mile (Ricketts et al., 1998). However, larger counties may have one or more metropolitan areas within driving distance of frontier communities, affecting the availability of goods and services. It was decided that additional criteria were needed. Therefore, the

TABLE 6.1 Rural Criteria

Originating Agency	Taxonomy	Criteria
Economic Research Service	RUCA Codes	Tract-level work commuting data
OMB	Metropolitan Taxonomy	Metropolitan, nonmetropolitan, and micropolitan
U.S. Census Bureau	Rural and Urban Taxonomy	Urbanized areas and urban clusters

OMB, Office of Management and Budget; RUCA, Rural–Urban Commuting Areas.

Source: Adapted from "Frontier/Remote, Island, and Rural Literature Review", by G. Hart, 2012, Center for Rural Health, University of North Dakota.

Department of Health and Human Services added two additional criteria to the frontier designation: (a) driving time to next level of medical care and (b) level of care at local hospitals (see Table 6.2). In 1997, another agency, the National Center for Frontier Communities (NCFC) in collaboration with the National Rural Health Association, developed a frontier scoring matrix; this iteration included a scoring mechanism (see Table 6.3).

More recently, the U.S. Department of Agriculture Economic Research Service (ERS) in partnership with the Federal Office of Rural Health Policy adopted a zip code-based methodology for determining which areas would be designated as frontier (Health Resources and Services Administration, 2012). Not only does this taxonomy account for rural counties with metropolitan population centers, it takes a four-level approach to determining how remote a frontier area is (see Table 6.4). The title for this latest frontier taxonomy is FAR, frontier and remote (Cromartie, 2015). Benefits of using the FAR taxonomy include the following:

- Accurately describes the phenomena based on a specific designation
- Accurately describes the participant sample based on a specific designation
- Allows for replication of the study
- Allows for conduction of comparative studies between different levels of the taxonomy

The limitations of the FAR taxonomy are that they only pertain to county data, and they are only useful in the United States.

The development of these frontier taxonomy schemes gives the frontier researcher options to define their research setting depending upon who or what is being studied.

TABLE 6.2 1986 Rural/Frontier Matrix

Parameter	Rural	Frontier
Driving time to next level of care	30 minutes	60 minutes or severe geographic and climatic conditions
Population density	Greater than six but less than 100	Less than six per square mile
Hospital	Small, 25–100 beds, may have swing beds	25 beds or less, or no hospital

Source: Data from Elison, G. (1986). Frontier areas: Problems for delivery of health care services. *Rural Health Care,* 8(5), 1–3.

TABLE 6.3 1997 Frontier Matrix

Density—Persons per Square Mile	POINTS
0–12	45
12.1–16	30
16.1–20	20
Note: Per county or per defined service area with Justification	
Total points density	

Distance—In Miles to Service/Market	
>90 Miles	30
60–90	20
30–60	10
Note: Starting point must be rational, either a service site or proposed site	
Total points distance in miles	

Travel Time—In Minutes to Service/Market	
>90 minutes	30
60–90	20
30–60	10
Note: Usual travel time; exceptions must be documented (i.e., weather, geography, seasonal)	
Total points travel time in minutes	

Total Points All Categories

Note: Total possible points = 105; minimum points necessary for frontier designation = 55; "extremes" = 55–105.

Source: Data from Cromartie, J. (2015). *Frontier and Remote (FAR) area codes: A preliminary view of upcoming changes*. National Center for Frontier Communities webinar, Washington, DC.

TABLE 6.4 FAR Criteria

FAR Level One	Zip code areas with majority populations living 60 minutes or more from urban areas of 50,00 or more people
FAR Level Two	Zip code areas with majority populations living 60 minutes or more from urban areas of 50,000 or more people *and* 45 minutes or more from urban areas of 25,000–49,999 people
FAR Level Three	Zip code areas with majority populations living 60 minutes or more from urban areas of 50,000 or more people; 45 minutes or more from urban areas of 25,000–49,999 people *and* 30 minutes or more from urban areas of 10,000–24,999 people
FAR Level Four	Zip code areas with majority populations living 60 minutes or more from urban areas of 50,00 or more people; 45 minutes or more from urban areas of 25,000–49,999 people; 30 minutes or more from urban areas of 10,000–24,999 people *and* 15 minutes or more from urban areas of 2,500–9,999 people

FAR, frontier and remote.

Source: Adapted from Health Resources and Services Administration. (2012). Methodology for designation of frontier and remote areas. *Federal Register, 77*(214), 25599. https://www.federalregister.gov/documents/2014/05/05/2014-10193/methodology-for-designation-of-frontier-and-remote-areas

For example, some counties are defined as entirely frontier, so a zip code-based designation system would be unnecessary. However, if you were studying nurses who worked at a specific site, using the zip code method would be appropriate. Therefore, the taxonomy used should fit the research question/purpose.

FRONTIER DEMOGRAPHICS

According to the NCFC (2012), there is a total of 812 frontier counties located in 38 states. In 2010, it was estimated that 5.6 million people in the United States live in frontier counties (Rural Health Information Hub, www.ruralhealthinfo.org/topics/frontier#how-much). Although the total numbers of people who live in the frontier is small, only about 3% of the U.S. population, the area on which they live is large. Frontier counties comprise approximately 46% of the land area in the United States. In addition, frontier lands contain 49% of the water area in the United States.

Although the majority of tribal land continues to be located in frontier areas (NCFC, 2012), frontier communities are becoming more ethnically diverse owing to regional migration patterns. During the 1990s and post-2000 period, the rural Hispanic population grew at the fastest rate of any racial or ethnic group, whereas the White population grew at the slowest rate (Johnson, 2006). The frontier population is also aging as more seniors plan to relocate to frontier communities upon retirement (NCFC, 2012).

Frontier dwellers have disparate access to healthcare due to geographic and economic factors that impact the availability of healthcare providers and services. Research indicates that the more rural the setting, the less access residents have to healthcare (Larson et al., 2020). Evidence also suggests that health status declines with increasing rurality (Singh & Siahpush, 2014).

QUANTITATIVE FRONTIER RESEARCH

In 2016, a quantitative study to determine the distribution of APRNs, family NPs, midwives, and certified nurse anesthetists, in U.S. frontier counties was conducted utilizing secondary data from the Nurses and the Population's Health Study (Jakobs & Bigbee, 2016). In addition, the investigators evaluated the relationship between the presence of APRNs and population health outcomes in those counties. As health indices were reported at the county level, the criterion of less than seven persons per square mile was the most appropriate method to determine a county's frontier designation. The numbers of APRNs in each frontier county was provided by each state's board of nursing. The study was the first attempt to link the concept of *nurse dose*, the number of APRNs in the county, to population health outcomes at the county level. However, due to small numbers of APRNs provided and missing county data, results were largely inconclusive, thus highlighting the challenges of conducting quantitative research in frontier areas.

Recruitment

Frontier areas have a relatively small pool of subjects in which to sample. Additionally, the more isolated and remote the community, the more difficult it may be to contact potential subjects. For quantitative studies that require recruitment efforts, post offices are often a point of social contact in rural, isolated communities (Pindus et al., 2010). The local post office may be an ideal place to post informational flyers about the research, or to distribute survey instruments. Another option is to find a local key player or players and enlist their help with recruitment (Johnston & Herzig, 2006). Additionally, medical providers are usually well respected in frontier settings and can be a valuable contact when trying to recruit in these sparsely populated settings, (Coyne et al., 2004; Loftin et al., 2005; Parra-Medina et al., 2004).

Small Populations

Quantitative research relies heavily on statistical analysis of data. A certain number of subjects are required to give the results enough power to be meaningful. The small sizes of frontier populations magnify the challenges of health disparities research, especially if the health condition in question is rare, as with certain genetic diseases or cancers (Sue & Dhindsa, 2006). For example, when researching the rate of disease spread or immunizations, the smaller the population the more likely that one case will translate to a very high rate of the condition being studied. For instance, if you have one case of measles in 1 year, and two cases of measles the following year, you could report a 100% increase of measles cases over the prior year. Therefore, if you're looking at specific rates of increase or decrease in a health problem or disease state, having a very small population can make the data look more powerful than it may actually be. When looking at the prevention measures that may cause a decline in the number of cases, the reverse would also be true. The percentage of change might seem significant, but there is little meaning to the data.

Due to low numbers, researchers need to be very transparent with their data and use data analysis methods appropriate for a small number of subjects. For example, in the APRN and distribution study, data on APRN distribution were available for only 308 frontier counties out of the 486 frontier counties in the coterminous United States. This limitation was noted in the discussion section of the article.

One method to increase sample size is *borrowing data* (Korngiebel et al., 2015). This method entails finding two or more frontier communities that are similar enough that you can combine data. For example, when looking at disease rates, data from areas with similar demographic and or economic characteristics might be combined to create a larger sample. For this technique to be credible, you would need to clearly describe the technique, rationale, and the similarities in the published work.

Small sample sizes may also hinder the researcher's effort to obtain grant funding as government agencies often fund research efforts that are generalizable to large populations (Etz & Arroyo, 2015). Frontier researchers may need to search for smaller grant opportunities, focusing on organizations that have an interest in either the condition/situation under study, or organizations that focus on rural populations.

Missing Data

The APRN and population health study evaluated the relationship of APRN presence and the most consistently reported frontier county health indices: premature death rate (mortality), the percentage of low birth weight births, sexually transmitted infection rates, and adult smoking rates. One issue with reporting mandates is that some frontier counties may not have a local health department. This became apparent when it was found that the only consistently reported health index in the study was the sexually transmitted disease rate. This index is not affected by rurality as it reported to the state's health department directly from the testing laboratory. Therefore, missing health index data from as many as 138 frontier county health departments limited the study's findings. This highlights the need to ensure the data you need to collect from the frontier setting in question is available prior to developing a research proposal. When utilizing secondary data, however, you must work with the information available.

QUALITATIVE FRONTIER RESEARCH

Recruitment

In 2015, a study was conducted to elicit narrative data from NPs working in frontier settings (Jakobs, 2017). The main purpose of the study was to develop a conceptual framework for educating NPs who plan to work in the frontier. The FAR methodology was utilized to locate clinics with a FAR level four designation, the most remote setting. Once a clinic was located, a search of their website revealed the name and credentials of the clinic providers. Oftentimes, clinics in these remote areas were satellite clinics of a larger health organization and could be located on the parent organization's website. If an NP was located, they were contacted by phone or email to determine their interest in study participation. This strategy yielded six participants in five different states. As qualitative research involves a more in-depth study of the participants, studies involving 6 to 10 participants are common and considered adequate. Small numbers of participants make qualitative research particularly fitting for remote settings/populations where the pool of possible participants is low.

Small Populations and Privacy Considerations

Due to the small number of residents in frontier communities, it is possible that many people are either related to one another, or know one another. In the frontier NP study, the locations of the NP practices were kept intentionally vague to rule out the possibility that community residents might recognize themselves or their communities in the published work. After transcription of the NP interviews at least one of the participants edited an answer that might have revealed too much about her community, which would make it recognizable to residents in that state. Another NP participant requested to be interviewed at a location outside her community, and out of view of its residents. All participants were very careful not to provide information that may somehow identify patients or community members.

TAKING RURAL NURSING THEORY TO THE FRONTIER

In 1989, Kathleen Ann Long and Clarann Weinert published results from their ethnographic study of rural residents in Montana (Long & Weinert, 1989; also see Chapter 2). The study was based on the assumption that healthcare needs are different in rural areas from that of urban areas. This meant that urban models were not appropriate or adequate for meeting the healthcare needs in rural areas. They also made the assumption that all rural areas are viewed as having some common health needs (Winters & Lee, 2018).

The authors interviewed rural nurses in Montana and identified concepts such as insider–outsider, role diffusion, and a lack of anonymity as characteristics of rural nursing practice. In addition, they also sampled rural residents regarding their health beliefs and practices. Based on their findings, Long and Weinert developed relational statements regarding healthcare characteristics of rural residents (Winters & Lee, 2018, p. 23). These statements can be summarized as follows:

1. Rural residents define health primarily as the ability to work or be productive.
2. Rural residents are self-reliant and resist accepting help or services from outsiders.
3. Healthcare providers in rural areas must deal with a lack of anonymity and much greater role diffusion than providers in urban or suburban settings.

The extent to which these statements can be generalized across rural settings is most likely affected by two factors: the rurality designation of the setting and the type of setting, that is, agricultural, recreational, and so on. Although their study participants represented a relatively narrow sample of rural dwellers and nurses, their research continues to be cited in the literature and represents the only widely accepted conceptual framework for rural nursing practice (Colledge, 2000; Guadron, 2008; Lauder et al., 2006; Senn, 2013; Sharp, 2010).

Use of Rural Nursing Theory in Frontier Research

In 2016, Long and Weinert's theory was validated for use with frontier populations (Jakobs, 2017). Although 25 years had lapsed since their study was published, it continued to prove valid and relevant to today's frontier population. In the following paragraphs, Rural Nursing Theory concepts are related to current frontier research.

HEALTH

In the theory of rural nursing, health is primarily defined as the ability to work, or be productive. Long and Weinert used an example of a farmer who didn't seek care for his illness until his work was done (p. 257). In the frontier NP study (Jakobs, 2017), one participant described an encounter whereby when herding cattle into a pen, a rancher's horse hit the side of the corral pinning the rancher's foot to the fence and fracturing his fibula and tibia. He did not seek care until after normal business hours because he couldn't leave the work undone (p. 76).

SELF-RELIANCE

The notion that rural residents are self-reliant was evident throughout the narratives. In the frontier setting the adage, *necessity is the mother of invention*, is applicable. This self-reliance is due to the lack of available resources and an independent spirit. One participant stated that while they started their clinic on a shoestring and did not have money for personal protective equipment, they had farm safety goggles and raingear (p. 72).

INSIDER/OUTSIDER

In Rural Nursing Theory, the concept of insider/outsider is related to both the skepticism that rural dwellers have about accepting help or services from outsiders, and the notion that healthcare providers, who are new to the community, are outsiders. In the case of NPs, the concept of outsider has broader implications as evidenced by one participant who said that prior to his arrival, "the community did not know what an NP was" (p. 65). He further went on to say that his credibility with the community increased when, on his first night in town, he responded to the scene of an accident where a car had gone down a steep embankment. He did not hesitate to climb down the embankment and treat the victim, even starting an intravenous (IV) and assisting with transport. He stated that the next day his actions were the talk-of-the-town, which really helped establish his NP practice in the community.

ROLE DIFFUSION

In Rural Nursing Theory, role diffusion was described as the need to function in multiple roles, not only in their professional life but in family and community life. For a rural nurse this may entail working across several hospital departments in one shift (Long & Weinert, 1989). Examples of this concept include (a) doing an EKG, (b) drawing labs, (c) delivering babies, or (d) cooking meals if the hospital was snowed-in (p. 266). This concept was exemplified by each participant in the frontier NP study. One participant stated that, "You have to wear many hats; you're the housekeeper, carpenter, the plumber, and the repairman" (p. 72). Other participants discussed doing all the administrative clinic work in addition to their NP practice, another mentioned acting as the de facto school nurse, and another mentioned teaching emergency medical technician (EMT) classes because there was no one else in the community qualified to do it.

LACK OF ANONYMITY

In frontier settings, a lack of anonymity may be broadly applied to include patient confidentiality. The frontier NPs interviewed by Jakobs (2017), are well-recognized community members. Most participants stated that it can be difficult to take off the NP *hat* when outside the clinic setting. At times, this can lead patients to inadvertently disclose private information in public settings. One participant dealt with the situation by wearing scrubs in the workplace and nowhere else (p. 76). Another participant had a standard response script when patient's approach her in public places and wanted to discuss their medical problems (p. 100).

CONCLUSION

Although a frontier community may fall under the umbrella term *rural*, there are population and geographic characteristics that make these communities unique; therefore, frontier communities should be identified as such. There are multiple methodologies to determine the rural status of a community, or to find a rural/frontier community in the geographic location of interest. The extant frontier research is sparse, situating new research in the frontier is important for healthcare policy, and could impact access to healthcare services.

The Rural Nursing Theory is an ethnographic theory that informs researchers about rural culture. It remains a valid and relevant contextual framework for rural and frontier nursing research. The theory can guide researchers, explain rural phenomena, and inform data analysis.

The disparate access to healthcare services makes frontier dwellers a vulnerable population. This issue alone makes research with frontier populations an important contribution to nursing knowledge. Despite the research challenges discussed in this chapter, well-designed and evaluated research studies are preferable to no research with these remote and underserved populations.

REFERENCES

Colledge, P. (2000). *Hardines as a predictor of nurse practitioners in rural practice*. PhD Dissertation, University of Idaho.

Coyne, C. A., Demian-Popescu, C., & Brown, P. (2004). Rural cancer patients' perspectives on clinical trials: a qualitative study. *Journal of Cancer Education, 19*(3), 165–169. https://doi.org/10.1207/s15430154jce1903_11

Cromartie, J. (2015). *Frontier and Remote (FAR) area codes: A preliminary view of upcoming changes*. National Center for Frontier Communities webinar, Washington, DC.

Elison, G. (1986). Frontier areas: Problems for delivery of health care services. *Rural Health Care, 8*(5), 1–3.

Etz, K. E., & Arroyo, J. A. (2015). Small sample research: Considerations beyond statistical power. *Prevention Science, 16*(7), 1033–1036. https://doi.org/10.1007/s11121-015-0585-4

Farmer, J., Munoz, S., & Daly, C. (2012). Being rural in rural health research. *Health & Place, 18*, 1206–1208. https://doi-org.hmlproxy.lib.csufresno.edu/10.1016/j.healthplace.2012.05.002

Guadron, M. (2008). *Identification of patterns of knowing used by rural community health nurses in decision-making.* PhD Dissertation, State University of New York at Binghamton.

Hart, G. (2012). *Frontier/Remote, island, and rural literature review* (pp. 1–37). Center for Rural Health, University of North Dakota.

Health Resources and Services Administration. (2012). *Methodology for designation of frontier and remote areas.* http://www.gpo.gov/fdsys/pkg/FR-2012-11-05/pdf/2012-26938.pdf

Jakobs, L. (2017). *The frontier nurse practitioner: A conceptual model for remote-rural practice.* Springer Publishing Company.

Jakobs, L., & Bigbee, J. (2016). U.S. frontier distribution of advanced practice registered nurses and population health. *Online Journal of Rural Nursing and Health Care, 2*(16), 196–218. http://dx.doi.org/10.14574/ojrnhc.v16i2.423

Johnson, K. (2006). Demographic trends in rural and small America. *Reports on Rural America, 1*(1), 23–26. https://dx.doi.org/10.34051/p/2020.6

Johnston, M. E., & Herzig, R. M. (2006). The interpretation of "culture": Diverging perspectives on medical provision in rural Montana. *Social Science & Medicine, 63*(9), 2500–2511. https://doi.org/10.1016/j.socscimed.2006.06.013

Korngiebel, D. M., Taualii, M., Forquera, R., Harris, R., & Buchwald, D. (2015). Addressing the challenges of research with small populations. *American Journal of Public Health, 105*(9), 1744–1747. https://doi.org/10.2105/AJPH.2015.302783

Larson, E. (2020). Supply and distribution of the primary care workforce in rural America: 2019. (Policy Brief #167). WWAMI Rural Health Research Center, University of Washington.

Lauder, W., Reel, S., Farmer, J., & Griggs, H. (2006). Social capital, rural nursing and rural nursing theory. *Nursing Inquiry, 13*(1), 73–79. https://doi.org/10.1111/j.1440-1800.2006.00297.x

Loftin, W. A., Barnett, S. K., Bunn, P. S., & Sullivan, P. (2005). Recruitment and retention of rural African Americans in diabetes research. *The Diabetes Educator, 31*(2), 251–259. https://doi.org/10.1177%2F0145721705275517

Long, K. A., & Weinert, C. (1989). Rural nursing: Developing the theory base. *Scholarly Inquiry for Nursing Practice, 3*(2), 113–127. https://doi.org//10.1891/0889-7182.3.2.113

National Center for Frontier Communities. (2012). *Resource maps: National center for frontier communities.* http://frontierus.org/resources/

Parra-Medina, D., D'Antonio, A., Smith, S. M., Levin, S., Kirkner, G., & Mayer-Davis, E. (2004). Successful recruitment and retention strategies for a randomized weight management trial for people with diabetes living in rural, medically underserved counties of South Carolina: The POWER study. *Journal of the American Dietetic Association, 104*(1), 70–75. https://doi.org/10.1016/j.jada.2003.10.014

Pindus, N., Brash, R., Franks, K., & Morley, E. (2010). *A framework for considering the social value of postal services.* Postal Regulatory Commission.

Ricketts, T., Johnson-Webb, K., & Taylor, P. (1998). *Definitions of rural: A handbook for health policy makers and researchers.*

Senn, J. F. (2013). Peplau's theory of interpersonal relations: Application in emergency and rural nursing. *Nursing Science Quarterly, 26*(1), 31–35. https://doi.org/10.1177/0894318412466744

Sharp, D. (2010). *Factors related to the recruitment and retention of nurse practitioners in rural areas.* PhD Dissertation, The University of Texas at El Paso.

Singh, G., & Siahpush, M. (2014). Widening rural–urban disparities in all-cause mortality and mortality from major causes of death in the USA, 1969–2009. *Journal of Urban Health, 91*(2), 272–292. https://doi.org/10.1007/s11524-013-9847-2

Smith, M., Dickerson, J., Wendel, M., Ahn, S., Pulczinski, J., Drake, K., & Ory, M. (2013). The utility of rural and underserved designations in geospatial assessments of distance traveled to healthcare services: Implications for public health research and practice. *Journal of Environmental and Public Health, 2013*, 960157. https://doi.org/10.1155/2013/960157

Sue, S., & Dhindsa, M. K. (2006). Ethnic and racial health disparities research: Issues and problems. *Health Education & Behavior, 33*(4), 459–469. https://doi.org/10.1177%2F1090198106287922

Winters, C. A, & Lee, H. (Eds.). (2018). *Rural nursing: Concepts, theory, and practice* (3rd ed.). Springer Publishing Company.

CHAPTER 7

Program of Research in Rural Settings[1]

Clarann Weinert, Elizabeth Nichols,
and Jean Shreffler-Grant

DISCUSSION TOPICS

- Identify two challenges experienced by the research team in the course of their "journey."
- How did the research team overcome the challenges identified in question #1?
- Discuss how the national focus on health literacy was utilized by the research team as an opportunity to advance their program of research.

INTRODUCTION

Sustaining a program of nursing research in a rural setting is a journey with many opportunities and challenges. The purpose of recounting the story of our journey is to share how a program of nursing research can thrive despite being conducted in low nursing research resource environments, across geographic distances, and with a limited patchwork of funding. We attribute our success to an active and astute research team, a topic of interest to all team members, the ability to work across long distances, and a large dose of persistence. In telling this story, only the highlights of our studies are presented. The full descriptions of these studies have been published previously.

THE RESEARCH TEAM

The early phase of this journey was launched by a senior administrator at the University of North Dakota (UND) and a senior investigator from Montana State University (MSU), institutions separated by 800 miles. A master's student and junior faculty member at UND rounded out the original team. Shortly into the research adventure, these two junior

---

1. From Weinert, C., Nichols, E., & Shreffler-Grant, J. (2015). A program of nursing research in a rural setting. *Online Journal of Rural Nursing and Health Care, 15*(1), 100–116. https://doi.org/10.14574/ojrnhc.v15i1.343. Reprinted with permission.

individuals moved on—the master's student into a doctoral program in another state, the faculty member to clinical practice. To replace the lost team members and enrich this two-institutional research team, the two senior investigators then sought additional members from each institution who were junior in their research roles but interested and competent. A junior investigator from MSU with an interest in complementary and alternative medicine (CAM) and previous rural research joined and was quickly mentored into the role of principal investigator. In addition, a senior faculty member from UND joined the team. These four researchers began a research collaboration that has continued for almost 20 years.

Depending on the needs of the research program, other investigators have joined the team for specific tasks. For example, two senior MSU investigators were hired: one to conduct interviews in an early study, and one to collect data in a more recent study. Graduate and undergraduate students enriched the research team and engaged in library searches, assisted with data collection and management, and helped with the preparation of manuscripts and presentations.

A significant challenge to the team was working over long distances—not only across states but also within the state of Montana. For example, the principal investigator's location is 200 miles from the main campus of MSU and the second MSU investigator. The key to successfully meeting this challenge has been ongoing and frequent communication among the members of the team, utilizing a variety of strategies. The increased ease of electronic and telephone communication facilitated productive meetings. Highly important were annual face-to-face meetings that promoted team cohesion, allowed for concentrated group work time, and resulted in the production of grant applications, publications, and presentations.

Over the course of the journey, the core research team has adapted to a variety of changes: new academic roles/status, the relocation of one of the North Dakota team members to Montana, and the death of the other North Dakota colleague. The remaining three core members continue to work successfully as an engaged research team.

IDENTIFYING THE FOCUS OF RESEARCH

Central to our program of research has been an emphasis on examining strategies for enhancing the health of older rural adults. Our early studies on the use of CAM by older rural dwellers were driven by the interests of the initial junior team members and that meshed well with the broader research endeavors of the senior investigators. Further, the cutting-edge studies by Eisenberg et al. (1993) and Eisenberg et al. (1998) on CAM use did not differentiate between urban and rural populations, our area of interest.

During the late 1990s and early 2000s, several well-known national studies were conducted that demonstrated the use of CAM among the general U.S. population was more common than previously thought. Further, researchers found that often there was limited communication between consumers and providers about treatment options and the consumers' use of CAM (Astin, 1998; Eisenberg et al., 1993). Researchers noted that CAM therapies were used more often for chronic than acute health problems. Use was more common among women, younger adults, those with higher incomes, more education, and those living in the western United States (Astin et al., 2000; Cherniack et al., 2001; Eisenberg et al., 1998). These investigators tended not to differentiate between rural and urban populations. However, when studies were designed to focus on the use of CAM among rural dwellers, the results were inconsistent. Vallerand et al. (2003) found that CAM use was less prevalent among rural dwellers than among urban. Yet, Harron and Glasser (2003) reported that the use of CAM was more common among rural residents.

Conversely, other researchers found that the prevalence of use among rural and urban dwellers was similar (Arcury et al., 2004).

Initial Studies on the Research Journey

The initial research on our journey included a series of studies with older adults living in rural areas to further understand the role of CAM in health decisions. The primary purpose was to explore the use of, and satisfaction with, CAM from the perspectives of older rural people. The team also sought to gain a better understanding of why CAM was used and what sources were used to obtain information about CAM therapies. Throughout these early studies, participants were recruited from counties in Montana and North Dakota that met the federal definitions for "rural" and "frontier." All studies discussed in this journey were approved by the universities' institutional review boards for protection of human subjects.

In the first study, 325 randomly selected older adults in 19 rural communities were interviewed by telephone. Participants had a mean age of 72 years and most (67.7%) reported having one or more chronic illnesses. Only 17.5% reported using complementary providers, whereas 35.7% used self-prescribed CAM practices, such as home remedies, nutritional supplements, and herbal products. Participants most often learned about the therapies from relatives and friends or consumer marketing rather than from healthcare professionals. Those most likely to use CAM were women who were fairly well educated, not currently married, and in their early older years. They had one or more significant chronic illnesses and lower health-related quality of life (Shreffler-Grant et al., 2005, 2007). From this survey, the research team gained an overview of who used CAM and what type they used, but it did not provide information about why they used CAM, or how much they knew about what they used.

To obtain more in-depth information, 10 older rural adults with a chronic illness who had reported using CAM in the initial interview were reinterviewed. Six of the 10 participants were women; eight were between the ages of 70 and 80; and two were between 60 and 70 years. Their mean education level was 12.5 years. They used self-prescribed CAM therapies primarily to compensate for perceived dietary deficiencies. For the most part, they were satisfied with the results they attributed to the CAM. It was clear, however, that some participants used the therapies in an inconsistent manner and did not understand the purpose of the products.

Participants attempted to use reputable sources for information; yet, few sought information from their allopathic providers due to a perception that the providers were too busy to answer their questions about CAM (Nichols et al., 2005).

It was of interest to the team that most of the respondents in the original study did not interact with CAM providers. The team questioned whether this phenomenon was related to the availability of providers in rural areas and concluded it merited further study. Internet and telephone directory searches were used to locate CAM resources in 20 small rural communities in Montana and North Dakota. Seventy-three providers, representing a wide variety of CAM therapies, were identified in these communities. The team also sought to ascertain the contribution of one type of CAM provider, naturopathic physicians, to rural healthcare (Nichols et al., 2006), through an online survey. Most naturopaths were located in population centers, but some offered outreach clinics to rural communities.

In summary, participants in all of these early studies tended to use self-directed or self-prescribed CAM rather than therapies provided by practitioners. Local availability of practitioners did not appear to be a factor in the use of CAM by older rural residents. The residents gleaned information about the therapies primarily by word of mouth or from the media. Some respondents used CAM inconsistently; others did not seek information about the effects or risks, and when they did, the information sources used were those generally considered unreliable.

CAM Health Literacy—A Detour

As on any journey, it is wise to be aware of changing circumstances and respond appropriately. On a road trip, if there is construction indicated ahead, one needs to be prepared to slow, stop, or perhaps take a detour. On our research journey, we became astutely aware of the growing national focus on the role of health literacy, that is, "the degree to which individuals have the capacity to obtain, process, and understand basic health information and services needed to make appropriate health decisions" (U.S. Department of Health and Human Services, 2000). Creating a health-literate populace had become a major priority in the nation's public healthcare policy, research, practice, and education arenas. The Institute of Medicine (IOM) included health literacy as one of 20 priority areas and noted that it is fundamental to improving self-management of health conditions (IOM, 2004). The IOM cited a critical need for more rigorous work to develop appropriate, reliable, and valid measures of health literacy (IOM, 2004). More specific to the teams' program of research, the IOM also noted that there was very little research on how American consumers obtain, understand, and evaluate information about the various CAM therapies (IOM, 2005). With the advent of these critical documents, there was a clear need for research in the area of CAM health literacy. It was evident to our team that a detour from our focus on informed CAM use was needed. In order to develop and test an intervention to enhance health decision-making related to CAM, a measure of CAM health literacy was essential. Prior to developing a measure, it was critical to have a definition and conceptual model of CAM health literacy.

CAM HEALTH LITERACY MODEL DEVELOPMENT

The team's working definition of CAM health literacy was the information about CAM that individuals need to make informed health decisions. The MSU Conceptual Model of CAM Health Literacy was constructed from a comprehensive review of the literature, the team's prior research, the definition of CAM health literacy, and input from national experts (Shreffler-Grant et al., 2013). There are three major components to the model: antecedents, structure, and outcome. The primary outcome of the model is informed self-management of health. Antecedents are factors that can affect the structural component. Four concepts: dose, effect, safety, and availability, compose the structural component and were the focus for the subsequent CAM health literacy instrument development. The MSU Conceptual Model of CAM Health Literacy is the first known attempt to conceptualize the essential elements of health literacy regarding CAM. Health literacy, in this model, is expanded in a context different from allopathic healthcare and goes beyond reading and computational skills (see Figure 7.1).

The development and refinement of the model was thoroughly discussed in an earlier publication (Shreffler-Grant et al., 2013).

INSTRUMENT DEVELOPMENT

Following the articulation of the conceptual model, the next segment of our research journey was the development of a measure of CAM health literacy. DeVellis' well-established and tested eight-step process for scale development was used to guide our efforts (DeVellis, 2012; see Table 7.1).

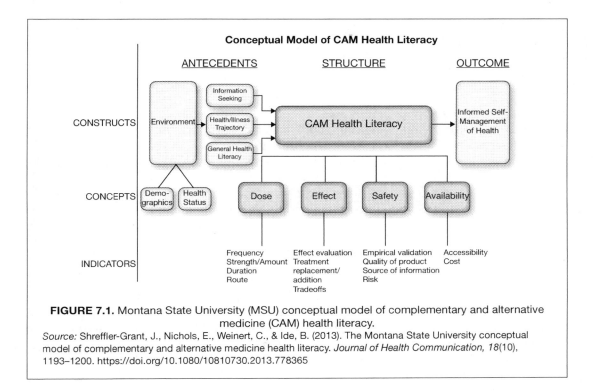

FIGURE 7.1. Montana State University (MSU) conceptual model of complementary and alternative medicine (CAM) health literacy.

Source: Shreffler-Grant, J., Nichols, E., Weinert, C., & Ide, B. (2013). The Montana State University conceptual model of complementary and alternative medicine health literacy. *Journal of Health Communication, 18*(10), 1193–1200. https://doi.org/10.1080/10810730.2013.778365

TABLE 7.1. DeVellis's Guidelines for Scale Development

Step 1	Construct determination
Step 2	Generate item pool
Step 3	Determine measurement format
Step 4	Review of item pool
Step 5	Consider validation items
Step 6	Administer to development sample
Step 7	Evaluate items
Step 8	Optimize scale length

The structural component of the newly developed model provided the constructs and concepts necessary to initiate the instrument development process. Empirical indicators were identified for each of the four major concepts, and two to seven items for each indicator were generated. A 6-point Likert scale response format with equally weighted items was selected to allow for a summed single scale score. To ensure that the items were clear and understandable, plain language principles (Plain Language, 2013) were used and medical jargon was avoided. Items were written at an eighth grade or less reading level based on the Flesch–Kincaid grade level (Readability Formulas, 2013).

To refine the item pool, a panel of experts in the areas of tool development and CAM therapy generously reviewed the items for consistency with the model and clarity of wording. They also suggested additional items. A revised item pool and response set was reviewed and critiqued by four focus groups. Two focus groups were composed of community-dwelling senior citizens and two of allopathic and complementary health-care providers. Recommendations from the experts and the focus groups resulted in the team's careful rereview of the item pool. At this point in the journey, the initial instrument consisted of 54 items with two versions of the measure. One version had a dichotomous response option of "agree/disagree"; the other version had a four-point response set with anchors of "agree strongly" to "disagree strongly."

REFINING THE INSTRUMENT

A professional research interview company was hired to administer the draft CAM health literacy instruments, obtain basic demographic data including CAM use, and a single item health literacy measure included for validity assessment: the participant's ease of completion of medical forms (Chew et al., 2004). Interviews were conducted with a random sample of 1,200 adults over the age of 55 from households in nonmetropolitan areas of the northwestern quadrant of the United States. One half of the sample ($n = 600$) completed the version with the four-point response set, the other half with the dichotomous response option.

DECISION POINT

The availability of resources required a team decision as to how to proceed with the initial data analysis. We had the skill and statistical programs necessary to analyze the four-response data set. However, to appropriately analyze the two-response set required different statistical resources and personnel. In addition, DeVellis, a consultant on the project, recommended focusing on the four-point response set. Thus, the decision was made to initially analyze only the four-point response set version. The analysis procedures were conducted on one half of that sample ($n = 300$), and then were validated by comparing the results with results of duplicate analyses from the second half of that data set. The procedures were then run on the data from the entire sample ($n = 600$). Standard exploratory factor analysis procedures with the number of factors (three) based upon parallel analysis were used. Principal components extraction with oblimin rotation was used to determine factors and item loadings. Items with weak loadings or that loaded on more than one factor were deleted. The reliabilities of each factor as well as each item's contribution to that alpha were also examined to determine which items to retain. This process continued until a stable solution with an adequate alpha was obtained. The final 21-item four-response set instrument had a Cronbach's alpha of 0.75. The correlation between the CAM Health Literacy Scale and the medical forms completion item was 0.174 ($p = .003$; Shreffler-Grant et al., 2014).

VALIDATION STUDY

The final leg of the instrument development detour was to conduct a study to further assess validity by comparing CAM Health Literacy Scale scores with those on a general health literacy measure. The validation procedures were implemented with a convenience sample of 110 community-dwelling older adults (average age 68). The data collection packet included the MSU CAM Health Literacy Scale and two health literacy measures: the Newest Vital Sign (Osborn et al., 2007) and one question about the ease of completion of medical forms (Chew et al., 2004). Also included were basic demographics, CAM use information, and presence of chronic illness. Sixty-six percent of the sample were women, 75% had more than a high school education, and 51% were currently married. Eighty-two percent indicated that they used CAM, and 51% said that they had no significant health problems. The alpha on the CAM Health Literacy Scale in this sample was 0.73. The correlation with the Newest Vital Sign was 0.221 ($p = .002$) and with the single medical forms completion question was 0.277 (p = .004; Shreffler-Grant et al., 2014). Now, with an instrument in hand, the team was ready to return to the main trail—how to improve the CAM health literacy of older rural dwellers and thus enhance the information they bring to bear on the management of their health.

FUNDING THE JOURNEY

Ideally, a program of research is continuously funded; however, life is not always ideal. Yet, there are times when the "financial planets" do align! The launching of our journey fortuitously coincided with the National Center for Complementary and Alternative Medicine becoming a funding agency. This center funded our first exploratory study and also our most recent work to develop the CAM Health Literacy Scale. Between the two grants, the research journey was sustained by small intramural grants, investigator dedication, the generosity of time and expertise donated by our nursing and nonnursing research colleagues, and the ongoing commitment of the team members. At times, we felt like "the little engine that could!"

LESSONS LEARNED ON THE JOURNEY

This research program has been a journey filled with twists and turns that are likely to continue as we travel down the CAM health literacy path. The success of this research team can be attributed to active, committed investigators, a topic of interest that has engaged all members, and, at least, occasional funding. Maintaining sufficient continuity in the research team while also being open to enlist help from additional investigators was critical to the development and sustainability of this program of research.

The importance of building from one study to the next was an ever-present precept. We invested significant time and energy reflecting, discussing, and "cogitating" about the results of each step of the research program in order to tease out the meaning from the data and identify remaining questions to be answered along with the most appropriate approaches to answer them.

Being alert to historical events that have relevance to the program of research is critical. The CAM health literacy "detour" was inspired by the IOM report that indicated a critical need for more rigorous work to develop appropriate, reliable, and valid measures of health literacy (IOM, 2004). In retrospect, what we thought was a detour may have been a main road on the map. From the outset of our research endeavors, the overall goal was the promotion of informed healthcare choices by older rural dwellers. Addressing the definition, model, and measurement of CAM health literacy has enlightened and enhanced our research program and is a genuine fit with our goal.

This research journey has not been without obstacles. The several definitions of health literacy complicated the task of developing the model of CAM health literacy. Further, it became clear that there were no markers on the trail, other than our own model, to guide the writing of items and the selection of the response option anchors. An additional challenge was the lack of an appropriate and mature measure of general health literacy against which to validate the MSU CAM Health Literacy Scale. Additional obstacles were the geographic distance between team members along with limited and inconsistent funding.

Reviewing the journey of a team of researchers over time, including the original intent, the challenges, and the detours, can be instructive to other teams as they travel on their own research journeys. The way is seldom straight nor paved with continuous funding, but persistence, a meaningful goal, and good working relationships have kept this team on task and energized.

ACKNOWLEDGMENTS

Research supported by National Institutes of Health/National Center for Complementary and Alternative Medicine R15 AT095-01, R15 T006609-01; National Institutes of Health/ National Institute of Nursing Research 1P20NR07790-01; Montana State University College of Nursing Block Grant; University of North Dakota College of Nursing Intramural Grant. Acknowledgment also to Bette Ide, PhD, RN, FAAN, Lompoc, California, a former research team member (deceased).

REFERENCES

Arcury, T., Preisser, J., Gesler, W., & Sherman, J. (2004). Complementary and alternative medicine use among rural residents in western North Carolina. *Complementary Health Practice Review, 9*(2), 93–102. https://doi.org/10.1177/1076167503253433

Astin, J. (1998). Why patients use alternative medicine: Results of a national study. *Journal of the American Medical Association, 279*(19), 1548–1553. https://doi.org/10.1001/jama.279.19.1548

Astin, J., Pelletier, K., Marie, A., & Haskell, W. (2000). Complementary and alternative medicine use among elderly persons: One-year analysis of a Blue Shield Medicare supplement. *Journal of Gerontology Series A, Biological Sciences and Medical Sciences, 55*(1), M4–M9.

Cherniack, E., Senzel, R., & Pan, C. (2001). Correlates of use of alternative medicine by the elderly in an urban population. *Journal of Alternative and Complementary Medicine, 7*, 277–280. https://doi.org/10.1089/107555301300328160

Chew, L. D., Bradley, K. A., & Boyko, E. J. (2004). Brief questions to identify patients with inadequate health literacy. *Family Medicine, 36*(8), 588–594.

DeVellis, R. (2012). *Scale development: Theory and applications* (3rd ed.). Sage.

Eisenberg, D., Davis, R., Ettner, S., Appel, S., Wilkey, S., Van Rompay, M., & Kessler, R. (1998). Trends in alternative medicine use in the United States, 1990–1997; Results of a follow-up national survey. *Journal of the American Medical Association, 280*(18), 1569–1575. https://doi.org/10.1001/jama.280.18.1569

Eisenberg, D., Kessler, R., Foster, C., Norlock, F., Calkins, D., & Delbanco, T. (1993). Unconventional medicine in the United States. *New England Journal of Medicine, 328*, 246–252. https://doi.org/10.1056/NEJM199301283280406

Harron, M., & Glasser, M. (2003). Use of and attitudes toward complementary and alternative medicine among family practice patients in small rural Illinois communities. *Journal of Rural Health, 19*(3), 279–284. https://doi.org/10.1111/j.1748-0361.2003.tb00574.x

Institute of Medicine. (2004). *Health literacy: A prescription to end confusion.* National Academies Press.

Institute of Medicine. (2005). *Complementary and alternative medicine in the United States.* National Academies Press.

Nichols, E., Sullivan, T., Ide, B., Shreffler-Grant, J., & Weinert, C. (2005). Health care choices: Complementary therapy, chronic illness, and older rural dwellers. *Journal of Holistic Nursing, 23*(4), 381–394. https://doi.org/10.1177/0898010105281088

Nichols, E., Weinert, C., Shreffler-Grant, J., & Ide, B. (2006). Complementary and alternative providers in rural locations. *Online Journal of Rural Nursing and Health Care, 6*(2), 40–46. http://rnojournal.binghamton.edu/index.php/RNO/index

Osborn, C. Y., Weiss, B. D., Davis, T. C., Skripkauskas, S., Rodrigue, C., Bass, P. F., & Wolf, M. S. (2007). Measuring adult literacy in health care: Performance of the newest vital sign. *American Journal of Health Behavior, 31*(Suppl. 1), S36–S46. https://doi.org/10.5993/AJHB.31.s1.6

Plain Language. (2013). *Plain language and information network (PLAIN).* U.S. General Services Administration. http://www.plainlanguage.gov

Readability Formulas. (2013). *The Flesch grade readability formula.* http://www.readabilityformulas.com/flesch-grade-level-readability-formula.php

Shreffler-Grant, J., Hill, W., Weinert, C., Nichols, E., & Ide, B. (2007). Complementary therapy and older rural women: Who uses and who does not? *Nursing Research, 56*(1), 28–33. https://doi.org/10.1097/00006199-200701000-00004

Shreffler-Grant, J., Nichols, E., Weinert, C., & Ide, B. (2013). The Montana State University conceptual model of complementary and alternative medicine health literacy. *Journal of Health Communication, 18*(10), 1193–1200. https://doi.org/10.1080/10810730.2013.778365

Shreffler-Grant, J., Weinert, C., & Nichols, E. (2014). Instrument to measure health literacy about complementary and alternative medicine. *Journal of Nursing Measurement, 22*(3), 489–499. https://doi.org/10.1891/1061-3749.22.3.489

Shreffler-Grant, J., Weinert, C., Nichols, E., & Ide, B. (2005). Complementary therapy use among older rural adults. *Public Health Nursing, 22*(4), 323–3311. https://doi.org/10.1111/j.0737-1209.2005.220407.x

U.S. Department of Health and Human Services. (2000). *Healthy People 2010, Section 11–2: Health communication objective.* http://www.healthypeople.gov.

Vallerand, A., Fouladbakhsh, J., & Templin, T. (2003). The use of complementary/alternative medicine therapies for the self-treatment of pain among residents of urban, suburban, and rural communities. *American Journal of Public Health, 93*, 923–925. https://doi.org/10.2105/AJPH.93.6.923

SECTION II

Rural Nursing Practice

Section II focuses on rural nursing practice. It opens with the seminal chapter by Jane Ellis Scharff, The Nature and Scope of Rural Nursing Practice: Philosophical Basis, which has appeared in the previous editions of this book. This classic work is followed by a qualitative study of the lived experience of rural nurses updated for this edition. Chapter 10 updates information on the experiences of nurses living in rural and frontier areas who chose to commute to urban medical centers for practice. Written by a director of a Family Nurse Practitioner (NP) program, the updated Chapter 11 provides insight into the contributions of NPs as healthcare providers in the rural setting. It includes a brief background on the NP role, a section on access to healthcare, and a look at the unique patient-centered care provided by NPs. Chapter 12 is new to this edition. It explores the use of registered nurses (RNs) as primary care providers in rural settings.

CHAPTER 8

The Distinctive Nature and Scope of Rural Nursing Practice: Philosophical Bases[1]

Jane Ellis Scharff

DISCUSSION TOPICS

- Describe from your perspective what it means to "be a rural nurse." Compare and contrast your meaning of being rural with your colleagues' meaning of being an urban nurse. How are they similar? How are they different?
- Design a project to explore rural nursing. How does rural nursing today compare with rural nursing described by Scharff?

INTRODUCTION

Plenty and little have changed in 10 years. Rural nursing practice seemed a dichotomous set of the routine and the extraordinary to me back then, as it does now. I was an insider, if not an old-timer, and my findings, although remarkable to some, seemed simply confirmatory to me. Already a budding pragmatist and not yet fully a scientist, I thought, at the time, it was enough to have empiric validation for the practice that I had known and in which my former workplace colleagues continued. For that reason and so many others, I did not publish the findings of my master's thesis in 1987. Subsequently, I have been cited frequently, misrepresented occasionally, and poached a time or two when it comes to references about the world of rural nursing. It is time to uphold my responsibility to nursing science and to set the record straight. The nature and scope of rural nursing is distinctive. I am now willing to be quoted on that. Furthermore, rural nursing can now be given a definition based on that distinctiveness.

Rural nursing practice, be it hospital practice, private practice, or community health practice, is distinctive in its nature and scope from the practice of nursing in urban settings. It is distinctive in its boundaries, intersections, dimensions, and even in its core. Ten years ago, I was loath to claim distinctiveness within rural nursing's core. It seemed

---

1. Seminal chapter first published in the first edition, *Conceptual Basis of Rural Nursing*, and subsequent editions of *Rural Nursing: Concepts, Theory, and Practice*.

too bold to proclaim that at the very level of essence, and not attributable to setting alone, rural nursing could be so different. Today, I am determined to claim it: The core of all nursing is care, and care is the substance of the relationship between nurse and patient; consequently, what happens at the core of rural nursing is something apart from what happens at the core of nursing anywhere else.

I am still a pragmatist; my job is to get readers as close to the experience as I can. Thankfully, my growth as a scientist makes the job easier than it was some years back. Although no longer in the practice, I understand rural nursing better today than I did then. The importance of rural nursing has not decreased as my worldview has expanded. On the contrary, the more I dissect and reconstruct my thoughts about life and truth and nursing science, the more clearly I see the beauty emanating from the nature and scope of rural nursing, and the more clearly I appreciate its relevance to all of nursing science.

From an ontological viewpoint, I will share some information about what it means to "be" a rural nurse, and from an epistemological viewpoint, I will express a little of what it means to "know" rural nursing practice. What came as primary expression to me, because I lived it, breathed it, and studied it, is secondary expression as I write it; I will do my best to translate the experience through common language. However, the story I tell will require imagination to transcend time and space and to gain a sense of the reality of rural nursing practice. The information for this chapter comes from my ethnographic study of rural hospital nurses in the Inland Northwest, completed in 1987, from dialogue with key informants before then and up until today, and from my personal experiences within rural healthcare systems over the past 20 years.

In the past 10 or 15 years, I have made some presentations about portions of this work to nurse clinicians, nurse researchers, and nonnurse healthcare audiences. Inevitably, following such presentations, I was approached by one or two individuals who had been rural nurses who wanted to tell me that the presentation struck a chord. I understood their need, which stemmed from the human desire to be recognized and understood. It stems from the frequent, albeit unintended, distortion of truth about rural nursing communicated by those who do not fully understand what it means to walk a mile in a rural nurse's duty shoes. I may not be able to change that, but I offer my perspective, nonetheless.

CONCEPTUALIZING RURAL NURSING PRACTICE

Being Rural

There was a wonderful line in the 1984 science fiction film *The Adventures of Buckaroo Banzai: Across the 8th Dimension* (Rausch, 1984). The line was delivered by the main character, Buckaroo, a multiskilled neurosurgeon, particle physicist, rock musician, and Zen warrior who, in the midst of chaos matter-of-factly declared, "No matter where you go, there you are." If this sounds simple, I would caution that it is hardly simple. Buckaroo was talking about being in the moment, so imagine for a moment what it means to have "gone rural." What of rural nursing identity? While the imagery may seem silly or surreal, the truth is real, authentic, important, credible, respectable, and as serious as any nursing practice anywhere. However, as indicated earlier, rural nursing practice is also distinctive from nursing anywhere else. Although I use the analogy of Buckaroo Banzai, hoping it will bring a smile, rural nurses will recognize the script of playing a cool and noble professional, simultaneously enacting multiple roles, and managing the continual transition from one part to another with the frankness of Buckaroo.

Being rural means being a long way from anywhere and pretty close to nowhere. Being rural means being independent or perhaps just being alone. Being a rural nurse means that when a nurse saves a life, everyone in the town recognizes that they were there; and when a nurse loses a life, everyone in the town recognizes that they were there. Being rural means turning inward for answers, because there may be nobody to turn to outward. Being rural means that when a nurse walks into the ED, it may be their spouse or child who needs a nurse, and at that moment, being a nurse takes priority over being anyone else. Being a rural nurse means being able to deal with what they had got, where they are, and being able to live with the consequences.

Knowing Rural

Certainly, every reader has heard that a little knowledge can be a dangerous thing. The adage was probably modified from what Alexander Pope (1711, as cited in Evans, 1978) said in the 17th century: "A little learning is a dangerous thing." I dispute it now and say that a little knowledge can be a lifesaving thing. The demarcation between danger and safety is the difference between having knowledge and using knowledge. From time to time, I have had conversations with academic colleagues about dangerous nurses. In these conversations, we have agreed that dangerous nurses are not those who know they do not know what they are doing—although there is certainly an element of danger in that scenario, which ultimately must be addressed. The greater danger, however, emerges with those nurses who think they do know, but actually do not know, what they are doing. Although I have no statistics on the prevalence of such nurses, it is my belief that they hide more easily in urban settings than they do in rural settings.

Knowing rural means knowing that what one knows may be all one has. Knowing rural means personally knowing everyone with whom one works and having knowledge about nearly everyone for whom one cares. As a rural nurse, knowing means sharing knowledge in an informal yet crucially important exchange with other professionals, where the addition of one mind can mean expanding the knowledge base by 100%. Although whom one knows can be important in any setting, the distinction between rural and urban dynamics of whom one knows is that in the urban setting whom one knows is more likely to be related to competitive advantage, whereas in the rural setting whom one knows is more likely to be related to cooperative advantage. Knowing rural means that knowledge can mean the difference between perishing, surviving, and thriving, and therefore knowing is inextricably connected to being when one is rural.

THE NATURE AND SCOPE OF NURSING

For practicality, a framework for the study of the nature and scope of rural nursing practice was sought to identify and describe the distinctive characteristics of practice in rural settings. The American Nurses Association (ANA) Social Policy Statement (1980) provided the framework for a logical sequence of investigation into details of rural nursing practice. The policy statement includes an organized and systematic approach to studying nursing nature and scope.

Nursing's Nature

Within the policy statement, the nature of nursing is characterized as a relationship between the nursing profession and the society that is mutually beneficial, and nursing itself is deemed an essential outgrowth of the society that it serves. Nursing is described as existing in response to society's needs. From that standpoint, my study of rural nursing was based on assumptions that rural nursing emerges from and is essential to rural society, and distinctions of rural nursing are due, in part, to distinctive interests and needs of rural society.

Nursing's Scope

The scope of nursing includes four definitive characteristics: intersections, dimensions, core, and boundary (ANA, 1980). These four characteristics became the conceptual foundation blocks for my study of rural nursing.

INTERSECTIONS

Nursing intersects with other professions involved in healthcare. These intersections are points at which nursing meets and interfaces with other professions and expands its practice into the domain of other professions as necessary.

DIMENSIONS

Characteristics such as philosophy, ethics, roles, responsibilities, skills, and authority are examples of nursing dimensions. These are qualities that add depth to nursing practice. They are characteristics underscored and influenced by interpersonal relationships and intimacy as well as the intrapersonal quality of nursing.

CORE

The concept of the core of nursing is complex and somewhat more difficult to discuss than are the other concepts. It is oversimplification to say that the needs of people are the core of nursing, although such is true. Nursing exists to deal with human response to health issues, and human response can be equated to human need with respect to health. The patients' needs and their responses are the outgrowths of who they are as human beings. The nursing care we provide is an outgrowth of who we are as human beings. The core of nursing is the dynamic of nursing care juxtaposed with human response.

BOUNDARIES

Nursing's boundaries change and expand in direct reflection of the intersections, dimensions, and core of practice. Boundaries are nebulous, unseen, intangible lines of demarcation between what is clearly within the nature and scope of nursing and what is questionably within nursing's scope. Unlike physical boundaries, nursing's boundaries are metaphysical, are relationally and contextually based, and sometimes have origins outside the control of nursing.

METHODS

In an effort to describe the nature and scope of rural nursing, it was determined that an ethnographic method, using participant observation and interviewing techniques, would yield the most pertinent data for analysis. Data were gathered throughout several stages of conceptualization concerning rural nursing phenomena. Field notations, printed news media, and taped interviews were employed. The study of rural hospital nurses included an exploratory phase in which eight rural nurses from northwest Montana were interviewed. These interviews were audiotaped, and from initial open-ended questions, a more refined interview guide was developed that contained both closed and open-ended questions. Twenty-six rural hospital nurses in one of four rural towns in eastern Washington, northern Idaho, or western Montana were interviewed. All interviews were audiotaped and then transcribed verbatim. The findings reported in this chapter are related to many aspects of rural nursing practice and are based on the responses of all 34 rural nurses, as well as several other key rural informants and my own observations. All samples were convenience, and all informants elected to be included in the studies.

FINDINGS

Informant Demographics

All of the informants were women ranging in age from 25 to 61 years with an average age of 40 years. The number of years actively employed as an RN was 3 to 35 years. The mean number of years spent working in rural hospitals was 8 years and, for most informants, was roughly half the total of their active nursing years. Most informants were originally diploma-prepared, seven were baccalaureate graduates, and four were associate graduates. Two informants had achieved a master's degree in nursing. Although informants were not asked about marital or parental status, nearly all said during the interview that they were married and were parents.

Most of the informants worked full time, and those who worked part time averaged 23 hours/week. In addition, many were placed "on-call" if they were not working. On-call status could be attributed to low census, high census, operating room call, cardiac care call, or ED call. Most informants reported 1 or 2 days of overtime per month. In almost every case, informants indicated a need to be flexible about their working schedules with regard to the events of the rural practice setting. Turnover rates were low at all facilities, and the most senior nurses had been on staff from 16 to 25 years.

Hospital Demographics

Information about the hospitals was obtained through interviews with nursing, fiscal, administrative, or other personnel, as well as from public records and the participant observation process. The hospital organizations were between 20 and 60 years in existence, the present structures were between 3 and 35 years old, and all had undergone some renovation over time. Ownership of the hospitals was stated as nonproprietary, public district, or community. Each hospital was governed by a board of directors of three to 10 individuals who held fiduciary and decision-making authorities and to whom the administration was accountable. Board membership was either self-perpetuating or community elected. One facility was accredited by what was then the Joint Commission on Accreditation of Healthcare Organizations (JCAHO). Administrative personnel said that there was little to be gained by small rural hospitals having JCAHO accreditation, especially in light of what the JCAHO charged for the process.

The hospitals had licensure ranging from 20 to 44 acute care beds, zero to three intensive or cardiac beds, five to seven newborn bassinets, and three to five swing beds for extended care. In every case, occupancy was at a fraction of licensure, and occupancy figures averaged to be about 20% to 40% for acute care beds. There was some variability in the use of the other services at each facility. Two had fairly active use of the cardiac or intensive care beds. Two had fairly active obstetrical departments. Three had active surgical departments. Emergency cases at these hospitals ranged from three to 13 per 24-hour day during the previous fiscal year. One relied on the constant occupancy of swing beds to maintain financial solvency. The number of physicians on medical staff ranged from three to 17. Typically, physicians who held admitting privilege at a given facility did not necessarily live within the community. Undoubtedly, the variety of medical practitioners on staff impacted the occupancy of each facility. Usually, nurses were expected to be able to float from medical–surgical areas to emergency, obstetrical, and intensive care areas, but not to the operating room, which seemed to be the one sacrosanct specialty area.

The Rural Communities

At the time of the study, I spent several weeks traveling to and about four separate communities in western Montana, northern Idaho, and eastern Washington to gather information regarding the nature and scope of rural nursing. Each of these towns fits the operational definition of being geographically isolated and of having less than 5,000 residents. Upon arrival in each community, time was taken to drive about, observe the local terrain, look for indicators of economy, walk around town to observe the pace and lifestyle, note the casual conversations taking place in public areas, and read each community's local weekly newspaper.

There were many similarities and few differences between the communities in terms of how they appeared to the outsider. Each town was located near railroad tracks, all of which were currently used. Three of the towns were on a river in forested mountain terrain and were logging or lumber mill towns. The fourth town was on an expansive plain and was an agricultural community. Each town was inhabited mostly by White residents, and each was laid out in typical western fashion with one main street and several auxiliary streets at which the center of the business district was found. Each town boasted the typical hardware stores, grocery stores, restaurants, farm or logging machinery shops, tool shops, post office, drug store, employment office, beauty shops, ice cream stands, feed stores, junk shops, small motels, bars, and churches. Each town had a well-kept appearance, although each had a few empty buildings or storefronts in the business district.

Residents in these communities were friendly and helpful. They recognized me as an outsider, and, although willing to answer my questions, were curious and wanted to know the purpose of my presence in their town. When I explained myself, the residents registered sincere interest and pleasure that their community had been targeted for this study. They acted like they felt privileged and eagerly conveyed their high regard for nurses in general and their nurses specifically. Never did these residents express animosity toward the community of nurses. Most of them had a story to tell about how a friend or relative's life was saved at the local hospital.

Rural Hospital Nurses

The rural nurses I observed and interviewed were a dynamic group of women who could certainly be called *expert generalists*. They moved quickly, and for the most part easily, from one role to another as circumstances required. They explained that most rural nurses have a great deal of knowledge regarding a variety of nursing practice areas. When beginning work in a rural hospital, many nurses suffer reality shock due to the variety of demands placed on them. One seasoned nurse told me, "Although you might start out and you don't have that wide knowledge, you better get it quickly." A relative newcomer nurse expressed admiration about the knowledge level of her rural colleagues, calling them "impressive." The nurses I interviewed routinely worked in three or four different specialty areas of nursing practice every week, and sometimes every day. When talking with one respondent about this phenomenon and how easy certain nurses made it look, she said, "The ones who are experienced in rural nursing seem to be very comfortable in switching back and forth between specialties."

Nursing Staff Tenure and Group Acceptance

At all facilities, nurses were heard to use the terms "new" or "newcomer" and "old" or "old-timer" in reference to a given nurse's tenure on the staff. There was no particular time limit identified when a nurse makes the transition from new to old, nor how one arrives at a level of acceptance. However, tenure of less than 2 years was apparently definitely considered "new," and tenure of 3 to 5 years in combination with competence generally constituted acceptance. Tenure beyond 10 years was considered "seasoned," and in special cases of achieving high proficiency or social acceptance, one of these nurses might be called an "old-timer," but usually this term was reserved for someone who had been around for 20 or more years. What I discerned was some gray area depending on a nurse's tenure, level of proficiency, and sociability related to group fit. It seemed that a nurse who was very skillful, flexible, and likeable might reach old-timer status sooner than a nurse who was lacking one of those characteristics.

Although I cannot pinpoint a typical rural nurse, certain characteristics were confirmed as traits of distinctive advantage for a rural nurse's success. For example, good common sense, good judgment ability, the ability to set priorities, good physical assessment skills, and physical and emotional strengths were considered of survival significance to these nurses due, in part, to the aloneness of their practices. They made comments such as, "You have to make all your own decisions. There's no one to do that for you." "You have to be able to be autonomous." "You can't go to somebody for concurrence with decision making." "At any time during your shift, your assignment may change drastically." "You can make the difference between life or death—the judgment calls are yours." All informants were adamant that the prevalent feeling of aloneness and serious responsibility were distinctive to the rural setting. None would concede that the feeling was anything like that experienced in an urban setting. These nurses expressed a very real and pervasive sense of responsibility that rural nurses bear for their patients. The nurses who do not have the ability consistently to carry the burden of such decisional responsibility are the ones who do not survive as rural nurses. Old-timers claimed they could often tell right away, or within a few weeks, if a newcomer was going to catch on or not. Old-timers based such predictions on their assessments of a newcomer's characteristics as mentioned earlier, combined with evidence of adaptation to the new environment.

Education and Professional Development

The burden for self-responsibility of education is greater in the rural setting than in the urban setting, and most rural nurses accept this burden. There is a wide variety of sources from which rural nurses receive their continuing education, such as out-of-town workshops or conferences, in-service education, journals, textbooks, practice sessions, physicians, and other nurses. The greatest educational needs voiced were in cardiac, trauma, maternal/child, and complex medical nursing.

Informants indicated a thirst for knowledge in accredited professional continuing education. Several respondents reported attending more than 10 continuing education events in a year. Most attended between three and 10 events annually. These events were developed and held locally, developed elsewhere but held locally, or developed and held in urban settings. Although expenses were a factor, they were not the central factor in respondents' attending continuing education events.

Nearly all informants also relied on journals for new information, read journals regularly, and reported the most popular journals to be *Nursing, American Journal of Nursing, RN, Journal of Nursing Administration*, and *Nursing Management*, in that order. Current journals were visible in each facility, and notations were seen hanging on bulletin boards in nursing report rooms or locker rooms with a suggestion from one nurse to others that everyone review a given recent journal article germane to a given current case.

Rural nurses, in fact, identify one another as their most important single source of information and education. This was often explained as information being imparted from a peer when it was needed most, so that learning occurred while doing, which tended to heighten the memory. Comments that supported these phenomena included, "We try to share everything we can with each other." "New nurses sometimes come in with great new information or real current ideas. It helps a lot." "Sometimes the new girls expect you to know things, and I don't, and it can be embarrassing. So, we look it up together." "When you've been around for a while, you develop camaraderie. We know what we can expect from each other."

Out-of-town workshops were identified as the next most important source of continuing education to rural nurses. Informants qualified this by stressing that the topic or presentation needed to be relevant to the rural environment. One informant said, "It's got to be meaningful. You know, you go up to the city and they tell you how to do something, and they don't realize how different the setup is."

Interpersonal Relationships and Nursing Practice

Rural nurses know everyone who works at the hospital, all of the physicians, and most of their patients. Rural nurses say that the interpersonal closeness of knowing everyone with whom they work and for whom they care generally has a positive influence on their practice. The intensity of this interpersonal dynamic is unique to the rural setting. Although it is likely that nurses in any setting develop close relationships, rural nurses are in the distinctive situation of being personally acquainted with all of those around them, so that the depth of interaction is potentially greater, and the accountability for interpersonal exchange is a constant that is simply not present in other settings. An informant explained the bond she felt with coworkers by saying, "It's nice to know the people you're working with. You work more together, you try harder, and you work closer." Another nurse shared that among many rewarding qualities of rural nursing, "The cooperation of the other nurses and the cohesiveness of the group is probably the biggest."

An old-timer at one hospital said, "I don't have to explain when I say something. They believe me, and they do it without wasting time." It was easy to verify this through observation. Certain old-timers could communicate a virtual reassignment of responsibilities through the tone of their voices as they disappeared momentarily to deal with a risen crisis, such as the admission of trauma victims in the ED. On occasions, it was like watching a dance, the motions of which were so well understood, each dancer so valued and respected, that without missing a step, workers would change places based on available expertise and would back each other up without visible cues. Even physicians were seen deferring to old-timer nurses at such times. Yet, the choreography depended heavily on the direction of the one in charge; and on other occasions, with an inexperienced newcomer directing, the dance was frantic and the flow chaotic.

Practicing Medicine

Rural nurses are understandably reluctant to admit that they practice medicine, but they know their boundaries are sometimes stretched by circumstance. "You take it upon yourself and do what has to be done to make sure the patient's stable before you can call the doctor," said one nurse to me. When patient crises occur, calling the physician is considered important, but it simply does not rank at the top of the list. The nurses I interviewed and watched used a standard A-B-C (airway, breathing, circulation) order of setting priorities to respond to patient needs. Thus, they often began written or unwritten medical protocols while the aide would be sent to summon the physician. Physician response times varied from 5 to 30 minutes at the rural hospitals, resulting in nurses being responsible for considerable decision-making during the time lapse. At each site, I heard or saw variations on the themes of nurses stabilizing cardiac or trauma victims and nurses managing precipitous births without the benefit of physicians present. In interviews, nurses were adamant that they had a responsibility to the patients to do whatever was required during an emergency, and although it sometimes felt uncomfortable, inaction would have constituted neglect. The words of one nurse summarize the collective opinion, "We do it because we have to, because it would be wrong if we didn't."

There were also circumstances of newcomer physicians relying on seasoned nurses for insight into or even direction regarding a given patient case. Per physician request, the nurse would literally advise what medications and treatments to order in cases where the doctor did not have the familiarity with a patient's history that the nurse did. This was especially true in after-hours situations of physicians covering for another's patients. My assessment of these circumstances is that each party acted within unseen lines of mutual trust and understanding with the dynamic of trust specific to a given relationship.

Another observation I made at these facilities, which struck me then and which I have informally reconfirmed on multiple occasions since, is that rural physicians seem more likely to read and respond to nurses' notes about patients than do urban physicians. Doubtless there is great individual variability, yet it is tempting to hypothesize that rural professionals have a better grasp than do their urban counterparts of pertinent information that is necessary to communicate to the healthcare team. Certainly, further study would be required to confirm the probability.

Rural Expertise: Aces and Pinch Hitters

Rural nurses generally believe that no one can be an expert in every area of rural nursing practice. However, a few nurses are extremely proficient in all clinical areas, and these nurses become role models and mentors to the other nurses with whom they work. At two study sites, many informants identified a colleague or two who fit this category. Interestingly, those who were identified by others as "aces" did not identify themselves as such. Each nurse was very modest about her own capability, but the pride toward aces among the staff was obvious. I was aware that talking to or watching these aces in action was as much an honor for the locals as it was for me as an investigating outsider.

All rural nurses interviewed agreed that they must be competent in more than one clinical area to be considered an acceptable staff member. The top four clinical areas deemed to be most important for competency were emergency nursing, obstetrical nursing, intensive or coronary nursing, and medical–surgical nursing. A supervisory nurse told me, "There's a difference between competent and expert. I think everybody who works in this hospital should be able to walk into any specialty area and function." But there was an expectation held by all informants that they be clinically strong, if not expert, in at least two of the above-named areas and be able to float to any other department and still function well in a pinch.

With regard to functioning in a pinch, in the early 1980s, two rural Montana nurse executives who are admitted baseball fans coined the Pinch Hitter Theory of Rural Nursing. One of those persons, Jean Shreffler, now an academic, is author of other chapters in this book. The second person, Maura Fields, was then and remains today the nurse executive at a rural hospital in Montana and is arguably one of the most innovative and masterful nurse leaders I have ever had the good fortune to know. Her rendition of the theory went like this:

> *In rural nursing, you have to be like a pinch hitter. You may not perform a task or procedure or work on a very specialized case but once a year. But when you go to do it, you have to do it like you do it every day. In baseball, a batting average of 300 is good. But the pinch hitter, well, you want them to be better than that, really, you want them to bat a thousand. That's what it's like for a rural nurse, when they go to work, you want them to bat a thousand. (Maura Fields, personal conversation, 1983)*

For those readers who are doubting that there can be that many instances in which the aforementioned theory becomes important, rest assured that it happens all the time. Industrial and recreational traumas are frequent in these communities. Rural citizens experience their share of severe burns, drug overdoses, cardiac arrests, head injuries, freak accidents, and critical illness. Although transfer to larger medical centers is sometimes preferred, stabilization is necessary first, and transfer is sometimes not possible. One hospital in this study is 90 road miles from the nearest medical center of any size and 150 road miles from a trauma center. Rotary blade or fixed wing aircraft are often used to transport cases that require more care than can be delivered locally, but northwest mountain weather conditions can be a significant factor in keeping aircraft grounded.

Although rural nurses do not expect an easy routine, frustration is common surrounding the conflict of trying to achieve expertise in such a complex practice. Boredom is rare as they face the constant variety of demands. One informant related the example of the prior day's evening shift. The informant was one of two RNs on duty at the time, assisted by one aide. The scenario she described began after change of shift report and went like this:

> *Just yesterday evening there were seven patients in the house with nothing going on. Within an hour, there was one admitted with a depression state, an OB came in, and there were four or five cases in the ER, one being a child with rectal bleeding, which makes you wonder about child abuse.*

Although two nurses and an aide would have no difficulty caring for seven stable medical–surgical patients, the admission of the depressed patient was a wrench in the works. Mental health diagnoses are among those for which rural nurses feel least appropriately prepared, and they lack confidence in rural physicians' ability to treat mental health patients appropriately, as well. The depressed patient required suicide precautions for a period of time, which meant that the aide was assigned to remain with the patient at all times. The pediatric patient in the ED required careful documentation, delicate interaction, and a social services consultation. The obstetrical patient admission required nurse assessment and individual care until it was determined that the patient was in early labor. One nurse moved back and forth between the ED and the general care unit; the other moved back and forth between the labor room, the depressed patient, and the general care unit.

Here is an account from another informant about another evening shift where three RNs were on duty but without assistance from an aide:

Not long ago we had an OB with a bad baby, small for gestational age; and at the same time, we got two ambulances 5 minutes apart, and they were both cardiacs with chest pain. While that was happening, there was surgery going on, and there was somebody in the unit. I don't know if god is watching you or what, but, for the most part, things seem to come out okay in the end.

In this case, one nurse was already assigned to the intensive care unit (ICU), and one was required to remain with the obstetrical patient to do monitoring and other procedures. When the first ambulance arrived, the third nurse was dispatched to the ED. Fortunately, some ambulance crew members were emergency medical technicians and could help with continued patient monitoring and calling in the physician, laboratory, and respiratory personnel. Also, fortunately, the physician arrived within 10 minutes and was designated to care for both patients. The final good fortune is that nothing went wrong on the general care unit while hell was breaking loose elsewhere.

Knowing Patients Personally

Most rural nurses subscribe to the belief that when they know patients personally, they can give better care. The possibility of experiencing fear when caring for family members or best friends notwithstanding, the rewards are considered rich. A gradual loss of anonymity occurs to rural nurses as they become immersed in and assimilated into rural society, making anonymity nonexistent for old-timers. "I can be more supportive emotionally when I know them," one said, and another elaborated, "Let's say in the ER, with chronic lungers, you know them, and they feel secure because they know we remember them." I saw instances of rural nurses informally calling to check on patients after discharge. As far as I know, patients were always glad to have these calls. The loss of anonymity is generally considered reassuring for those professionals who are comfortable with rural life, but it can be constricting as well. It should not be assumed, however, that negative aspects of anonymity loss are necessarily related to poor patient outcomes. On the contrary, one informant told me,

I know of several situations where knowing my OB patients who had poor outcomes made a difference to them, where I was really able to help them get through the experience. It's a real emotional drain, but you're ahead of the game because the trust is there.

The argument could be made that patients perceive their care to be better based on the close personal contact that is often made in the rural setting. A nurse who believes that her relationship to a patient made a difference in the patient's outcome said,

I recovered my little neighbor girl after her surgery. Most little kids are scared when they wake up, but when she woke up she knew me and wasn't afraid and recovered really fast. Because fear generates pain, but she wasn't afraid, she recovered faster than usual.

It is a cultural expectation of many rural people to be taken care of by someone they know. This differs from the expectation in urban settings. For the most part, informants agreed that rural people do expect to have their medical needs met, even though they live far from a major medical center. However, one informant said that rural patients often wait until they are "half dead" before they seek intervention and are "grateful for what they get." Another nurse said, "People have told me they were glad I was on when they were here, that if I said it was going to be okay, then it was going to be okay."

Nearly all rural nurses could confirm that sometimes they had patients from out of town who had previously experienced urban hospital admissions. These patients, whether vacationing in the rural setting or passing through the rural area, ended up in rural hospitals for reasons not important to this story. Their comments about the care they received in rural hospitals are important. The nurses were told by these patients that the care was of better quality, that they felt more cared for, that the rural nurses took more time to listen, that care was accomplished more quickly and smoothly, and that they felt more like people and less like numbers in the rural hospital than they did in any urban hospital. The outsider patients often expressed surprise at the high level of competence they encountered in the rural setting.

DISCUSSION

Rural Nursing's Distinctive Nature and Scope

Analyses of the reports of rural nurses show that the nature and scope of rural nursing are clearly distinctive. Using a framework to focus the discussion, the distinctions can apparently be categorized as those pertaining to rural nursing's nature, as well as the four components of rural nursing's scope, those being intersections, dimensions, core, and boundary.

THE NATURE OF RURAL NURSING

Most rural nurses have difficulty in defining their practice, although they can describe it. Their descriptions are a variety of rich, thoughtful, colorful, and articulate responses. Rural nursing is generalist nursing, not to be mistaken for mundane, and includes an intensity of purpose that makes it distinctive. Rural nurses may feel misunderstood and poorly recognized by the larger nursing community, but they are nonetheless a proud lot.

THE SCOPE OF RURAL NURSING

The intersections of rural nursing are distinctively marked and fluid. Rural nurses consistently and necessarily practice well within the realm of other healthcare disciplines, the most notable being respiratory therapy, pharmacy, and medicine. The intersection between nursing and medicine has the most extensive implications. It is a gray area that hinges on circumstances and relationships, and the most complex intersections occur during emergent situations, "until the doctor gets there." Some rural nurses embrace this intersection more willingly than others, but none do it casually. Reflective concern is apparent in comments related to this intersection. One informant said, "It means putting your neck out there on the line, but you have to make the judgment and go on." Another told me, "It sometimes feels uncomfortable, but it's part of my responsibility to the patient."

It is evident that the practice of rural nursing is dimensionally distinctive. Rural nurses embrace an ethic of openness and honesty that is pervasive. The dimension of interpersonal knowing is viewed as a positive feature of rural practice, and it exists between nurses and patients as well as among coworkers. A nurse administrator shared with me that, "in terms of practice outcomes, your accountability is right in front of your face." Rural nurses talked about being able to accomplish goals more quickly with their patients and said that guidance, teaching, and counseling behaviors are automatic to their practice in the rural environment. Communication patterns in the rural setting are more direct and suffer less obfuscation than do those in urban settings. There are fewer barriers to go through when imparting messages from one to another. As a result, there are probably fewer errors of omission and commission related to practice in the rural setting than there are in the urban setting. Confronting and managing conflict is more common in the rural setting, avoidance being an unacceptable dynamic for group cohesiveness that stems from mutual concern and regard for one another. Independent decision-making is given in rural practice, but rural nurses are aware of their limitations. One said, "You have to know when you don't know, and you have to know where to go to find out." Rural nurses are mindful, if not fully informed, about the legal dimensions of their practice. However, with respect to questions of patient safety and survival, rural nurses sometimes decide that their ethical obligation to do what is right for their patients carries more weight than their legal responsibility to uphold the law. These cases generally become lessons of learning, are scrutinized and discussed by the group, and are entered into memory for future reference.

Human responses, which nurses diagnose and treat, are the core of nursing. Some sources have suggested, and informants in this study agreed, that rural dwellers are known to delay health seeking and tend to define health as the ability to get out of bed and go to work. Thinking in terms of nursing diagnosis, one might call this behavior "dysfunctional perceptual orientation to health," which requires distinctive intervention at nursing's core. Rural nurses are faced with determining an appropriate line of demarcation between a rural dweller's rugged individualism and stubborn disregard for health. Inextricable from rural nursing's core are the relational issues of what it means to be rural. As noted earlier in this chapter, from an ontological standpoint, rural nursing is distinctive at its very core.

Boundary being dependent on the intersections, dimensions, and core of nursing, there can be no question as to rural nursing's distinctive boundary. Rural nursing is constantly changing in response to complex intersections and dimensional intricacies distinctive to rural society. The boundary is therefore neither smooth nor even static. When nurses come to a rural setting from an urban setting, they are very aware that the boundary of their practice changes. The transitional period for these nurses is not always easy, and boundary expansion can be accompanied by ambivalence, anxiety, and frustration. Newcomers must become adjusted to the rural culture to function effectively, and not all survive. Rural experts can play a key role in the success of newcomer transition, and those aces who invest themselves in the orientation and mentoring of newcomers know the importance of the payoff.

DEFINING RURAL NURSING

Rural nursing is a special variety of nursing in which the nurse must have a wide range of advanced knowledge and ability, in combination with commitment, to practice proficiently in multiple clinical areas simultaneously along the career trajectory. The practice requires constant and continual personal and professional adaptation in developing identity. A rural nurse has both an ontological sense of being and an epistemological sense of knowing that connect the nurse with the surrounding community, and through which the rural nurse creates a reality of rural professional nursing practice. In no other setting is a nurse's practice so thoroughly and integrally a constant factor in a nurse's life. In a society where separating one's private life from one's professional life is considered obligatory, rural nurses are singularly challenged, stripped of their own anonymity while simultaneously charged with protecting their patients' privacy.

CONCLUSION

The newcomer practices nursing in a rural setting, unlike the old-timer who practices rural nursing. Somewhere between these spectral extremes lies the transitional period of events and conditions through which each nurse passes at their own pace. It is within this temporal zone that nurses experience rural reality and move toward becoming professionals who understand that having gone rural they are not less than they were, but rather they are more than they expected to be. Some may be conscious of the transition and others may not, but in the end, a few will say, "I am a rural nurse."

REFERENCES

American Nurses Association. (1980). *Nursing: A social policy statement*. Author.

Evans, B. (Ed.). (1978). *Dictionary of quotations*. Avenel Books, Delecorte Press.

Rausch, E. M. (Screenplay Author). (1984). *The adventures of Buckaroo Banzai: Across the eighth dimension* *[Film]*. Vestron Video.

CHAPTER 9

Understanding the Lived Experiences of the Rural Bedside Nurse: A Global View

Judith Paré, Polly Petersen,
and Dayle Sharp

DISCUSSION TOPICS

- What strategies should healthcare administrators implement to support the recruitment and retention of rural nurses?
- How can mobile technology be better utilized in rural settings to enhance options for continuing and advanced education of rural nurses? What are the three potential funding sources that would support the costs of these technologies?
- The concept of a situation or locale-specific theory and its relationship to the larger body of nursing knowledge must be seriously considered (Winters, 2013). Reflect upon the geographic locality and how the concepts of Culture Care Theory and Sunrise Enabler Model support nursing care and profession in these locations.
- Compare and contrast the theory of Transcultural Care Diversity and Universality and the Rural Nursing Theory related to rural nursing practice.

INTRODUCTION

Rural and remote areas exist across the world. The difference in how rural and remote areas are defined is specific for many countries. The U.S. Census Bureau (2017) defines rural as those areas that encompass all population, housing, and territory not included within an urban area. Urban areas include geographic areas that are highly developed and populated with residential, commercial, and other nonresidential land uses. In many countries, it is simply the comparison of rural and urban related to population density. The World Health Organization (WHO) notes that those populations that live in urban areas have a higher standard of living (United Nations Statistics Division, 2020). Rural communities have a lower number of people, resulting in diminished economic, political, and cultural resources and support. This also results in the inability to look past the potential for growth and expansion in such areas as healthcare. Many rural residents do not have the desire to change the way things currently are as that is the way it has always been done, therefore there is no reason to make a change. Rural nurses are reluctant to make changes within their own practice as they are typically confident with the care they deliver. Subsequently, such healthcare systems may indirectly (and sometimes directly) affect the health status of residents who live there and influence healthcare delivery systems and services in those regions (Bushy, 2003). Those who practice in these rural and remote settings encounter values, beliefs, and cultural mores that necessitate self-reflection to ensure that the nurse is delivering culturally competent care. This chapter examines the lived experience of nurses working in critical access/rural and remote settings through the lens of phenomenology.

THEORETICAL FOUNDATION

Leininger (1974) first identified that culture, social structure, kinship, religion, and family directly influence nursing values and practice. The central thesis of the theory is that "varied cultures perceive, understand, and deliver care in varied ways, although there are some commonalities about care among all cultures across the globe" (Fawcett, 2002, p. 131). The Culture Care Theory supports the notion that culturally congruent care can be achieved by nurses who study the local views of residents and the emic knowledge dimensions that are derived from the people (McFarland & Webhe-Alamah, 2015). It is the synthesis of this knowledge that allows nurses the ability to deliver culturally congruent care (Leininger, 1978, 2005, Leininger & McFarland, 2002; McFarland, 2018). Tenets of this theory include the following:

- Care diversities and universalities exist among and between cultures in the world.
- Worldview and social structure factors, such as religion, economics, education, technology and kinship, environment, language and generic care, and professional care factors affect culture care meanings, expressions, and patterns in various cultures.
- The third theoretical tenet focuses on generic (emic or insider's view) and professional (etic) health factors in diverse environmental contexts greatly influence health and illness outcomes and therefore need to be taught, studied, and brought together into care practices for satisfying care for clients, leading to improved health and well-being.
- The fourth tenet includes the conceptualization of the three major culture care decisions and action modes used to plan culturally congruent care for clients' general health and well-being or to help them face death or disabilities (Leininger & McFarland, 2002, p. 78).

These four tenets add importance, strength, and precision to the overall focus of Culture Care Theory and provide a path for a greater depth of understanding of the nurse's obligation to deliver culturally competent care.

Research indicates that the lived experiences of nurses who practice in rural/remote settings are considerably different than those nurses in urban settings. Providing direct patient care in these settings may pose unique opportunities and challenges even for the most experienced urban nurses. Rural and remote practice requires that the RN cares for a variety of patients who may be family and friends in different circumstances. The Rural Nursing Theory (RNT) identifies rural dwellers as self-reliant and resistant to help from outsiders (Long & Weinert, 2018, Chapter 2). Likewise, many rural residents seek their healthcare from insiders, people who they know and are familiar within their community. This correlates with the Culture Care Theory that outlines practices of culture mainly from an emic, an insider, or an individual with a local perspective and an etic, an outsider's perspective (Leininger, 1998). Leininger (1995, p. 4) described transcultural nursing as an "essential area of theory and practice centered on comparative cultural care (caring) values, beliefs, and practices of individuals, or groups of similar or different cultures … with the aim to provide culture-specific and universal nursing care practices for the health and well-being of rural nurses" (Leininger & McFarland, 2002, p. 148). This definition of transcultural nursing provides important concepts when analyzing phenomenological data related to the lived experiences of rural and remote nurses. These concepts include the focus on assimilating to the culture, the care values of rural residents and communities, their system of beliefs, and practices or specific cultures or subcultures that provide assistance to meet the physical health, mental health, and spiritual needs. According to Leininger (2005, Chapter 15), culture refers to the shared and communicated knowledge of values, beliefs, norms, and life practices of a particular group that are generally transmitted intergenerationally and influence thinking, decisions, and actions in patterned ways (Leininger, 1995, p. 27; McFarland & Wehbe-Alamah, 2015, Chapter 9, p. 303). The nurses who provide direct care to rural and remote residents may or may not have been raised in that culture. For those who have been lifelong residents, they have shared life experiences and values. For those who have come from urban areas or transferred from other rural settings, they may experience enhanced feelings of isolation, loneliness, and cultural blindness.

Cultural Care

The Sunrise Enabler Model depicts dimensions of cultural care diversity and universality (Leininger, 1988, p. 157). Leininger considered the notion of nursing interventions as being intrusive to culturally competent care. She appreciated the ability of the nurse to recognize the values, mores, and beliefs of individuals in a holistic fashion, as a powerful tool to support evidence-based care. The updated Sunrise Enabler Model (see Figure 9.1) from McFarland and Wehbe-Alamah (2018) includes biological factors as a dimension of cultural and social structure factors and integrative care as a new construct.

In 2002, Leininger added the concept of integrative care to the Sunrise Enabler (McFarland & Wehbe-Alamah, 2019), thus extending cultural care as a holistic approach for all healthcare professionals and patients. Rural nurses need to respect the culture of care while also providing evidence-based care. Leininger believed nurses needed creative and different approaches to offer cultural and meaningful care to help patients. Although each of these decisions and action modes were established related to the culture of the patient, they can also be utilized for the culture of rural nursing. In the Culture Care Theory, Leininger proposed three modes of care decisions and actions: culture care preservation and/or maintenance; culture care accommodation and/or negotiation; and culture care repatterning and/or restructuring.

Culture Care Preservation and/or Maintenance

A common theme identified in research by rural and remote nurses is professional isolation (Paré, 2015; Petersen et al., 2017). Professional isolation is the result of limited team members to collaborate with in the healthcare setting. Rural nurses can experience isolation in a variety of ways. Isolation can be geographic, such as living in an area that is a

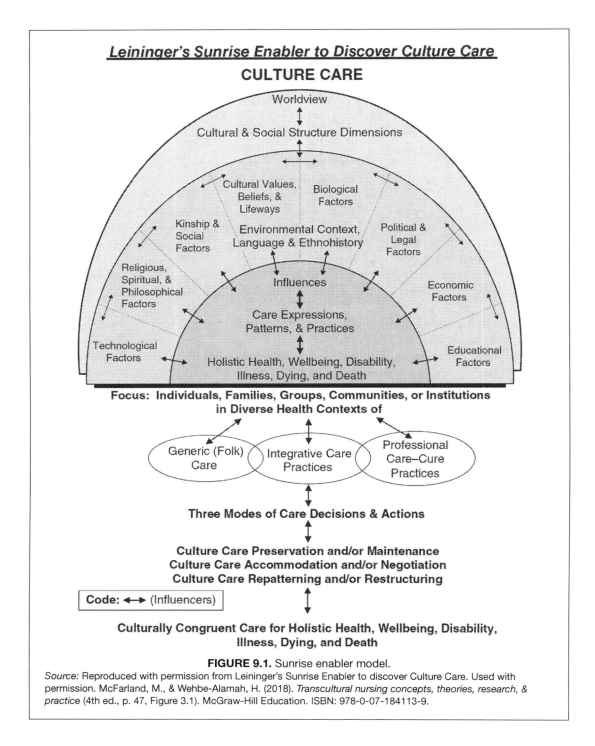

FIGURE 9.1. Sunrise enabler model.

Source: Reproduced with permission from Leininger's Sunrise Enabler to discover Culture Care. Used with permission. McFarland, M., & Wehbe-Alamah, H. (2018). *Transcultural nursing concepts, theories, research, & practice* (4th ed., p. 47, Figure 3.1). McGraw-Hill Education. ISBN: 978-0-07-184113-9.

great distance from family, friends, and services. Professional isolation becomes a reality for the nurse when they are unable to contact other members of the healthcare community for consultation or support. Isolation can affect professional growth; nurses can experience limited access to continuing education opportunities. Nurses often expressed feelings of isolation from both local and distant colleagues in the nursing community.

Participant "Julie," a 24-year-old woman who works in a critical access hospital, described her situation "I am very happy with my professional peer group, but there are times that I struggle to connect with them, especially in the bad weather. It simply is not possible to attend a seminar or meeting of a professional organization if the roads are closed or if the hospital is not adequately staffed. These are realities we deal with often but our peers who work in larger medical settings never experience." Julie and other participants completed interviews at the critical access hospital.

Another form of isolation often mentioned was staffing levels that do not allow for a nurse to actually leave the unit to participate in educational offerings. Nurses often do not have the opportunity to view this offering within the unit or perhaps even accessing it at a convenient time. When the number of nurses is limited, the idea of exclusion from social and professional development situations only further contributes to a sense of isolation. Isolation that some in rural/remote areas feel can be related to lack of support from the medical providers and/or management. Nurses often stated they felt unsupported by management and other healthcare providers (Sharp et al., 2020), stating there is a "lack of support from management and access to specialist medical advice" (Sharp et al., 2020, p. 11). Often, when nurses felt they were not supported by management, they cited that the culture of nursing within the institution was unsupportive (Paré, 2015; Petersen et al., 2017). The realities of such varied expectations including high levels of accountability while coping with fewer resources, higher levels of regulation, and stressors among care providers and administrators that too often lead to conflicts among and between groups (McFarland & Wehbe-Alamah, 2018, Chapter 2). Rural nurses generally see patients of all ages with a variety of needs; rural residents are typically stoic, often not wanting to be a bother, leading to the nurse having to address rural cultural aspects. They may also be challenged by staffing shortages, geographical obstacles, and barriers posed by technological limitations to find appropriate mentors who can model the tenets of transcultural care and diversity.

A second theme of isolation can be viewed as a lack of connectedness and, in the absence of formal or informal mentoring, this isolation can erode nurses' resilience and ability to perform transformative care. Mentors are essential to guide and transform traditional nursing practice to be congruent with the cultural mores, values, and beliefs (Leininger & McFarland, 2002, Chapter 1, p. 14). The art and science of mentoring allows nurses to shift from a focus of task-oriented care to one that is holistic, culturally focused, and based upon the resilience of the recipient of that care. Mentors can support new graduates in thinking of new ways to approach professional situations (Fawcett, 2002). An unintended consequence of lack of mentoring resources poses a barrier to culture care preservation and/or maintenance including professional actions and decisions that help people retain their culture and preserve relevant care values to assist in maintaining their well-being. However, with limited numbers of experienced nurses in these settings, mentors are rare. Mentoring assists in the transformation from traditional nursing practice to practice that fits rural culture. Mentors are needed to encourage new nurses to use holistic, culturally based practices to see people broadly and yet as individuals (Fawcett, 2002). Nurses often stress the value of mentoring, despite the absence of an approved mentoring/preceptor program (Paré, 2015).

CULTURE CARE ACCOMMODATION AND/OR NEGOTIATION

Culture care accommodation and/or negotiation includes professional actions to assist individuals from a culture to adapt to, negotiate with others, to accommodate for a beneficial, or satisfying health outcome. Two themes identified by nurses are personal isolation and personal connections or relationships within the community. Many rural/remote nurses have connections with their community. Some nurses recommend before practicing in a rural setting to ensure a rural lifestyle is what you want, the new nurse should relocate to a rural setting then make the most of serving the community to the best of their ability. Rural nurses need to build strong relationships with allied health, doctors, paramedics, and others to serve the community with limited resources. Understanding the culture that you are practicing requires recognizing your role in a small town is not just something you do; "you are part of the fabric of the town" (Sharp et al., 2020, p.12).

Some rural nurses experience barriers to their professional development that include a lack of a career ladder, promotion opportunities not correlated to advanced level of education, and a lack of tuition reimbursement. Despite limited funding and career advancement, many nurses continue to feel an obligation to remain current in yearly competencies. Nurses felt they were accountable for their own learning. "Each nurse must have self-motivation to want to stay current, improve, and learn. Each nurse should believe that they need to better herself in order to better serve her patients" (Petersen et al., 2017, p. 112). Nurses employed various techniques to continue their learning and to remain current in their skills.

Culture Care Repatterning and/or Restructuring

Culture care repatterning and/or restructuring assists patients to modify their lifeways through mutual decisions while respecting the patient's cultural values and belief for beneficial health outcomes. When applying this repatterning/restructuring to nurses who have become part of the community, many felt practicing in a rural setting is worth it.

Participant "Audrey," a 45-year-old woman from Australia, described her professional situation as worth the effort; challenging, always changing, occasionally slow but not boring. Participant "Cynthea," a 28-year-old woman who works in a remote area of Australia states that "it's a challenge but a brilliant experience." Audrey and Cynthea completed online interviews.

Many nurses across geographical locations accept the opportunity to treat patients with whom they have a personal relationship offering the opportunity for individualized care. Committing to a rural area allows building a "strong therapeutic relationship with the community that builds trust and respect" (Paré, 2015, p. 3).

Having a connection to the community has a positive impact on the nurse and the community members. When these patients have a relationship with the nurse, there can be more compassion because of the bond (Paré, 2015). Rural nurses report knowing how a patient will handle a hospital admission and the type of support they will have, if any post-hospitalization. If the patient is lacking a support network, a rural nurse will know what community resources they can alert to provide essential care. This requires that rural nurses possess a broad knowledge base and a sense of resiliency regardless of the circumstances. Helping community members can lead to supporting family members; one nurse spoke about saving a patient multiple times, which led to nurses being able to engage in intimate conversations with family members related to allowing for the patient to have a peaceful death. Nurses related their thoughts of extreme responsibility for patients, family members, and colleagues while providing acute and chronic care to persons recovering from trauma, systemic disease, pregnancy, and end-of-life or palliative care. Nurses' protocols included:

The persons who seek care in our hospital are friends, neighbors, colleagues, and sometimes, even our relatives. They are vital members of our town. It really takes a village to provide the best nursing care, and that is who we are (Paré, 2015, p. 4).

Isolation can also be felt when the nurse does not have a relationship with the community. Having an understanding of the community can be both positive and negative. Some nurses in rural areas find they are lost and are not a part of the community. Having an understanding of the community members can guide the nurse's interventions. This supports nurses who demonstrate social responsibility by meeting the social and health needs of the community (International Council of Nurses, 2012) while respecting the patient's cultural values and beliefs. Due to the close ties in rural communities, lack of extended services, and social injustice, it can be assumed that rural nurses engage more with their patients and community than their urban counterparts. "Socially responsible nurses should have professional self-confidence" (Faseleh-Jahromi et al., 2014, p. 292). Social responsibility contributes to the deep connectedness that rural nurses feel toward the patients they come across. One nurse stated:

"We need to let our patients know that we want to know about them, what they do for a living, tell us what is bothering them, we need to show patients that we care enough to communicate and that their lives and health are important to us. Caring for the community expands to offering shelter to community members in need" (Petersen et al., 2017, p. 113).

CONCLUSION

Rural nursing is defined as the provision of healthcare by nurses to persons living in sparsely populated areas (Long & Weinert, 2018, see Chapter 2). Rural nurses commonly express strong job satisfaction, stressing the realities of professional autonomy, the ability to serve a variety of patients with acute and chronic needs and the ability to preserve close community ties (Bigbee et al., 2009). Rural nurses must be skilled and ready to manage the care of any patient situation that presents in their practice setting (Petersen et al., 2017). They approach their professional responsibility with a general knowledge primarily based on an associate degree education (Newhouse et al., 2011). Rural nurses are motivated by an unwavering desire to make contributions to a patient population that they often know as family, neighbors, and friends. The lack of social boundaries and the outsider/insider construct are valued by rural nurses who preserve their personal roots as rural residents (Long & Weinert, 2018, see Chapter 2). Rural Nursing Theory supports the process of understanding commonalities and differences in rural care in order to support the delivery of evidence-based care to rural residents. Leininger's Culture Care Model (McFarland & Wehbe-Alamah, 2019, Chapter 1) adds support to the need for nurses practicing in rural and remote settings to be able to acknowledge both the cultural care nurses provide for their patients but also the impact of the rural/remote culture on their professional life.

REFERENCES

Bigbee, J.L., Gehrke, P., & Otterness, N. (2009). Public health nurses in rural/frontier one-nurse offices. *Rural Remote Health, 9*(4), 1282.

Bushy, A. (2003). Considerations for working with diverse rural client systems. *Lippincott's Case Management, 8*(5), 214–223. https://doi.org/10.1097/00129234-200309000-00007

Faseleh-Jahromi, M., Moattari, M., & Peyrovi, H. (2014) Iranian nurse's perception of social responsibility: A qualitative study. *Nursing Ethics, 21*(3), 289–298. https://doi.org/10.1177/0969733013495223

Fawcett, J. (2002). The nurse theorists: 21st-Century Updates-Madeleine Leininger. *Nursing Science Quarterly, 15*(2), 131–136. http://doi.org/10.1177/08943180222108787

International Council of Nurses. (2012). *The ICN code of ethics for nurses.* http://www.icn.ch/images/stories/documents/about/icncode_english.pdf publications/free_publications/Code_of_Ethics_2012.pdf

Leininger, M. M. (1974). The leadership crisis in nursing: A critical problem and challenge. *Journal of Nursing Administration, 4*(7), 28–34. https://doi.org/10.1097/00005110-197403000-00022

Leininger, M. M. (1978). *Transcultural nursing: Concepts, theories, and practice* (1st ed.). John Wiley & Sons.

Leininger, M. M. (1988). Leininger's theory of nursing: Cultural care diversity and universality. *Nursing Science Quarterly, 1*(4), 152–160. https://doi.org/10.1177/089431848800100408

Leininger, M. M. (1995). *Transcultural nursing: Concepts, theories, research, and practice.* McGraw-Hill College Custom Series.

Leininger, M. M. (1998). Special research report: Dominant culture care (emic) meanings practices and findings from Leininger's theory. *Journal of Transcultural Nursing, 9*(2), 45–49. https://doi.org/10.1177/104365969800900207

Leininger, M. M. (2005). Culture care diversity and universality: A worldwide nursing theory. In M. M. Leininger & M. R. McFarland (Eds.), *Culture care diversity and universality* (2nd ed., pp. 1–41). Jones & Bartlett Publishing.

Leininger, M. M., & McFarland, M. (2002). *Transcultural nursing: Concepts, theories, research, and practices* (3rd ed.). McGraw-Hill.

Long, K. A., & Weinert, C. (2018). Rural nursing: Developing the theory base. In C. A. Winters & H. Lee (Eds.), *Rural nursing: Theories, concepts, and practice* (5th ed., pp. 17–30). Springer Publishing Company.

McFarland, M. R., & Wehbe-Alamah, H. B. (2015). *Leininger's transcultural nursing: Concepts, theories, research & practice* (3rd ed.). McGraw-Hill Education.

McFarland, M. R., & Wehbe-Alamah, H. B. (2018). *Leininger's transcultural nursing: Concepts, theories, research & practice* (4th ed.). McGraw-Hill Education.

McFarland, M. R., & Wehbe-Alamah, H. B. (2019). Leininger's theory of culture care diversity and universality: An overview with a historical retrospective and a view toward the future. *Journal of Transcultural Nursing, 30*(6), 540–557. https://doi.org/10.1177/1043659619867134

Newhouse, R. P., Morlock, L., Pronovost, P., & Breckenridge Sprout, S. (2011). Rural hospital nursing: Results of a national survey of hospital executives. *Journal of Nursing Administration, 41*(3), 129–137. http://dx.doi.org/10.1097/NNA.0B013e31820c7212.

Paré, J. (2015). Understanding the lived experiences of nurses working in critical access hospitals. *American Research Journal of Nursing, 1*(5), 1–6.

Petersen, P., Sharp, D., & Paré, J. (2017). A story of emergent leadership: Understanding the lived experiences of nurses working in a rural hospital setting. *Online Journal of Rural Nursing and Health Care, 17*(2), 103–125. https://dx.doi.org/10.14574/ojrnhc.v17i2.454

Sharp, D., Petersen, P., & Paré, J. (2020). *The lived experiences of rural and remote nurse caregivers in Australia.* Unpublished manuscript, Department of Nursing, University of New Hampshire.

United Nations Statistics Division. (2020). *Population density.* https://unstats.un.org/unsd/demographic/sconcerns/densurb/densurbmethods.htm

United States Census Bureau. (2017). *American community survey.* https://www.census.gov/acs/www/data/data-tables-and-tools/data-profiles/2017/

Winters, C.A, (2013). (Ed.). *Rural nursing: Concepts, theory, and practice* (4th ed.). Springer Publishing Company.

CHAPTER 10

Experiences of Nurses Living in Rural Communities Who Commute for Employment

Laurie Johansen

DISCUSSION TOPICS

- List several circumstances that give rise to nurses experiencing a blurring of personal and professional boundaries as they live in a rural community.
- What are some challenges nurses face, related to their visibility and lack of anonymity, as they live and practice nursing in rural communities?
- How do the connections nurses make with their coworkers differ when working in a rural healthcare facility, compared to working in a nonrural healthcare setting?
- Describe how RNs experience feeling valued as professional nurses in their rural, home communities.

INTRODUCTION

Maintaining access to quality healthcare services is a significant problem facing many rural communities. Factors affecting access to healthcare are complex. One distinct factor affecting access is the shortage of healthcare professionals (National Rural Health Association, 2016). Deliberate strategies are needed to create and maintain an adequate number of healthcare professionals providing care to the rural population. Successful strategies must be based on a clear understanding of the challenges faced by rural healthcare providers.

A qualitative study completed in 2017 explored the experiences of RNs living in rural communities who commuted to nonrural healthcare settings for employment (Johansen, 2017). This chapter provides information about a portion of the findings from that study, which leads to greater understanding of RNs' experiences and the potential implications for rural populations. Background information, study method, and findings are found within this chapter as well as implications of the study.

BACKGROUND

One factor that contributes to the lack of availability of healthcare professionals for the rural population is the increasing number of RNs driving away, or commuting away, from their rural, home communities for employment (Skillman et al., 2006). Using 2004 data from the National Sample Survey of Registered Nurses (NSSRN), Skillman et al. (2012) reported approximately 37% of RNs living in rural communities commuted for employment. In fact, the percentage of RNs commuting from rural, home communities for employment increased from 14% in 1980 to 37% in 2004. No further commuter trend data is available due to discontinuation of the NSSRN survey data collection until recently. However, there is no evidence the commuter trend of RNs has stabilized or diminished. Additionally, in the literature, there is no focus on the impact of commuter trends of RNs on the availability of nurses working in rural healthcare settings.

Little is known about the experiences of RNs commuting for employment and the impact of those decisions. However, there are assumptions that higher wages in larger healthcare settings are a driving force of RNs' employment decisions (Skillman et al., 2012). It is known that the per capita rate of RNs residing in rural areas is lower than urban areas in the United States, with rural areas having 852.7 RNs per 100,000 people, compared to 934.8 RNs per 100,000 people in urban areas (Health Resources and Services Administration, 2013). This per capita rate of RNs considers only the residences of RNs, not the per capita rate of RNs working in rural areas. Probst et al. (2019a) reports the salary averages of rural nurse is nearly $4,500 less on average, per year, than urban nurses, which may impact rural nurse employment decisions. When considering the rural population's access to healthcare, it is important to consider the impact of a continued trend of RNs commuting away from rural communities, adding to the potential for inadequate numbers of RNs practicing in rural healthcare settings. The looming nursing shortage (Snavely, 2016), coupled with decisions of RNs to commute for employment, potentially decreases access to quality healthcare in rural communities.

METHOD

A descriptive phenomenological study approach (Dahlberg et al., 2008) guided a description of RNs' experiences living in rural communities while commuting to nonrural healthcare settings for employment. The sample selection process sought to recruit currently licensed RNs with varied experiences surrounding the phenomenon of commuting away. Specifically, the sample included RNs living in rural communities with critical access hospitals located within those rural communities ("rural" defined as less than 2,500 residents), with those RNs commuting to nonrural healthcare settings for employment. Purposeful sampling with snowballing allowed the researcher to seek variations in the RNs' experiences, including experiences practicing as a nurse, number of years practicing nursing, levels of education, types of worksites, length of residence in a rural community, and experiences with commuting for employment. In the end, 16 nurses participated in this study.

FINDINGS

Findings revealed the core meaning, or essence, of the phenomenon of commuting away for RNs who live in rural communities, and commute away to nonrural healthcare settings, to be *commuting to achieve personal and professional goals while being a nurse in a rural community*. One major component of the essence was identified as *being a nurse in a rural community*, which is the focus of this chapter.

Being a Nurse in a Rural Community

Nurses shared a wide array of experiences living in rural communities, some unique to each nurse and others like other nurses. However, whether the nurses had lived in their home communities their entire lives, or had recently moved to the rural community, all the nurses experienced *being a nurse in a rural community*. Discussion of these findings follows, weaving connections in the literature to the understanding of *being a nurse in a rural community*.

PRACTICING NURSING IN THE RURAL COMMUNITY

While *being a nurse in a rural community*, nurses had varying experiences working as healthcare professionals in rural healthcare settings. Some had practiced in rural healthcare settings as a nurse, an emergency medical technician, or perhaps a nursing assistant, whereas others had never practiced as a healthcare professional in any rural healthcare setting. Irrespective of their previous experiences, they all had perceptions about what it would be like to be a rural nurse. Rural nurses were described as "jacks of all trades" with diverse roles that required vast knowledge bases. Such role diffusion was supported within the rural nursing theory (Long & Weinert, 1989).

Nurses in this study had differing perceptions about the skills used by rural nurses, with some believing rural nurses used their professional skills more fully in rural healthcare settings, compared to skills used in nonrural healthcare settings. Other nurses had opposing perspectives, believing nurses would lose nursing skills if they practiced in rural healthcare settings because certain skills would not be used often enough. It is valuable to understand all perspectives about what it would be like to be a rural nurse. Differing perceptions surrounding the value of the roles of all nurses, including the rural nurse, have been found in the literature. Jackman et al. (2010) found the need for all roles of the nurse to be perceived, and represented, as important without diminishing the role of the rural nurse, in order to prevent negative influences on rural healthcare. Medves et al. (2015) went on to report the need to illuminate the opportunities for rural nurses to use all their nursing skills, as nurse specialists in rural nursing, to retain nurses in rural healthcare settings. In the end, differing perceptions were found, surrounding the perceived skills needed to practice rural nursing, and the subsequent impact on employment decisions.

As nurses shared their varying perspectives of skills needed to practice as rural nurses, it became evident that not all nurses felt comfortable with the role diffusion required to practice successfully as a rural nurse. Nurses shared their sense of discomfort and anxiety related to feeling unsure of their own ability to function as a rural nurse. The idea of leaving their practice in a nonrural healthcare setting to return to rural practice was daunting for some. Nurses in this study are not alone with such feelings. In 2009, Hunsberger et al. found similar findings, with nurses being uncomfortable and stressed practicing rural nursing with skills that they did not use on a routine basis. Additionally, Probst et al. (2019b) report nurses in rural practices felt less prepared academically then their peers in urban or suburban healthcare settings. In the end, in this study, it was understood that a wide range of experiences, perceptions, and feelings surround rural nursing.

The perception about the type of care given to the people served in rural healthcare settings is different from care provided in nonrural healthcare settings. The rural environment was experienced as being more intimate, with nursing practice being more hands on in a caring and personal setting. One nurse said, "I just feel that it's not just numbers in and out … I love the more caring atmosphere that I think rural nursing brings to the table." Similar descriptions of care provided in rural healthcare settings were reported by Baernholdt et al. (2010) with rural nurses creating settings that made patients "feel at home" (p. 1350) where "nurses cared about me" (p. 1349). Individualized, hands-on patient care was found to be a hallmark of rural nursing for Baernholdt et al., as well as this study.

CARING FOR PEOPLE YOU KNEW AND/OR PEOPLE WHO KNEW YOU IN RURAL COMMUNITIES

As nurses practiced in rural healthcare settings, they experienced providing care for people they knew and people who knew them, with patients including community members, neighbors, friends, or family. Like the study by Scharff (2018), nurses working in rural healthcare settings within their home communities regarded themselves to be more connected to their home communities and the people served within those communities. Nurses got to know their patients better, noticing that patients were more receptive to them, finding, "Families could talk to me easier … They respond to you better." However, a lack of separation existed between the personal and professional lives of these nurses. Patients would ask about the personal life of the nurse, including information about who their family members were and details about their family as found in the rural nursing theory (Long & Weinert, 1989). The acceptance of the nurse was, at times, dependent on the concept of outsider/insider, with the familiarity between patients and their healthcare providers being a key component in the patient's acceptance of help from the medical professional.

One concern that surfaced about practicing rural nursing was the fear of caring for family and friends who needed urgent treatment. Being the primary person responsible for assisting a neighbor or family member in an emergency was daunting. As noted by Scharff (2018), fear also arose as the nurses contemplated future interactions that would occur in the community as the nurse communicated with family and community members. One nurse in this study shared:

> I don't want my neighbor and my family coming into the emergency room and I have to work on them [in rural, home community]. That scared me terribly. It still does. I don't want to be that first person that sees them and has to do that … And then you're seeing those people, whether it turns out good or bad, all the time, and it's hard … You're with those people all the time and so what if things don't go right? Then you have that where people hold you accountable for that whether you could have done something different or not, and I just think its way, way, way more personal and hard.

By the same token, findings revealed that not all nurses were comfortable knowing about patient outcomes in these situations, such as the death of a patient, before the family knew.

> Ninety-five percent of the patients you run into you know, both personally, community, you know them. That's very hard … always knowing the patients and you see them at vulnerable times … There is a death … You know before their family even knows.

Along with the connections experienced between nurses and patients came nurses' concerns surrounding the maintenance of patient confidentiality, due to a lack of separation between the personal and professional lives of rural nurses. Caring for someone with whom the nurse socially interacted in the community brought challenges in maintaining privacy for patients. The feelings nurses experienced regarding the blurring of personal and professional lives in these situations ranged from contented or neutral feelings, to feelings of being uncomfortable.

Finally, due to the distinctive nature of the blurring of personal and professional lives between nurses and their patients in rural communities, nurses living in rural communities felt uncomfortable dealing with situations that involved legal aspects of the lives of their patients. One nurse shared:

I had a situation where it was a neighbor … and there was alcohol involved. By law, I have to report it, and I knew that if I did, [the neighbor] would be in a lot of trouble again, and it was really hard … It was really hard … I was like, "I have no choice. I have to notify the police." I remember hugging [the neighbor's spouse], and I started crying … Sometimes the community would say, "How could you do that?" I'm like, "Oh, you just don't understand."

The providing of care to patients in rural healthcare settings is distinctive, as healthcare professionals care for people they know and people who know them. The beauty of this context parallels the challenges faced by nurses as they live *being a nurse in a rural community*.

CONNECTION TO COWORKERS

The blurring of the lines between nurses' personal and professional lives extended beyond patient care to include the connections nurses made with their coworkers, while working in a rural healthcare setting. Nurses knew everyone with whom they worked on a personal and professional level, creating a feeling of being a part of a family with these people, including medical providers and ancillary staff. Scharff (2018) summarized the connections between coworkers in rural settings, stating that "rural nurses are in the distinctive situation of being personally acquainted with all of those around them" (p. 116). These connections create the potential for added depth to interfaces between coworkers with the potential for added accountability not found outside of rural healthcare settings.

In this study, the resulting connections between coworkers in rural healthcare settings led to feelings of obligation to each other. One nurse in this study stated, "The relationship that you had with the rest of your staff, it was a tighter bond, because there were a smaller number of you, and you knew that you needed to be there for each other." Feelings of concern for their coworkers and patients followed the nurses into their personal lives and their time away from work. Also, with the nurses' residences being relatively close to the healthcare facility, it was convenient for nurses to get called back in to work when needed. It was not unusual for the nurses to feel obligated to go back to work when needed during their time off because there were so few nurses working at the facility. MacKusick and Minick (2010) found that feelings of obligation were correlated with nurses leaving clinical practice due to nurses being called in to work on their time off and nurses feeling as though they never recover from the strain of working as a nurse. Similar feelings were expressed by participants in this study:

When I worked in … [rural home community], it was almost too easy for me to pick up [hours] because I was too convenient, and that's where I burned myself out … because I was five blocks away. I was way too accessible … It was too easy for me to say yes, and I got too involved.

Thus, the experiences brought about by the connections to coworkers in rural healthcare settings had the potential to bring about feelings of obligation for the rural nurse. Just as the nurses' experiences working in rural healthcare facilities varied, nurses' feelings about connections to coworkers varied. Some nurses appreciated feeling like part of a family working in a rural healthcare facility and missed those connections as they commuted to nonrural healthcare settings for employment. Other nurses appreciated feeling more disconnected from their coworkers as they commuted for employment, valuing a more distinct boundary between personal and professional lives and fewer feelings of obligation.

One last consideration found in this study regarding coworker connections in rural healthcare settings was the impact that currently employed people in a rural healthcare setting had on prospective employees. As nurses thought about seeking employment in a rural healthcare facility, they knew that they would be working with every professional in that healthcare facility. Thus, if there was an individual in that rural healthcare facility with whom the nurse would prefer not to work, their employment decision may have been swayed. One nurse discussed this, stating:

> *There is also the fact that you know who works there [in rural facility], and you maybe don't want to necessarily work with them, and you know you're going to work with them all the time … You don't want to go to work every day and just cringe to go to work … because there are only a few people that work there.*

Nurses shared many experiences *being a nurse in a rural community*, including the blurring of the lines between their personal and professional lives. While working in rural healthcare settings, connections nurses made with their coworkers created varying feelings about the subsequent benefits, as well as challenges, in their personal and professional lives.

CONNECTIONS TO RURAL COMMUNITY

As nurses shared their experiences *being a nurse in a rural community*, they not only had a variety of experiences, or perceptions, of practicing nursing in a rural community, they also had a variety of connections to their rural communities. All the nurses in this study lived in a rural community. The nurses' social connections to their rural community were a key part of their lives, which is not exclusive to this sample of nurses. Historically, social networks in rural communities have been found to enrich the social well-being of nurses, as well as their job satisfaction in the rural community (Kulig et al., 2009). Richards et al. (2005) found that healthcare providers, which included nurses, who lived and practiced in a rural community, felt like they were more a part of that community. However, as they commuted for employment to nonrural communities, they felt less connected to their home communities. Similar findings came from this study. As nurses in this study sample commuted for employment, they too experienced changes in their connections to their rural communities, feeling less tied to the community. Some nurses were saddened by this disconnect; others appreciated this experience. Understanding the nurse's experiences with connections to their rural communities led to the following themes.

EVERYBODY KNOWS EVERYBODY

A common statement made by many nurses was that, in a rural community, everybody knows everybody. People living in rural communities had a high level of information about their neighbors and community members. One nurse commented, "People knew everybody's business. They knew who came in [to the hospital] before you even did."

Rural community members were also familiar with who the nurses were in their communities, as well as the nurses' families.

Rural community members knew how important the role of the nurse was to their community. Thus, due to the community members being familiar with the nurses and their families, they were willing to help care for the nurses' families. One nurse spoke about feelings of appreciation for such help, sharing the following experience:

> One time, there was an emergency, and I had to go in, and I didn't have anybody for my youngest, and he was three. So, I just brought him with me, and the kitchen staff took him so I could help with the emergency … They just fed him brownies and juice for three hours. But that wouldn't happen in a different place.

Several nurses believed that the expectations of their community members required their professional roles as a nurse to extend into personal events, such as attending church or going to a ballgame. As one nurse said, "I'm a nurse in this community. So, at church when somebody faints, you know, everybody runs to me." Community members also came to the nurses' homes requesting assistance with their medical needs, such as assistance with a blood sugar check. Some nurses appreciated these interactions with community members, whereas others voiced discomfort. Community members did not always consider the areas of expertise that a nurse may, or may not have, when asking for assistance, and some nurses felt unprepared to offer assistance when it was out of their area of expertise. Then again, even if the community members were requesting assistance within an area of expertise for the nurse, the situation could be unnerving for the nurse, as one nurse shared:

> [In] rural communities … everybody knows what everybody does. So, your phone might ring. When I was getting my hair cut, she's like, "I told the … [medical provider] that if I go into labor, because I have quick labors, I was going to pick her up," and she said, "Oh no, you're not. You're going to pick up [nurse participant in this study] on the way because she's the one that does that." So you're like, "Are you really going to call me?" Just different things like that.

Even though the familiarity of community members with the nurse in the rural community was appreciated at times, for many nurses, this familiarity also created difficult situations. Nurses sensed judgments as well as social and professional expectations from community members, because of their role as a nurse in the community. Some social expectations interfered in the personal lives of the nurses and their families. As one participant noted,

> When you work in the area you grew up in, you know almost all the people and their families, and certain situations are uncomfortable. And seeing them out—like, the older nurses never went to a bar. They never went to the VFW in town, because they worked at the hospital, and they wanted people to respect them. And I kind of felt the same way, so we just didn't go out.

Professional expectations from the rural community also surfaced about the nurses' employment decisions, with nurses feeling judged about their decisions to commute for employment elsewhere. One participant noted,

> The hospital needs help, why aren't you helping? Why are you going someplace else? You should be here. Quit your job and come here now, because that would be the thing that you should do. You get that strong opinion from the people that say that to you, "Why are you not here?"

The rural community members' familiarity with everybody not only exposed the nurse to judgments, but judgment fell on the nurse's family members as well, which leaked into the rural workplace. One nurse passed on the following experience:

> *People know you, and they know who you are, and they know what kind of person you are ... In a small town, people judge your kids based on your actions. If they like you, they like your kids. If they don't like you or something that you did, they don't like your kids. Or if your kids did something that was way out in left field, you're going to hear about it first ... I would hear things at work before I ever heard it from my kids or from anybody else.*

In the end, within a rural community, the familiarity of everybody knowing everybody can create a kinship between community members, including nurses within those communities. However, concerns can arise regarding the role of nurses within the community, interfering in the nurses' personal lives.

FAMILY CONNECTIONS

Family connections to the rural community impacted the decision for many of the nurses to live in their rural community. Having family members in the community, some of the nurses had spent their entire lives in their rural community, whereas other nurses' residential histories ranged from having recently moved to the rural community, having lived in the rural community for several years, or having moved back after being gone for many years.

> *It was more of a personal, private, family decision that we wanted to have our kids raised in a smaller, safer town. We both are from ... small towns ... We definitely have always had that in the back of our minds that we want to be in a smaller town, not in a larger city ... We wanted to get back closer to family.*

The impact of family on the nurse living in a rural community is not new to the nurses in this study. Previous literature has supported the influence of family connections to nurses. Molanari et al. (2011) studied rural nurses' employment choices and lifestyle preferences, finding that ways of living found in rural communities impacted decisions to seek employment in rural communities. Being close to family was one lifestyle preference sought living in a rural community. Similarly, being close to family was a lifestyle consideration for many of the nurses in this study.

VISIBILITY IN THE RURAL COMMUNITY

With the familiarity of everybody knowing everybody in the rural community, nurses faced a lack of anonymity while living in a rural community. The inevitable blurring of boundaries between the nurses' personal and professional lives resulted in nurses facing challenges preserving anonymity and privacy, not only for themselves and their families but also their patients as well. Social interactions were common between nurses and community members. Community members frequently contacted the nurses, asking for advice, opinions on health-related problems, or assistance with their medical needs. Such contacts may have been by phone, by community members stopping by a nurse's home, or while a nurse was out and about in the community.

> *They can ask you a lot. "What do you think of this?" or "What should I do about that?" ... "I was told this. What do you think?" or "This is what's happening," and they want you to say ... They know you're a nurse ... they expect you to know everything.*

Frequently, confidentiality concerns arose when community members asked the nurses about patients in the rural communities. The nurses desired to maintain patient confidentiality for their patients, but found, "It's hard even when somebody says, 'How is so-and-so doing?' You can't say anything … They'll still ask, knowing that we can't say anything, but they'll still ask anyway, and it just makes it very difficult." Encounters with community members asking about patient information, or personal advice, occurred regularly at common locations within the community, such as the grocery store, church, or school activities. "You couldn't go to the grocery store without, 'Oh, did you work today? I saw you … [at work].' It was definitely a challenge."

Nurses also encountered their patients in their rural communities. At times, patients would disclose their own personal, medical information to the nurse and the group of people surrounding the nurse. In these circumstances, the nurses may have felt pleasure in the acknowledgment of the care they had provided. However, they were also put in a precarious position, as they continued to try to maintain their responsibility to assure patient confidentiality. One nurse explained:

> That's up to them if they want to come up to you in public and acknowledge that you were their nurse … It's that "thank you so much for your help" or "for helping my parents." There is that, too, which is kind of nice in a way because you know them and you've got that connection then.

Nurses faced an additional challenge of maintaining patient confidentiality. As nurses lived and worked in their rural, home community, they found it impossible to be able to come home and talk to family and friends about what had been taking place at work. The nurses knew that if they talked about work, even if they did not use specific names of people, the familiarity of everybody knowing everybody in the rural community could lead to family members or friends identifying who was being talked about. In the end, the nurses were unable to get the support they desired from those nearest and dearest to them, experiencing an inability to talk about the joys and burdens of their work. These nurses were not alone with these feelings, with Evanson (2006) finding similar experiences with public health nurses working in rural settings.

Lack of anonymity is a specific concept within the rural nursing theory (Long & Weinert, 1989) and has been commonly reported among other studies including rural nurses. In this study, nurses' feelings about their visibility in their communities ranged from neutral feelings, with a lack of anonymity just being part of a rural life, to this visibility being inconvenient and undesirable. For some nurses in this study, the discomfort with this visibility contributed to their decision to commute for employment outside of their rural, home communities. One nurse shared feelings of relief while commuting:

> I go home and nobody [patients] knows what I do at night after [I go home] … I like that people don't know what time I go home at night, and where I live, or what my home phone number is, or anything like that.

The blurring of the personal and professional lives of nurses in rural communities is commonplace. It is important to consider the implications of the visibility of nurses in rural communities and the impact a lack of anonymity may play in nurses' decisions to commute for employment.

RESPECT, TRUST, AND CONFIDENCE IN COMPETENCE

As stated earlier, all the nurses had different experiences living and practicing nursing in the rural community. One noteworthy finding from this study was that, whether the nurses had lived in the rural community their entire lives or had recently moved to the rural community, whether the nurses had worked in the rural community in the past or had never worked in the rural community, all the nurses in this study felt valued by their rural community members. The feeling of being valued came to be through the nurses' perceptions of being respected, trusted, and/or competent as nurses. By virtue of their roles as nurses and being members of the nursing profession, the connections to the close-knit rural community created a context where trust and respect developed.

> I feel like I'm respected, that's for sure. They trust you. Everybody's very trusting in a small town. When you make little connections and things like that in a small town, they remember you. Just the trust and the confidence that they have in you. Even though I was a new nurse at the nursing home, and I had like no experience whatsoever, they just trusted me. If something was wrong, they felt confident that they could tell me, and they felt confident that I would pass things on to the doctor or whoever to get resolved. Even the aides, I think they could sense that too. Families could talk to me a lot easier than some of the pool nurses that were coming in … They just trust you a lot more, and they know that you know what they're talking about, and you know kind of their background better … Definitely I feel that people trust me being a nurse, and the confidence they put in me is really nice, too.

Nurses appreciated this sense of feeling valued. For some nurses, this sense of value continued within their rural, home communities even as they commuted for employment. However, this was not experienced within the communities to which the nurses commuted for employment.

Further Study Findings Beyond Being a Nurse in a Rural Community

The findings from this study revealed *being a nurse in a rural community* to be one key component of the essence of *commuting to achieve personal and professional goals while being a nurse in a rural community*. The remainder of the study results is not described in detail in this chapter. However, to summarize, although nurses experienced *being a nurse in a rural community*, there was an inability to get all their personal and professional goals met in their rural, home communities. This, along with some of the experiences nurses faced by *being a nurse in a rural community*, led to nurses commuting to nonrural communities for employment, allowing them to experience different professional connections.

IMPLICATIONS

Findings from this study can influence recruitment and retention efforts to address the shortage of healthcare professionals in rural healthcare facilities. Unique, individualized strategies to recruit and retain rural nurses need to be developed to benefit the rural population, nursing practice, and employers of nurses in rural healthcare settings. Recruitment and retention policy development should focus on job motivators for nurses, as well as job satisfaction. Additionally, academic settings need to prepare new nurses for future clinical practices in rural settings. We continue to need to understand the experiences of rural nurses through further research of this important topic.

CONCLUSION

Nurses living in rural communities have rich personal and professional experiences. Understanding the complex layers of living as a nurse in a rural community adds depth to the understanding of nurses' decisions to commute away from their rural home communities for employment. This new knowledge can be used to create future recruitment and retention strategies for nurses practicing in rural settings. Successful interventions can alleviate the potential for a scarcity of RNs in the rural United States, diminishing barriers the rural population face accessing healthcare.

REFERENCES

Baernholdt, M., Jennings, B. M., Merwin, E., & Thornlow, D. (2010). What does quality care mean to nurses in rural hospitals? *Journal of Advanced Nursing*, 66(6), 1346–1355. https://doi.org/10.1111/j.1365-2648.2010.05290.x

Calleja, P., Adonteng-Kissi, B., & Romero, B. (2019). Transition support for new graduate nurses to rural and remote practice: A scoping review. *Nurse Education Today*, 76, 8–20. https://doi.org/10.1016/j.nedt.2019.01.022

Dahlberg, K., Nyström, M., & Dahlberg, H. (2008). *Reflective lifeworld research*. Studentlitteratur.

Evanson, T. A. (2006). Intimate partner violence and rural public health nursing practice: Challenges and opportunities. *Online Journal of Rural Nursing and Health Care*, 6(1), 7–20. http://rnojournal.binghamton.edu/index.php/RNO/article/view/162

Health Resources and Services Administration, Bureau of Health Professions, National Center for Health Workforce Analysis. (2013). *The U.S. nursing workforce: Trends in supply and education*. https://bhw.hrsa.gov/sites/default/files/bhw/nchwa/projections/nursingworkforcetrendsoc013.pdf

Hunsberger, M., Baumann, A., Blythe, J., & Crea, M. (2009). Sustaining the rural workforce: Nursing perspectives on worklife challenges. *The Journal of Rural Health*, 25(1), 17. https://doi.org/10.1111/j.1748-0361.2009.00194.x

Jackman, D., Myrick, F., & Yonge, O. (2010). Rural nursing in Canada: A voice unheard. *Online Journal of Rural Nursing and Health Care*, 10(1), 60–69. http://rnojournal.binghamton.edu/index.php/RNO/article/view/74

Johansen, L. (2017). Commuting away: The experiences of RNs who live in rural communities and commute away for employment in non-rural communities. *Nursing Capstones*, 236. https://commons.und.edu/nurs-capstones/236

Kulig, J. C., Stewart, N., Penz, K., Forbes, D., Morgan, D., & Emerson, P. (2009). Work setting, community attachment, and satisfaction among rural and remote nurses. *Public Health Nursing*, 26(5), 430–439. https://doi.org/10.1111/j.1525-1446.2009.00801.x

Long, K. A., & Weinert, C. (1989). Rural nursing: Developing the theory base. *Research and Theory for Nursing Practice*, 3(2), 113–127.

MacKusick, C. I., & Minick, P. (2010). Why are nurses leaving? Findings from an initial qualitative study on nursing attrition. *MEDSURG Nursing*, 19(6), 335–340. http://amsn.inurse.com/sites/default/files/documents/practice-resources/healthy-work-environment/resources/MSNJ_MacKusick_19_06.pdf

Medves, J., Edge, D., Bisonette, L., & Stansfield, K. (2015). Supporting rural nurses: Skills and knowledge to practice in Ontario, Canada. *Online Journal of Rural Nursing and Health Care*, 15(1), 7–41. http://rnojournal.binghamton.edu/index.php/RNO/article/view/337

Molanari, D. L., Jaiswal, A., & Hollinger-Forrest, T. (2011). Rural nurses: Lifestyle preferences and education perceptions. *Online Journal of Rural Nursing and Health Care*, 11(2), 16–26. http://rnojournal.binghamton.edu/index.php/RNO/article/view/27

National Rural Health Association. (2016). *About rural health care*. http://www.ruralhealthweb.org/go/left/about-rural-health

Probst, J. C., McKinney, S. H., & Odahowski, C. (2019a). *Rural registered nurses: Educational preparation, workplace, and salary.* Rural & Minority Health Research Center. https://www.sc.edu/study/colleges_schools/public_health/research/research_centers/sc_rural_health_research_center/documents/ruralregisterednurses.pdf

Probst, J. C., McKinney, S. H., & Zahnd, W. (2019b). *Perceived facilitators and barriers to rural nursing practice.* Rural & Minority Health Research Center. https://www.sc.edu/study/colleges_schools/public_health/research/research_centers/sc_rural_health_research_center/documents/perceivedfacilitatorsandbarrierstoruralnursingpracticed.pdf

Richards, H., Farmer, J., & Selvaraj, S. (2005). Sustaining the rural primary healthcare workforce: Survey of healthcare professionals in the Scottish Highlands. *Rural and Remote Health, 5*(1), 1–14. http://www.rrh.org.au/publishedarticles/article_print_365.pdf

Scharff, J. E. (2018). The distinctive nature and scope of rural nursing practice: Philosophical bases. In C. A. Winters & H. J. Lee (Eds.), *Rural nursing: Concepts, theory, and practice* (5th ed., pp. 107–123). Springer Publishing Company.

Skillman, S. M., Palazzo, L., Doescher, M. P., & Butterfield, P. (2012). *Characteristics of rural RNs who live and work in different communities.* http://depts.washington.edu/uwrhrc/uploads/RHRC_FR133_Skillman.pdf

Skillman, S. M., Palazzo, L., Keepnews, D., & Hart, L. G. (2006). Characteristics of registered nurses in rural versus urban areas: Implications for strategies to alleviate nursing shortages in the United States. *The Journal of Rural Health, 22*(2), 151–157. https://doi.org/10.1111/j.1748-0361.2006.00024.x

Snavely, T. M. (2016). A brief economic analysis of the looming nursing shortage in the United States. *Nursing Economics, 34*(2), 98–100.

CHAPTER 11

The Nurse Practitioner as Rural Healthcare Provider

Jana G. Zwilling

DISCUSSION TOPICS

- What are some barriers to full scope-of-practice for nurse practitioners (NPs) in rural areas? How might these differ by state? By healthcare system?
- Discuss the benefits and detriments to NP practice in the rural area where you grew up.
- What economic benefits might be provided to rural areas with an NP-led primary care model? How might this benefit the patient? Community?
- Self-reliance and independence are hallmarks of the rural patient populations. Discuss the benefits and detriments of these traits when attempting to provide chronic disease management. How might the benefits and detriments differ with the provision of health promotion or prevention components?

INTRODUCTION

In a keynote address to the National Organization of Nurse Practitioner (NP) Faculties (NONPF), Dr. Loretta Ford stated, "Patients will be in control, as they always have been. This is something nurses have always understood" (Ford & Gardenier, 2015, p. 577). Rural patients see themselves as self-reliant and independent. No one knows this better than an NP in a rural clinic. In these days of relative value units (RVUs) and quality measures (QMs) for healthcare reimbursement, there is something lacking: the patient. Yes, QMs attempt to consider the patient's voice, but health indicators measured by prescribed standards do not always demonstrate the high quality of care in a collaborative patient–provider relationship. For example, the American Diabetes Association (ADA) might recommend that a patient's A1C needs to be less than or equal to 6.5% (ADA, 2020). The NP in a rural setting might see a farmer present for a large wound obtained during harvest. The farmer needs to "get sewn up quick" so he can get back out in the fields. This farmer also happens to have type 2 diabetes and has not had an A1C checked for 2 years; his last one being 7.5%. The NP engages in a conversation and education regarding the patient's diabetes, while suturing the patient's wound. The patient agrees to have labs drawn prior to leaving the clinic and schedules an appointment for "after harvest." The fact that this farmer even had his labs drawn should be marked as a high QM. The give and take between the patient and the NP can make small, incremental improvements toward target measures and greatly benefit the patient; however, these are not captured with the current QM model.

NPs have been steadily increasing in number and are working to break down the barriers to a full scope-of-practice. Evidence supports full-scope NP practice and the ability of APRNs to lead the way in formulating new and better primary care models. There have been many innovations over the past 50-plus years in the healthcare arena, none as disruptive as that of the NP. "If the natural process of disruption is allowed to proceed, we'll be able to build a new system that's characterized by lower costs, higher quality, and greater convenience than could ever be achieved under the old system" (Christensen et al., 2000, p. 2).

Ever since Drs. Ford and Silver envisioned the NP role, NPs have been chipping away at barriers to the provision of affordable, accessible quality care to meet the needs of the general healthcare consumer, especially those in rural and underserved populations. This chapter provides insight into the contributions of NPs as healthcare providers in the rural setting and includes a brief background on the NP role, a section on access to healthcare, and a look at the unique patient-centered care provided by NPs.

BACKGROUND

NPs have been the recognized healthcare providers in the United States since 1965. The NP role was the vision of rural pediatric public health nurses in Colorado. These nurses were advocating for their patients and wanted to provide more services while performing home visits in rural areas. Often the only healthcare provider in the county, these nurses believed their patients should not have to wait on assessments or orders from a physician to obtain the needed care. Thus, the first NP training program was born out of necessity to provide more and better services for the rural and underserved populations (American Association of Nurse Practitioners [AANP], n.d.[a]).

The NP role has continued to evolve since 1965, in both educational preparation and practice. Currently, NPs must have either a master's or doctoral degree in nursing practice (DNP). Most NP programs require applicants to practice as an RN for a minimum of 1 year prior to applying for graduate school. Each NP must pass a national certification exam specific to the NP role (family, psychiatric, pediatric, adult, etc.), and hold an active RN and APRN license to practice. There are also continuing education requirements that differ based on the state and national certification organization. According to the AANP (n.d.[b]), "NPs assess patients, order and interpret diagnostic tests, make diagnoses, and initiate and manage treatment plans, including prescribing medications." NPs perform their roles as independent practitioners, without physician supervision or collaboration in 23 states and the District of Columbia, with legislative efforts in many other states to insure full-scope-of-practice (AANP, n.d.[a]).

There are presently 290,000 licensed NPs in the United States (AANP, 2020). Approximately 90% of these NPs are certified in a primary care area such as family or adult care (AANP, n.d.[a]), and often practice in rural and underserved populations. Between 2008 and 2016, the number of rural practices including an NP increased by over 43%, whereas physician practices in rural areas decreased by almost 12% (Barnes et al., 2018).

A study of the geographic distribution of primary care clinicians demonstrated an average of 5.8 more NPs and 24 fewer physicians per 100,000 patient population in rural versus urban areas (Graves et al., 2016).

Rural Healthcare Access

Access to healthcare is defined as "the timely use of personal health services to achieve the best health outcomes" (Millman, 1993, p. 4). Getting *good access* to healthcare requires entrance into the healthcare system and access to facilities with necessary services and providers who meet the individual needs of the patient. Access is measured by the presence of health insurance, a physical healthcare facility, healthcare utilization measures, and patients' own assessment of how readily they can access care (Agency for Healthcare Research and Quality [AHRQ], n.d.). Isolation and distance from other towns, neighbors, or healthcare resources may be viewed differently by urban and rural persons. Living in an urban area where all necessities are located within a few city blocks, one might view having to drive 100 miles for a healthcare appointment ludicrous. However, if you grew up with your nearest neighbor 2 miles away, your mom driving an hour and a half to work 3 days per week, and your school bus ride taking 2 hours, traveling 100 miles for healthcare would not be out of the ordinary. The view of healthcare accessibility, therefore, can differ greatly by population. A rural patient may perceive easy access and the effective receipt of needed services as one acute care appointment during the year for which they drove 50 miles one way to their appointment.

Rural Healthcare Providers

The United States has long attempted to attract healthcare providers, especially primary care physicians, to rural areas. Medicare provides a large sum of money for graduate medical education (GME). The Medicare Prescription Drug, Improvement, and Modernization Act (2003) sought to redistribute unused Medicare-funded medical residencies and expand training in rural areas. A study conducted in 2013 showed that, of 3,000 residencies participating in this redistribution, only 12 were in rural areas. The growth of primary care residencies did improve; however, specialty care residencies grew larger by twice the number of primary care (Chen et al., 2013).

Less than 33% of physicians work in a primary care area defined as family medicine, general practice, internal medicine, pediatrics, and geriatrics (AHRQ, 2012). Only 11% of physicians practice in rural areas (AHRQ, 2018). Conversely, the NP workforce has shown a strong commitment to primary care and rural practice. Over 60% of NPs work in a primary care area defined as pediatrics, family, or internal medicine (Chattopadhyay et al., 2015). Nationwide, approximately 15% of NPs practice in rural areas with a per capita ratio of rural NPs at 21.8 per 100,000 population in those areas.

Rural locales demand an experienced clinician with a broad array of skills. Typically, the NP in rural areas is a family NP. Training as a family NP provides the broadest scope-of-practice, highly desired by rural healthcare systems that strive to reduce the need for multiple specialists. Rural NPs usually work more and longer hours, see more patients on an average day, perform more procedures, and refer out to specialists significantly less than their urban counterparts (Brown et al., 2009). Many NPs working in rural areas of the United States have additional privileges that are either not available or not necessary for their urban colleagues. In critical access hospitals (CAH) or other small rural hospital settings, NPs likely have hospital admitting privileges as well as long-term care–admitting privileges and all the responsibilities associated with caring for patients within those facilities.

Health Professions Shortage Areas, CAHs, and NPs

Health professional shortage areas (HPSAs) are designations that indicate healthcare provider shortages in primary care, dental health, or mental health. Primary care HPSAs are identified by the Health Resources and Services Administration (HRSA) based on applications submitted by each state's primary care officials (2020). Primary care HPSAs are roughly defined as a patient to physician ratio of 3,000:1 (or greater). Primary care providers include physicians in general or family practice, general internal medicine, obstetrics and gynecology, or pediatrics (Salinsky, 2010). APRNs are not considered when determining the HPSA for primary care.

A CAH is a facility that has applied for and met specific criteria to gain CAH designation. Some requirements of this designation are having no more than 25 inpatient beds, maintaining an annual average length of stay no more than 96 hours for acute inpatient care, offering 24-hour, 7-day per week emergency care, and being located in a rural area at least 35 miles away from any other hospital or CAH (Social Security Administration, 2006). For CAH status, a physician must be associated with the facility; however, there is no requirement for that provider to be on-site. In many cases, one physician is associated with multiple CAHs while NPs independently provide the ongoing care at the CAH. As an exemplar, North Dakota has 36 CAHs spread across 69,000 square miles and a population distribution of 9.7 persons per square mile (U.S. Census Bureau, 2010). Based on a review of North Dakota CAH websites, NPs outnumber physicians approximately 2:1 and physician assistants 5:1 as permanent employees of these facilities.

The CAH requirements support a focus on common outpatient conditions and immediate needs of the patient, while referring patients with complex conditions to larger facilities with more resources. It is of utmost importance for CAHs to keep costs low. This focus on high-quality care at a low cost is consistent with the tenets of NP scope-of-practice. One case study identified significant cost savings, as much as 28% for a CAH, by employing salaried and benefited NPs in their ED as opposed to contracting with either local or locum tenens physicians (Henderson, 2006).

Medicare and Medicaid, although beneficial for some populations, can have a negative effect on the financial health of rural areas. Although the patient may be covered for health services, to some extent, reimbursement rates to rural healthcare facilities can be lacking. For example, NPs are reimbursed at 85% of the rate of physicians, even when providing the same service (Medicare Learning Network, Center for Medicare & Medicaid Services, and Department of Health and Human Services, 2020). With many rural healthcare facilities employing primarily, or only, NPs, this lower reimbursement rate can be crippling. Furthermore, primary care practices bill largely for outpatient office visits or consultations as opposed to billing for individual procedures, a common practice among specialists. Reimbursement rates for office visits are significantly lower than procedural costs, hence another barrier to income production for rural facilities (Zismer et al., 2015). The 2017 Medicare Payment Advisory Commission (MedPAC) report cited negative average Medicare margins for rural healthcare facilities, with declines expected to continue (MedPAC, 2017).

Rural Patient-Centered Care

The rural patient population can be challenging to care for due to a multitude of reasons. Rural populations tend to be older, have higher rates of poverty and unemployment, depend heavily on Medicare or Medicaid, and are likely to live in an area designated as an HPSA (Parker et al., 2018). The rates of suicide and accidental death in rural populations are also higher than in urban populations (Garcia et al., 2017; Ivey-Stephenson et al., 2017). Farming and ranching, two major industries in rural America, have the second highest occupational fatality rate at 23 per 100,000 full-time equivalent (FTE; Bureau of Labor Statistics, U.S. Department of Labor, 2019). Many farms and ranches are family- or privately owned and often not able to supply employer-paid health insurance. Accessing resources can also be a challenge for rural patients and providers alike due to long distances, lack of public transportation, and poor travel conditions common in rural areas. One study cited that rural patients, on average, travel 113 miles for a primary care visit with an NP (Brown et al., 2009).

The Rural Nursing Theory outlines four primary concepts of rural populations that can affect healthcare (Long & Weinert, 1989; also see Chapter 2). Rural persons tend to assess their own health based on their ability to perform their jobs or daily work activities. If they can work, healthcare intervention is seen as unnecessary. The isolation and distance of rural populations could be construed as a barrier to healthcare access, but it has been found that rural inhabitants do not view themselves as isolated, nor do they see health services as inaccessible. The rural population is also seen as self-reliant and independent. Self-reliance can be a necessity in geographically isolated rural areas but can be a barrier to effective health promotion and disease management activities. Rural residents are known to seek services for acute illness or injury when self-care fails and are reluctant to rely on healthcare providers for health promotion and disease management services. Finally, the lack of anonymity and outsider/insider concepts can affect the provision and acceptance of rural healthcare services and providers.

The insider–outsider conundrum of rural culture can be a difficult barrier to overcome, especially when attempting to gain trust and establish a productive provider–patient relationship. According to the Agency for Healthcare Research and Quality (AHRQ, 2013), "good access" includes "providers ... with whom patients can develop a relationship based on mutual communication and trust" (n.d. para 2). With the cultural differences outlined in the Rural Nursing Theory (Long & Weinert, 1989; also see Chapter 2), provision of care within a trusting patient–provider relationship where communication is paramount can be difficult since many rural persons distrust outsiders, preferring a provider with whom they are familiar. Fortunately, nurses are seen as trusted professionals and have ranked first in the Gallup Poll for honesty and ethics for the past 18 years (Reinhart, 2020). There is also an abundance of evidence demonstrating that NPs have superior interpersonal skills and can produce excellent patient outcomes (Caldwell, 2007; Horrocks et al., 2002; Leipert et al., 2011).

Rural communities are often like a large family where everyone knows everyone else and is involved in each other's lives. "Culturally beneficial nursing care can only occur when cultural care values, expressions, or patterns are known and used appropriately and knowingly by the nurse providing care ... beneficial, healthy, satisfying, culturally based nursing care enhances the well-being of clients" (Leininger, 1991, pp. 44–45). Healthcare providers entering the community for a short period of time, for example, National Health Service Corps (NHSC) loan repayment participants are frequently met with skepticism and mistrust as these providers traditionally enter and leave the communities quite frequently (Pathman et al., 2004). Much time is needed to integrate a new *family member*. Fortunately, NPs commonly *grow where they are planted*, meaning they are members of the community and began work as RNs in the local healthcare facility. After obtaining their advanced degree, NPs often stay in their home communities to care for their friends, neighbors, and family. Although it is not always the case that NPs have resided in the area in which they currently practice, NPs are educated to consider the whole person versus merely the disease process. This thought process is so ingrained that NPs are typically found to quickly establish a nurturing rapport. Horrocks et al. (2002) found NPs, overall, spent more time with their patients, provided more guidance on self-care and management, and communicated better, when compared to physicians. Ultimately, patients were more satisfied with the NP encounter as compared to physician encounters (Horrocks et al., 2002). NPs can easily overcome the insider/outsider barrier typical of rural communities by becoming engaged in the community and focusing on patient-centered care. Rural healthcare facilities could benefit from educating local RNs as NPs in order to provide culturally competent care to their residents.

Madeleine Leininger (1991, p. 48) proposed that health be defined as "a state of wellbeing that is culturally defined, valued, and practiced, and which reflects the ability of the individuals or groups to perform their daily role activities in culturally expressed, beneficial, and patterned lifeways." Dr. Leininger's definition provides the underpinnings in describing the phenomenon of health in rural populations. Culturally speaking, as noted previously, rural persons tend to view their own health in terms of their individual work ability. Essentially, if they can perform their regular daily duties, they do not seek healthcare. However, if an illness or injury decreases or prohibits their ability to work, they will be first in line at the clinic. Numerous examples of this can be seen in a rural NP practice. A rural farmer whose wife is trying to get him to have his cholesterol checked, says it will have to wait until after planting is done. However, when the farmer's prize bull steps on his foot and he cannot push the pedals in the tractor, that farmer wants a quick fix so he can get back into the fields. The NP, knowing the futility of discussing preventive care and health promotion with the farmer, treats the fractured foot and provides direction for self-care, including written instructions for care and follow-up the farmer can take to his wife. Knowing the cultural background of a patient, as well as their personal concept of health, can lead to proper treatment and while maintaining a professional patient–provider relationship.

Encounters with rural patients often require the NP to strike a bargain or make some sort of compromise with the patient to achieve the desired health outcomes. This, fortunately, can be advantageous for both parties. Working in partnership with the patient versus using an authoritarian relationship can be very encouraging to that patient. When patients are emboldened to participate in their own healthcare, often they feel more in control and may be more apt to adhere more closely to provider guidance, especially with rural populations where self-reliance and independence are a common theme. "Promoting involvement in self-care, for example, often depends on the nurse's ability to use communication to create an identity for the client as someone who is capable of active participation in healthcare" (Kasch et al., 1998, p. 276). As an example, a rural mail carrier who has had type 2 diabetes for over 5 years attends annual physical exams with his primary provider but his A1C has been steadily increasing. Originally, the NP had recommended him to check his blood sugar twice each day. The patient admits to checking it "rarely" or "maybe once a week." The NP asks the mail carrier about the schedule that would work best for him. The patient is rather taken aback by this as he is used to being reprimanded by healthcare providers and family members for not taking better care of himself. He decides he can easily check his sugars first thing in the morning, but "the rest of my day is usually up in the air." The pair compromises on daily fasting sugars and checking postprandial sugars twice each week. The NP is satisfied as the patient will be checking his blood sugar and the patient is satisfied because he was the one to set the schedule, making him feel more in control.

The best healthcare providers will recognize that "patients will always be in control" (Ford & Gardenier, 2015, p. 577). Certainly, patients need evidence-based guidance and best practices to assist their decision-making, but ultimately, the decision is their own.

CONCLUSION

Guiding and supporting, as well as advocating for patients, have always been a hallmark of nursing. In this time of exploding healthcare expenditures, provider shortages, geographical distribution issues, and significant numbers of underserved populations, our system of healthcare is ripe for an upheaval. Christensen et al. (2000) apparently had a crystal ball to be so accurate about future *disruptive innovations* in healthcare. NPs are a definite innovation who can not only cut healthcare costs but also provide superior, patient-centered care while circumventing primary care provider shortages in rural America.

REFERENCES

Agency for Healthcare Research and Quality. (n.d.). *Topic: Access to care*. https://www.ahrq.gov/topics/access-care.html

Agency for Healthcare Research and Quality. (2012). *The number of practicing primary care physicians in the United States*. U.S. Department of Health & Human Services. http://www.ahrq.gov/research/findings/factsheets/primary/pcwork1/index.html

Agency for Healthcare Research and Quality. (2013). *National healthcare quality report*. https://archive.ahrq.gov/research/findings/nhqrdr/nhqr13/chap10.html

Agency for Healthcare Research and Quality. (2018). *The distribution of the U.S. primary care workforce*. https://www.ahrq.gov/research/findings/factsheets/primary/pcwork3/index.html

American Association of Nurse Practitioners. (2020). *NP fact sheet*. https://www.aanp.org/about/all-about-nps/np-fact-sheet

American Association of Nurse Practitioners. (n.d.[a]). *Historical timeline*. https://www.aanp.org/about-aanp/historical-timeline

American Association of Nurse Practitioners. (n.d.[b]). *All about NPs*. https://www.aanp.org/all-about-nps

American Diabetes Association. (2020). Standards of medical care in diabetes-2020. *Diabetes Care*, 43(Suppl. 1), S1–S2. https://doi.org/10.2337/dc20-Sint

Barnes, H., Richards, M. R., McHugh, M. D., & Martsolf, G. (2018). Rural and nonrural primary care physician practices increasingly rely on nurse practitioners. *Health Affairs*, 37(6), 908–914. https://doi.org/10/1377/hlthaff.2017.1158

Brown, J., Hart, A. M., & Burman, M. E. (2009). A day in the life of rural advanced practice nurses. *Journal for Nurse Practitioners*, 5(2), 108–114. https://doi.org/10.1016/j.nurpra.2008.10.013

Bureau of Labor Statistics, U.S. Department of Labor. (2019). *News release: National census of fatal occupational injuries in 2018*. https://www.bls.gov/news.release/pdf/cfoi.pdf

Caldwell, D. (2007). Bloodroot: Life stories of nurse practitioners in rural Appalachia. *Journal of Holistic Nursing: Official Journal of the American Holistic Nurses' Association*, 25(2), 73–80. https://doi.org/10.1177/0898010106293610

Chattopadhyay, A., Zangaro, G. A., & White, K. (2015). Practice patterns and characteristics of nurse practitioners in the United States: Results from the 2012) national sample survey of nurse practitioners. *Journal for Nurse Practitioners*, 11(2), 170–177. https://doi.org/10.1016/j.nurpra.2014.11.021

Chen, C., Xierali, I., Piwnica-Worms, K., & Phillips, R. (2013). The redistribution of graduate medical education positions in 2005) failed to boost primary care or rural training. *Health Affairs*, 32(1), 102–110. https://doi.org/10.1377/hlthaff.2012.0032

Christensen, C. M., Bohmer, R. M. J., & Kenagy, J. (2000). Will disruptive innovations cure health care? *Harvard Business Review*, 78(5), 102–112, 199. https://hbr.org/2000/09/will-disruptive-innovations-cure-health-care

Ford, L. C., & Gardenier, D. (2015). Fasten your seat belts—It's going to be a bumpy ride. *Journal for Nurse Practitioners*, 11(6), 575–577. https://doi.org/10.1016/j.nurpra.2015.03.012

Garcia, M. C., Faul, M., Massetti, G., Thomas, C. C., Hong, Y., Bauer, U. E., Iademarco, M. F. (2017). Reducing potentially excess deaths from the five leading causes of death in the rural United States. *Morbidity and Mortality Weekly Report*, 66(2), 1–7. Centers for Disease Control and Prevention. https://www.cdc.gov/mmwr/volumes/66/ss/ss6602a1.htm?s_cid=ss6602a1_w

Graves, J., Mishra, P., Dittus, R., Parikh, R., Perloff, J., & Buerhaus, P. (2016). Role of geography and nurse practitioner scope-of-practice in efforts to expand primary care. *Medical Care*, 54(1), 81–89. https://doi.org/10.1097/mlr.0000000000000454

Health Resources & Services Administration. (2020). *Health professional shortage areas (HPSAs).* https://bhw.hrsa.gov/shortage-designation/hpsas#:~:text=Health%20Professional%20Shortage%20Areas%20(HPSAs)%20are%20designations%20that%20indicate%20health,dental%20health%3B%20or%20mental%20health.&text=A%20shortage%20of%20providers%20for,within%20a%20defined%20geographic%20area

Henderson, K. (2006). TelEmergency: Distance emergency care in rural emergency departments using nurse practitioners. *Journal of Emergency Nursing*, 32(5), 388–393. https://doi.org/10.1016/j.jen.2006.05.022

Horrocks, S., Anderson, E., & Salisbury, C. (2002). Systematic review of whether nurse practitioners working in primary care can provide equivalent care to doctors. *British Medical Journal*, 324(7341), 819–823. https://doi.org/10.1136/bmj.324.7341.819

Ivey-Stephenson, A. Z., Crosby, A. E., Jack, S. P. D., Haileyesus, T., Kresnow-Sedacca, M. (2017). Suicide trends among and within urbanization levels by sex, race/ethnicity, age group, and mechanism of death – United States, 2001-2015. *Morbidity and Mortality Weekly Report Surveillance Summaries*, 66(18), 1–16. Centers for Disease Control and Prevention. https://www.cdc.gov/mmwr/volumes/66/ss/ss6618a1.htm

Kasch, C. R., Kasch, J. B., & Lisnek, P. (1998). Women's talk and nurse-client encounters: Developing criteria for assessing interpersonal skill, including commentary by Moccia, P. *Scholarly Inquiry for Nursing Practice*, 12(3), 269–287.

Leininger, M. M. (1991). The theory of culture care diversity and universality. In M. M. Leininger (Ed.), *Culture care diversity and universality: Theory of nursing* (pp. 5–68). National League for Nursing.

Leipert, B., Wagner, J., Forbes, D., & Forchuk, C. (2011). Canadian rural women's experiences with rural primary health care nurse practitioners. *Online Journal of Rural Nursing & Health Care*, 11(1), 37–53. http://rnojournal.binghamton.edu/index.php/RNO/article/view/8

Long, K. A., & Weinert, C. (1989). Rural nursing: Developing a theory base. *Scholarly Inquiry for Nursing Practice: An International Journal*, 3, 113–127.

Medicare Learning Network, Center for Medicare & Medicaid Services, and Department of Health and Human Services. (2020). *Advanced practice registered nurses, anesthesiologist assistants, and physician assistants.* https://www.cms.gov/Outreach-and-Education/Medicare-Learning-Network-MLN/MLNProducts/Downloads/Medicare-Information-for-APRNs-AAs-PAs-Booklet-ICN-901623.pdf

Medicare Payment Advisory Commission. (2017). *Report to the congress: Medicare payment policy* (pp. xi–xxiv). http://medpac.gov/docs/default-source/reports/mar17_entirereport224610adfa9c665e80adff00009edf9c.pdf?sfvrsn=0

The Medicare Prescription Drug, Improvement, and Modernization Act of 2003, 42 U.S.C. 1301 *et seq.* (2003). https://www.congress.gov/108/plaws/publ173/PLAW-108publ173.htm

Millman, M. (Ed.). (1993). *Access to health care in America.* National Academies Press.

Parker, K., Horowitz, J., Brown, A., Fry, R., Cohn, D., & Igielnik, R. (2018). *What unites and divides urban, suburban, and rural communities.* Pew Research Center. https://www.pewsocialtrends.org/2018/05/22/demographic-and-economic-trends-in-urban-suburban-and-rural-communities/

Pathman, D. E., Konrad, T. R., Dann, R., & Koch, G. (2004). Retention of primary care physicians in rural health professional shortage areas. *American Journal of Public Health*, 94, 1723–1729. https://dx.doi.org/10.2105%2Fajph.94.10.1723

Reinhart, R. J. (2020, January 6). *Nurses continue to rate highest in honesty, ethics.* Gallup. https://news
.gallup.com/poll/274673/nurses-continue-rate-highest-honesty-ethics.aspx

Salinsky, E. (2010). Health care shortage designations: HPSA, MUA, and TBD [Background paper
no. 75.] *National Health Policy Forum.* http://www.nhpf.org/library/background-papers/BP75_
HPSA-MUA_06-04-2010.pdf

Social Security Administration. (2006). *Compilation of the social security laws, medicare rural hospital flexibility program.* (Sec. 1820. [42 U.S.C. 1395i–4]). https://www.ssa.gov/OP_Home/ssact/title18/1820
.htm

U.S. Census Bureau. (2010). *Quick facts: North Dakota.* https://www.census.gov/quickfacts/table/
PST045215/38

Zismer, D. K., Christianson, J., Marr, T., & Cummings, D. (2015). *An examination of the professional services
productivity for physicians and licensed, advance practice professionals across six specialties in independent and integrated clinical practice: A report by the School of Public Health, University of Minnesota,
for the Medicare Payment Advisory Commission.* http://www.medpac.gov/docs/default-source/
contractor-reports/an-examination-of-the-professional-services-productivity-for-physicians-and-
licensed-advance-practic.pdf?sfvrsn=0

CHAPTER 12

Using RNs in Primary Care: Opportunities and Challenges for Rural Clinics

HEIDI A. MENNENGA, ROBIN J. BROWN, BETH WALSTROM, AND LINDA BURDETTE

DISCUSSION TOPICS

- What are some examples of RNs practicing to the full scope of their license in the primary care setting?
- What are the benefits of utilizing RNs in the primary care setting?
- What are some challenges related to utilizing RNs in the primary care setting?

INTRODUCTION

This chapter explores the topic of using RNs in primary care. Many primary care clinics, particularly in rural settings, are struggling with having an adequate number of healthcare providers. RNs who are practicing to the full scope of their license may help alleviate this challenge. There are many benefits to utilizing RNs in the primary care setting; however, there are also several challenges that need to be overcome. These opportunities and challenges will be discussed along with implications for leaders and nurses in the practice setting and the academic environment to encourage the use of RNs in primary care.

BACKGROUND AND LITERATURE REVIEW

RNs play an essential role in the healthcare setting, especially in rural primary care. The role of RNs in primary care has emerged and changed over the last century. The most significant change is the national movement of RNs practicing to the full scope of their license in the primary care setting (Bodenheimer & Mason, 2017). RNs provide a unique set of clinical and management skills, and when these skills are used to the fullest potential, the outcomes lead to better primary care teams and improved patient care (Flinter et al., 2017; Martinez-Gonzalez et al., 2014).

Primary care and the expanded role of nursing are deeply rooted in nursing's history (Keeling, 2015). Florence Nightingale, founder of modern nursing, indicated money should be spent on maintaining health in communities rather than inside hospital buildings (Bodenheimer & Mason, 2017). Another historical record of nurses in an expanded role is Lillian Wald's work with the Henry Street Settlement in 1893. Lillian Wald and her colleagues demonstrated how nurses worked to the full extent of their training to provide care to thousands of Americans by conducting home visits (Keeling, 2015). In the mid-20th century, healthcare moved from homes and communities to hospitals, which led to more nurses working in hospitals (Bodenheimer & Mason, 2017). In addition, primary care settings eliminated RN staff and replaced with licensed practical nurses (LPNs) and medical assistants due to the cost of RNs and the competition with hospitals.

There is a movement back toward community-based primary care. Leading this change is the Institute of Medicine (IOM; 2011) report, *The Future of Nursing: Leading Change, Advancing Health.* The report focused on the importance of nurses practicing to the full scope of their education and training and fully partnering with other healthcare providers (IOM, 2011). Additionally, the Josiah Macy Jr. Foundation hosted two conferences: in 2010, *Who Will Provide Primary Care and How Will They Be Trained,* and in 2016, *Preparing Registered Nurses for Enhanced Roles in Primary Care.* Several papers were commissioned because of the 2016 conference and compiled by Bodenheimer and Mason (2017). The IOM report and the Josiah Macy Jr. Foundation conferences ignited a movement for change in primary care, partially due to the shortage of providers in primary care and the complex needs of patients in the primary care setting.

In the United States, primary care in rural settings is also changing. According to Sinsky et al. (2013), the traditional primary care model is unsustainable. There is a need for changes in primary care due to the aging population, increasing healthcare costs, and the enactment of the Patient Protection and Affordable Care Act, which emphasized the importance of primary care (Smolowitz et al., 2015). In addition, there is a growing shortage of primary care providers, increased prevalence of chronic diseases, and dissatisfaction in the existing primary care environment (Association of American Medical Colleges [AAMC], 2019; Bauer & Bodenheimer, 2017; Flinter et al., 2017; Smolowitz et al., 2015). By 2032, the estimated shortage for primary care physicians is between 21,100 and 55,200 (AAMC, 2019).

Fortunately, RNs can help meet the healthcare needs in rural primary care settings. There are more than 3.2 million RNs nationwide employed in nursing (United States Department of Labor, 2019). Only 16% of RNs are employed in rural settings (Health Resources and Services Administration [HRSA], 2013) and fewer than 10% of RNs are employed in primary care (Auerbah et al., 2013). According to Martinez-Gonzalez et al. (2014), care provided by RNs is equally as good as care provided by physicians. In addition, nurse-led care has a positive effect on patient satisfaction, hospital admissions, healthcare costs, and mortality (Martinez-Gonzalez et al., 2014).

When employed in primary care, RNs frequently are not practicing to the full scope of their license (Bauer & Bodenheimer, 2017; Flinter et al., 2017). In primary care, the RN role has been primarily limited to telephone triage, education, immunizations, and medication administration (Flinter et al., 2017; Smolowitz et al., 2015). Although these roles and responsibilities do not encompass all RN duties practiced in primary care settings, the literature suggests a need for expanding the role and independence of the RN in primary care to address issues of access, provider shortages, and promote better work environments with higher interprofessional collaboration efforts (Flinter et al., 2017; Smolowitz et al., 2015). Additionally, utilizing RNs who practice to the full scope of their license in primary care can provide not only cost savings, but may also improve the quality of patient care (Martinez-Gonzalez et al., 2014).

Opportunities

RNs practicing to the full scope of their license hold many opportunities for expanding the typical role of an RN and enhancing primary care practice to benefit not only patients, but the entire healthcare team. Practicing to the full scope of the RN license may include, but is not limited to, conducting independent RN visits using standing orders for acute or chronic conditions, medication management, leading complex care management teams for patients with multiple diagnoses, and coordination of care between hospital, primary care setting, and home (Bauer & Bodenheimer, 2017; Flinter et al., 2017).

EXPANDED ROLES OF THE RN IN PRIMARY CARE

The changes occurring to address the needs in primary care settings ignites a call for RNs to learn and practice to the full scope of license by building on the traditional roles and responsibilities of the RN in primary care. Expanding the role of the RN addresses growing concerns and challenges facing primary care settings, including the shortage of primary care providers (e.g., physicians, nurse practitioners, and physician assistants) and the increasing need of primary care services by a growing population to manage chronic diseases (Bauer & Bodenheimer, 2017). Fortunately, RNs represent the largest healthcare occupation in the United States (United States Department of Labor, 2019). The large number of RNs working in the United States, along with the supply and demand issues facing primary care, encourages a shift in primary care practices to incorporate more RNs to play a key role in the delivery of primary care (Bauer & Bodenheimer, 2017). In practices already implementing RNs in a team-based capacity with expanded roles, three new major responsibilities emerged as part of the RN role:

1. Chronic disease management (Bauer & Bodenheimer, 2017)
2. Complex care management and care coordination (Bauer & Bodenheimer, 2017; Lamb et al., 2015)
3. Independent nurse visits (Flinter et al., 2017)

Chronic Disease Management

Managing care for patients with chronic diseases falls under the scope of the RN license. RNs leading chronic disease management efforts utilize assessment skills in primary care to identify the signs indicating early intervention needs for patients. Other duties led by RNs managing patients' chronic disease(s) include medication reconciliation (Smolowitz et al., 2015) or providing medication management services based on established orders provided by the primary care provider or facility. Medication reconciliation efforts by the RN allows for collaboration between patients, the patient's family members, and the healthcare team to ensure adherence to the medication regime and provide a safety net to avoid errors or unintended interactions between various medications or supplements (Barnsteiner, 2008; Smolowitz et al., 2015). Along with medication reconciliation, RNs have the capacity to provide medication management for patients per existing primary care provider orders. Examples of medication management for patients with chronic disease(s) may include titrating blood pressure medications or modifying a patient's diabetes medication (Bauer & Bodenheimer, 2017). When working in chronic disease management, the RN can communicate findings with primary care providers in a timely manner to determine new treatment strategies and reduce the number of hospital visits (Smolowitz et al., 2015). Even though RNs are acknowledged as effective chronic disease managers, they do not typically fill this role in the current primary care system (Bodenheimer & Bauer, 2016).

Complex Care Management and Care Coordination

Enhancing the role of RNs in primary care settings sets the stage for RNs to take on leadership responsibilities in providing complex care management and care coordination. RNs hold the potential to lead complex care management teams in primary care settings by overseeing unlicensed personnel providing care for patients (Bauer & Bodenheimer, 2017). The RN works closely with other team members as well to address the social factors that may inhibit the patient reaching established health goals. In some primary care settings, RNs practice to this capacity of leadership by fulfilling the RN care manager role. RN care managers typically serve a defined set of patients with a certain condition, comorbid factors, or when requested by the provider (Flinter et al., 2017). The RN care manager plays a critical role in coordinating assigned patients' care between primary practices and additional healthcare entities such as hospitals, therapies, and other specialty services (Lamb et al., 2015). With proper care coordination efforts by the RN and continued support provided to the patient and family members, the RN care manager can reduce the costs of care for high-need patients and prevent unnecessary hospital visits (Bauer & Bodenheimer, 2017; Smolowitz et al., 2015). Specific duties carried out by the RN care manager to lower hospital readmission and associated outcomes include providing patient and family support during the transition to home, medication management services, and creating clearly defined care plans for primary and specialty care needs of the patient (Smolowitz et al., 2015). Flinter et al. (2017) reemphasize the role of RN care managers in discharge services, adding the responsibility of the RN in conducting home visits for the patient. These home visits occur to assess and address the unmet needs of the patient and determine whether the environment is adequate to promote continued healing and care. The RN care manager is also responsible for reintegrating the patient into primary care services to continue managing illnesses or conditions post hospitalization (Flinter et al., 2017).

Independent Nurse Visits

Independent nurse visits allow RNs to provide relief for other primary care providers by working to the full scope of the RN license and assuming part of the patient load in primary care settings. According to Flinter et al. (2017), RNs can conduct independent nurse visits in a variety of ways. The first type of visit Flinter et al. (2017) established falls under the traditional roles and responsibilities of RNs in primary care, including patient education, care coordination, patient monitoring, and communicating with patient and family members to address health concerns and treatment questions. Other examples of the types of duties RNs might conduct during these visits involve new parent and/or lactation support, monitoring newborn weights, chronic illness monitoring, or diabetes education (Flinter et al., 2017).

The second way in which RNs conduct independent visits involves the RN taking on more responsibility for the patient via preestablished standing orders set forth by a licensed medical provider. Standing orders allow RNs to provide a variety of services for patients, but with access to medical providers if necessary. Examples of duties within the RNs scope of practice that can be performed with standing orders include assessment, management, and treatment of conditions with well-defined symptoms such as urinary tract infections or upper respiratory conditions, management of tuberculosis infections, testing and treatment for sexually transmitted infections, asthma education/support and testing, immunizations and vaccines, contraception counseling and support, lactation support, and routine prenatal care. Another variation of standing orders, distinguished as delegated by order sets, provides RNs with more autonomy and decision-making capabilities. Delegated by order sets allow primary care providers to create an individualized set of orders for specific patients based on the patient's response to treatment. With the delegated order sets, the RN independently conducts follow-up patient visits to reduce the frequency of unnecessary visits with the primary care providers, while also monitoring the patient on a regular basis to provide proper care (Flinter et al., 2017).

Finally, collaborative primary care providers and RN visits to conduct warfarin management are identified as a third type of independent RN visit by Flinter et al. (2017). In a collaborative warfarin management visit, the RN is responsible for taking patient history, conducts the examination, reviews systems, performs medication reconciliation, and reviews visit follow-up instructions with the patient. The primary care provider then reviews and confirms the findings by the RN, determining a final diagnosis and creates the treatment plan (Flinter et al., 2017). The process of the collaborative visit allows the RN to perform duties within the scope of the RN license, which saves the primary care provider's time and allows them to focus on diagnosis and treatment.

In addition to the responsibilities of the RN in various types of independent nurse visits identified by Flinter et al. (2017), another potential area impacted by nurse-led visits in primary care involves the opioid epidemic. Federally qualified health centers in Massachusetts utilize nurse care managers to support physicians in opioid use disorder treatment with Medicaid reimbursing nurse care manager services. Under this model, the nurse care manager is responsible for performing the screening, intake, and education of patients on opioid use disorders. The nurse care manager then assists in scheduling the patient with a physician to confirm the opioid use disorder diagnosis, and the physician comanages the patient's opioid use disorder treatment with the nurse care manager (Korthuis et al., 2017).

Benefits of RNs Practicing to the Full Scope of License in Primary Care

RNs in primary care settings practicing to the full scope of the RN license allows for many benefits for patients and health systems. As previously mentioned, the use of RNs in primary care addresses the issue of provider shortages and growing patient populations with chronic illnesses seeking care (Bauer & Bodenheimer, 2017). RNs acting autonomously and in leadership roles assist in the smooth operations of the primary care facility by providing continuity of care when primary care providers are unavailable, and participate in quality improvement initiatives (Smolowitz et al., 2015). Regarding patient care, the literature suggests care managed by nurses enhances patient and provider satisfaction and lowers hospital admission rates (Martinez-Gonzalez et al., 2014; Smolowitz et al., 2015).

RNs working as care managers assist patients in transitions between medical entities, preventing avoidable ED visits and hospitalizations by monitoring patients closer in the primary care setting and intervening in a timely manner. Telephone triage services led by RNs in primary care settings also prevents unnecessary ED visits and readmissions by providing patients with proper referrals based on symptoms and needs discussed. Enhanced primary care ultimately decreases ED visits, saving the patient and healthcare systems money (Smolowitz et al., 2015).

Along with lower readmission rates, RNs practicing in primary care settings provide other financial benefits for the facility and patients. Smolowitz et al. (2015) found although RNs require higher pay than LPNs and medical assistants, with the RN practicing to the full scope of license and becoming more autonomous, facilities see increased patient volumes and revenue. RNs free up primary care providers' time and efforts by taking on more responsibilities that fall under the RN scope of practice. Since RNs alleviate primary care providers' patient load, facilities can host more same-day appointments for patients with either the primary care providers or RNs leading independent nurse visits. In combination with increasing the number of patients seen, RNs conducting independent visits or practicing to the full scope of license provides more opportunities for patient education and prevent adverse medical events. Due to the many roles and responsibilities of the RN practicing to the full scope of license, the RN in primary care generates income for facilities and saves health systems and patients money by preventing unnecessary or additional medical care. Overall, the revenue generated by the RN practicing to the full scope of license in primary care and high patient and provider satisfaction offsets the higher pay of RNs (Smolowitz et al., 2015).

Challenges

To fully utilize RNs practicing to the full scope of their license, there are several challenges that must be overcome. These challenges exist both in the education of nurses and the practice of nurses in primary care.

CHALLENGES IN NURSING EDUCATION ABOUT PRIMARY CARE

The role of the RN in primary care also requires skills not taught in most nursing education programs. Wojnar et al. (2017) reported faculty buy-in, limited clinical sites, shortage of RN role models, students' expectations for acute care clinical placement, a belief that undergraduate programs prepare students to work in acute care, and lack of focus on primary care content on NCLEX as challenges to implementing primary care content into nursing curriculums. As previously identified by Bodenheimer and Mason (2017), many nursing education programs utilize acute care settings. The lack of focus on providing education on primary care knowledge, skills, and rural primary care clinical experience often leaves the RN unprepared to work in the primary care setting (Flinter et al., 2017; McCoy, 2009).

CHALLENGES FOR RNs IN PRIMARY CARE PRACTICE

In the primary care setting, RNs may be underutilized due to several issues including, but not limited to, difficulties in recruitment, salary challenges, reimbursement regulations, and practice changes. Each of these challenges will be discussed in further detail.

Difficulties in Recruitment

Barriers to recruitment of nurses in primary care may include limited professional development opportunities, lack of access to higher education, mentors/role models, resources, and salary differences. Access to continuing education for rural primary care RNs may be restricted due to travel time and distance, cost, work schedule, and time away from family and work (Hunsberger et al., 2009; McCoy, 2009; Mester, 2018; Rohatinsky & Jahner, 2016). In addition, rural facilities may lack resources to create education opportunities or offer financial incentives (Calleja et al. 2019). In a study by Cosgrave et al. (2018), turnover was influenced by job role, workplace relationships, and level of access to continuing professional development. These findings were also identified in an integrated literature review of nurses' experiences working in rural hospitals (Smith et al., 2019).

Salary Challenges

Salary is perceived to be a challenge for recruitment and retention for rural nurses in primary care. Probst et al. (2019) reported RNs across all rural practice settings, regardless of nursing education level, were making approximately $4,500 per year less than their urban counterparts. Rural physician office nurses, regardless of educational preparation, averaged a salary of $43,961 versus rural hospital nurse's average salary of $54,472. Rural associate degree–prepared nurses in a physician's office had the lowest average salary per year compared to their urban counterparts ($37,273 vs. $40,752). However, the average salary for rural bachelor-prepared nurses in physician offices is slightly higher than their urban counterpart ($53,460 vs. $53,184; $p = .9418$). Rural bachelor-prepared nurses working in the hospital setting had an average salary of $58,659 versus RNs working in rural physician offices who averaged $53,460 in salary. Determining salary differences for nurses working in primary care is difficult due to the lack of data. For example, the National Council of State Boards of Nursing (NCSBN; 2017) Nursing Workforce Survey does not identify a primary care or provider office as a practice setting. Ambulatory care is identified as a practice setting; however, no definition is provided. Furthermore, there is a lack of data illustrating the salary differences between RNs in the primary care setting and the other practice settings; however, anecdotal conversations with leadership in primary care settings suggest salary is a barrier, making it difficult to hire RNs in primary care positions.

Reimbursement Regulations

A major challenge to utilizing RNs more in the primary care setting is related to current reimbursement processes. Many primary care practices are reimbursed using a fee-for-service model. This model undervalues other members of the healthcare team, rarely providing compensation for services provided by anyone other than the primary care provider (Bauer & Bodenheimer, 2017). Oftentimes, this results in administrators who view RN work as an expense rather than a source of revenue for the primary care facility. Bodenheimer and Mason (2017) indicated some public and private insurers are beginning to pay for services performed by RNs. Additionally, Medicare has introduced fee-for-service payments for RNs conducting wellness visits and chronic care management services (Bodenheimer & Bauer, 2016). A nationwide reform is needed to universally provide reimbursement for services provided by RNs and other members of the healthcare team.

Practice Changes

As the RN role changes in primary care, the roles of other healthcare teams must change as well. Practice changes that occur must include buy-in from all members of the healthcare team to achieve high-functioning teams that provide high-quality patient care. Primary care providers must be supportive of giving RNs more responsibilities related to patient care and allowing all team members to practice to the full scope of their respective licenses. If RNs are conducting independent nurse visits, standing orders or protocols must be developed. Policies and procedures may need to be developed or revised and education may need to be provided for the entire primary care team. Physical space may also need to be evaluated and revamped to allow for optimal function (American Academy of Ambulatory Care Nursing, 2017).

IMPLICATIONS FOR NURSING PRACTICE, RESEARCH, AND EDUCATION

Leaders in healthcare facilities and nursing education share the responsibility for changing the RN role in the primary care setting. In the primary care setting, leaders should advocate to use RNs to the full scope of their license. Restructuring the roles of the interprofessional team to allow all team members to practice to their full abilities also falls under the responsibilities and actions of primary care administrators. In the educational setting, leaders should provide theory content about the enhanced role of the RN in primary care and primary care clinical experiences for students. Additionally, research could be conducted regarding the knowledge, skills, and abilities of RNs related to primary care nursing.

Recommendations from the Josiah Macy Foundation

The Josiah Macy Foundation (Bodenheimer & Mason, 2017) proposed six recommendations for nursing practice and education. The first recommendation is focused on changing the culture of healthcare. Primary care facilities should recognize and provide opportunities for the enhanced role of the RN in clinical practice. This requires changes among the entire interprofessional healthcare team and a shift in typical roles. Additionally, leaders in nursing schools should emphasize education in primary care.

The second recommendation is focused on transforming the practice environment. RNs are often underutilized in primary care, sometimes due to facility preference and sometimes due to state and federal regulations. Advocating for payment models that support RNs practicing to the full scope of their license is essential in broadening the RN role in primary care settings (Bodenheimer & Mason, 2017).

The third recommendation is focused on educating nursing students in primary care. In many schools of nursing, emphasis is often placed on acute care clinical settings, overlooking the role of the RN in primary care. Nursing students may graduate without knowledge about the role of RNs in primary care (Bodenheimer & Mason, 2017). By providing education related to the RN role in primary care, primary care facilities can seamlessly onboard new nurses who are equipped with the skills to practice in these roles.

The fourth recommendation is focused on supporting the career development of RNs in the primary care setting. Although lifelong learning is important in all practice settings, it is imperative in the primary care settings. Since many nurses may not have received formal education about the role of the RN in primary care, they may be hesitant to fill these roles and feel underprepared (Bodenheimer & Mason, 2017). An example of this situation in the primary care setting involves the RN practicing as a generalist, providing care to patients across the life span with diverse healthcare needs. The generalist role is essential in rural nursing practice where the nature, scope, and dimensions of rural nursing practice present specific and unique challenges (Scharff, 2018; also see Chapter 8). However, primary care facilities may need to provide additional education for RNs who are interested in stepping into a primary care position yet may need career development to do so.

The fifth recommendation is focused on developing faculty members who are experts in primary care. Since many nurses may not have received formal education about the role of the RN in primary care, nursing faculty may be lacking in knowledge as well. For faculty who practiced or currently practice in primary care, the role of the RN in primary care may vary widely in practice so experiences among faculty may differ greatly (Bodenheimer & Mason, 2017).

The sixth recommendation is focused on increasing interprofessional education opportunities (Bodenheimer & Mason, 2017). With the emphasis on high-functioning teams in the primary care setting, nursing students must witness and experience interprofessional education opportunities to prepare them for their role in the primary care team.

An Educational Approach

To expand knowledge and education about the RN role in primary care, faculty members at South Dakota State University implemented the Impacting Models of Practice and Clinical Training for Registered Nurses and Students (IMPACT-RNS) program. (This project was supported by HRSA of the U.S. Department of Health and Human Services under grant number UK1HP31729 and titled Nurse, Education, Practice, Quality and Retention—Registered Nurses in Primary Care.) The main objectives of IMPACT-RNS led the project team in development and implementation of providing new educational opportunities for undergraduate nursing students and practicing RNs, while also promoting partnerships between academia and primary care facilities.

Undergraduate nursing students were provided the opportunity to participate in a new clinical experience through the IMPACT-RNS program by completing 150 hours of clinical in a rural primary care setting. Since students do not currently receive this type of clinical experience, the IMPACT-RNS project allowed select students interested in pursuing a career in primary care the opportunity to learn the importance and roles of RNs in primary care. The remaining students who did not participate in the clinical experience received didactic training through new curriculum educating students on RNs in primary care. Practicing RNs were also educated on the ways in which RNs can practice to the full scope of license through continuing education modules developed by the project team. Through partnerships developed between academia and primary care facilities, the project team was able to create new placements for students to complete the IMPACT-RNS clinical experience. The partnerships also provided the opportunity for the project team to work with facility administrators and RNs to create and work toward goals to enhance RNs practicing in these primary care facilities. Overall, students were exposed to a variety of roles held by RNs in primary care and gained an awareness of the importance of the RN on the primary care team. Additionally, the new partnerships that were formed between academia and primary care facilities aided in the betterment of primary care education for nursing students.

CONCLUSION

With the changes in primary care, including the shortage of primary care providers and the increase in patients with complex chronic conditions, advocating for the use of RNs in primary care is essential. RNs who are practicing to the full scope of their license can assist in meeting patient and facility needs as well as improve patient outcomes. Nurses and leaders in both the academic and practice settings must contribute to the education and utilization of RNs in primary care.

ACKNOWLEDGMENT

The authors would like to acknowledge the other members of the IMPACT-RNS project team: Alham Abuatiq, Leann Horsley, Cassy Hultman, Valborg Kvigne, Christina Plemmons, and Marie Schmit.

REFERENCES

American Academy of Ambulatory Care Nursing. (2017). *American Academy of Ambulatory Care Nursing position paper: The role of the registered nurse in ambulatory care.* https://www.aaacn.org/sites/default/files/documents/RNRolePositionPaper.pdf

Association of American Medical Colleges. (2019, April 23). *New findings confirm predictions on physician shortage.* https://news.aamc.org/press-releases/article/workforce_report_shortage_04112018/

Auerbah, D., Staiger, D., Muench, U., & Buerhas, P. (2013). The nursing workforce in an era of health care reform. *New England Journal of Medicine, 268,* 1470–1472. https://doi.org/10.1056/NEJMp1301694

Barnsteiner, J. (2008). Medication reconciliation. In R. G. Hughes (Ed.), *Patient safety and quality: An evidence-based handbook for nurses* (pp. 459–472). Agency for Healthcare Research and Quality. https://www.ncbi.nlm.nih.gov/books/NBK2648/

Bauer, L., & Bodenheimer, T. (2017). Expanded roles of registered nurses in primary care delivery of the future. *Nursing Outlook, 65,* 624–632. https://doi.org/10.1016/j.outlook.2017.03.011

Bodenheimer, T., & Bauer, L. (2016). Rethinking the primary care workforce–An expanded role for nurses. *The New England Journal of Medicine, 375,* 1015–1017. https://doi.org/10.1056/NEJMp1606869

Bodenheimer, T., & Mason, D. J. (2017). *Registered nurses: Partners in transforming primary care.* Josiah Macy Jr. Foundation. https://macyfoundation.org/assets/reports/publications/macy_monograph_nurses_2016_webpdf.pdf

Calleja, P., Adonteng-Kissi, B., & Romero, B. (2019). Transition support for new graduate nurses to rural and remote practice: A scoping review. *Nursing Education Today, 76,* 8–20. https://doi.org/10.1016/j.nedt.2019.01.022

Cosgrave, C., Maple, M., & Hussain, R. (2018). An explanation of turnover intention among early-career nursing and allied health professionals working in rural and remote Australia-Findings from a ground theory study. *Rural and Remote Health, 18*(3), 4511. https://doi.org/10.22605/RRH4511

Flinter, M., Hsu, C., Cromp, D., Ladden, M., & Wagner, E. (2017). Emerging new roles and contributions to team-based care in high-performing practices. *Journal of Ambulatory Care Manager, 40*(4), 287–296. https://doi.org/10.1097/JAC.0000000000000193

Health Resources and Services Administration. (2013, April). *The U.S. nursing workforce: Trends in supply and education.* https://www.ruralhealthinfo.org/assets/1206-4974/nursing-workforce-nchwa-report-april-2013.pdf

Hunsberger, M., Baumann, A., Blythe, J., & Crea, M. (2009). Sustaining the rural workforce: Nursing perspectives on worklife challenges. *The Journal of Rural Health, 25*(1), 17–25. https://doi.org/10.1111/j.1748-0361.2009.00194.x

Institute of Medicine. (2011). *The future of nursing: Leading change, advancing health.* https://www.ncbi.nlm.nih.gov/pubmed/24983041

Keeling, A. (2015). Historical perspectives and activities on an expanded role for nursing. *The Online Journal of Issues in Nursing, 20*(2), 2. https://doi.org/10.3912/OJIN.Vol20No02Man02

Korthuis, T., McCarty, D., Weimer, M., Bougatsos, C., Blazina, I., Zakher, B., Grusing, S., Devine, B., Chou, R. (2017). Primary care-based models for the treatment of opioid use disorder: A scoping review. *Annals of Internal Medicine, 166*(4), 268–278. https://doi.org/10.7326/M16-2149

Lamb, G., Newhouse, R., Beverly, C., Toney, D., Cropley, S., Weaver, C., Kurtzman, E., Zazworsky, D., Rantz, M., Zierler, B., Naylor, M., Reinhard, S., Sullivan, C., Czubaruk, K., Weston, M., Dailey, M., & Peterson, C. (2015). Policy agenda for nurse-led care coordination. *Nurse Outlook, 63*(2015), 521–530. http://dx.doi.org/10.1016/j.outlook.2015.06.003

Martinez-Gonzalez, N., Djalali, S., Tandjung, R., Huber-Geismann, F., Markun, S., Wensing, M., & Rosemann, T. (2014). Substitution of physicians by nurses in primary care: A systematic review and meta-analysis. *BMC Health Services Research*, *14*, 214. https://doi.org/10.1186/1472-6963-14-214

McCoy, C. (2009). Professional development in rural nursing: Challenges and opportunities. *The Journal of Continuing Education in Nursing*, *40*(3), 128–131. https://doi.org/10.3928/00220124-20090301-08

Mester, J. (2018). Rural nurse recruitment. *Nursing Management*, *49*, 51–53. https://doi.org/10.1097/01.NUMA.0000544468.98484.b7

National Council of State Boards of Nursing. (2017). *National nursing workforce study*. https://www.ncsbn.org/workforce.htm

Probst, J., McKinney, H., & Odahowski, C. (2019). *Rural registered nurses: Education preparation, workplace, and salary*. Rural & Minority Health Research Center. https://www.sc.edu/study/colleges_schools/public_health/research/research_centers/sc_rural_health_research_center/documents/ruralregisterednurses.pdf

Rohatinsky, N., & Jahner, S. (2016). Supporting nurses' transition to rural healthcare environments through mentorship. *Rural and Remote Health*, *16*, 3637. https://doi.org/10.22605/RRH3637

Scharff, J. (2018). The distinctive nature and scope of rural nursing practice: Philosophical bases. In C. A. Winters & H. J. Lee (Eds.), *Rural nursing concepts, theory, and practice* (5th ed., pp. 107–124). Springer Publishing Company.

Sinsky, C. A., Willard-Grace, R., Schutzbank, A. M., Sinsky, T. A., Margolius, D., & Bodenheimer, T. (2013). In search of join in practice: A report of 23 high-functioning primary care practices. *Annals of Family Medicine*, *11*(3), 272–278. https://doi.org/10.1370/afm.1531

Smith, S., Sim, J., & Halcomb, E. (2019). Nurses' experiences of working in rural hospitals: An integrative review. *Journal of Nursing Management*, *27*, 482–490. https://doi.org/10.1111/jonm.12716

Smolowitz, J., Speakman, E., Wojnar, D., Whelan, E., Ulrich, S., Hayes, C., & Wood, L. (2015). Role of the registered nurse in primary healthcare: Meeting healthcare needs in the 21st century. *Nursing Outlook*, *63*, 130–136. https://doi.org/10.1097/JAC.0000000000000193

United States Department of Labor. (2019, May). *Occupational employment statistics: Registered nurses*. U.S. Bureau of Labor Statistics. https://www.bls.gov/oes/current/oes291141.htm#(1)

Wojnar, D., & Whelan, E. (2017). Preparing nursing students for enhanced roles in primary care: The current state of prelicensure and RN-to-BSN education. *Nursing Outlook*, *65*, 222–2323. https://dx.doi.org/10.1016/j.outlook.2016.10.006

Healthcare Delivery in Rural and Frontier Settings

The focus of Section 3 is the delivery of healthcare in rural and frontier settings. Eight chapters are included in this section. New to this edition are chapters on emergency medical services in frontier settings (Chapter 16) and rural youth suicide (Chapter 19). Six chapters that appeared in the previous edition of the text were updated for the sixth edition. The updated chapters address a model explicating the timeline and decision-making used by rural persons to respond to illness (Chapter 13), acceptability as one component of choosing a rural healthcare provider (Chapter 14), telehealth care delivery (Chapter 15), palliative care of rural residents (Chapter 17) and veterans (Chapter 18), and health literacy (Chapter 20).

CHAPTER 13

Beyond the Symptom–Action–Timeline Process: Explicating the Health–Needs–Action Process

ANDREA D. SKROCKI, CHARLENE A. WINTERS,
AND CHAD O'LYNN

DISCUSSION TOPICS

- Select a rural subpopulation for these exercises.
    - Explore perceptions and responses to health needs.
    - Analyze the findings and discuss the fit with the Symptom–Action–Timeline (SATL), Symptom Action Process (SAP), and Health–Needs–Action Process (HNAP) models.
- Identify the responses to health needs in rural men and younger individuals to support the revised HNAP model in these populations.

INTRODUCTION

There is an important study in the first (1998) and subsequent editions of this book (2006, 2010, 2013) by Buehler et al. who proposed an initial model detailing how rural dwellers recognize health symptoms and the processes rural dwellers go through in relieving those symptoms. As Buehler et al. noted, the significance of such a model is the provision of a framework from which healthcare providers can better assess an individual's interpretation and response to symptoms and then work with them to more accurately interpret symptoms and choose responses that optimize health outcomes. The model also offers healthcare providers a framework to better assess all resources available to individuals (such as self-care or lay resources) that might be tapped to resolve health problems and provide emotional support during illness. The authors recommended additional research to validate the use of their *Symptom–Action–Timeline* (SATL) process model for rural dwellers.

O'Lynn (2006, 2010) examined the SATL process and made several recommendations that would allow the model to be used in other studies. O'Lynn's literature review supported the SATL process; however, he proposed a revised model titled the *Symptom Action Process* (SAP). The SAP model was intended to be more inclusive of the various rural subgroups and their health behaviors and holistic health needs. In addition, O'Lynn theorized that findings from studies using the new SAP model would provide health professionals and policy makers a better understanding of how health needs are manifested and interpreted in rural settings.

In this chapter, we report the findings of a literature review designed to examine the level of support for the SATL process (Buehler et al., 1998, 2006, 2010, 2013) and O'Lynn's (2006, 2010) SAP model. We specifically address the recommendations proposed by O'Lynn to (a) expand the definition of symptom to include psychological symptoms; (b) expand the definition of symptom to be more reflective of a health need so that self-care measures to prevent illness or promote health are included; (c) recognize that intentional disregard of a health need is a type of self-care action, especially when mental health needs are involved; (d) embed the model within an environmental context external to the decision tree to account for demographic variables, access to resources, and so on; and (e) design the model to be more circular in nature, allowing for sequential or concurrent health-related actions.

Based on the findings from our review of the literature, we recommend the SAP model be expanded and renamed the *Health–Needs–Action Process* (HNAP) model to incorporate all holistic aspects of the above. We further propose additional studies be conducted with rural populations, both domestically and internationally, to explore support for the revised model.

REVIEW OF THE SATL PROCESS AND THE SAP MODEL

The SATL Process

We present a brief review and graphic depiction of the SATL in this section; however, we refer the reader to previous editions of this text (Buehler et al., 1998, 2006, 2010, 2013) for more details about the SATL process. The SATL process and SAP model (O'Lynn, 2006, 2010) will be compared in a graphic description later in the chapter.

The SATL process encompasses four phases: (a) symptom identification, (b) self-care, (c) lay resources, and (d) professional resources (Figure 13.1). The process is preceded by the occurrence of a symptom, defined as an alteration in the usual state of health that requires action. Unless that symptom is recognized by an individual (symptom identification), the SATL process does not continue. It is important to note that *symptom* was defined as a negative entity (Buehler et al., 1998, 2006, 2010, 2013) and the SATL process as one of resolving a problem.

Symptoms are characterized by three general components: (a) physical signs and sensations, (b) degree of interference with the person's usual or desired level of functioning, and (c) intensity and duration of the symptom (Buehler et al., 1998, 2006, 2010, 2013). These three characteristics, coupled with an individual's prior experience of and knowledge of the symptom, are used in assigning meaning to the symptom. Based on this meaning, an individual will decide whether to act. According to Buehler et al., self-care is the first action taken after identifying a symptom.

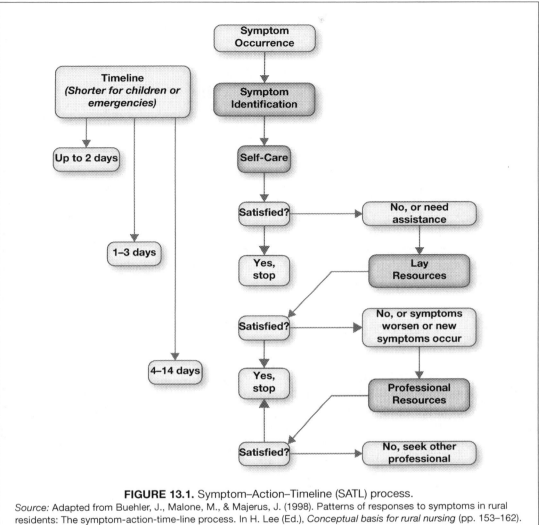

FIGURE 13.1. Symptom–Action–Timeline (SATL) process.
Source: Adapted from Buehler, J., Malone, M., & Majerus, J. (1998). Patterns of responses to symptoms in rural residents: The symptom-action-time-line process. In H. Lee (Ed.), *Conceptual basis for rural nursing* (pp. 153–162). Springer Publishing Company.

Self-care refers to the myriad activities initiated by and performed by an individual to relieve a symptom (Buehler et al., 1998, 2006, 2010, 2013). For individuals relying upon others for their health needs (e.g., dependent children and elders), family members or other caretakers would be responsible for initiating activities to address an identified symptom. Self-care activities include applying home remedies, taking over-the-counter medications and herbal preparations, using the Internet, and reading reference books to learn more about the symptom and symptom resolution. Self-care activities, as well as all other actions taken in the SATL process, are evaluated by the individual in terms of efficacy, and a decision is made whether to proceed through the SATL process, alter actions, or cease activities.

If self-care activities do not resolve a symptom to the individual's satisfaction, family, friends, and neighbors are consulted. These lay resources are used to provide (a) validation of symptom interpretation, (b) advice and emotional support, and (c) physical care

(Buehler et al., 1998, 2006, 2010, 2013). Although not defined by Buehler et al., unlike professional resources, lay resources are not financially reimbursed for their services. If symptoms do not resolve, if symptoms intensify, or if additional symptoms occur, professional resources are then sought. If professional resources do not lead to symptom resolution, individuals may seek other professional resources.

The time one takes to navigate the SATL process (Buehler et al., 1998, 2006, 2010, 2013) is influenced by the intensity and duration of a symptom and the degree to which the symptom interferes with usual functioning. Actions are implemented more quickly when a symptom is particularly intense, greatly interferes with usual functioning, or children are involved. If the symptom is interpreted as an emergency, the individual may seek professional care immediately and bypass the early phases of the SATL process. However, if the SATL process is completed in its entirety, the time from symptom identification to self-care can take up to 2 days; from symptom identification to lay resources can take from 1 to 3 days, and from symptom identification to professional resources can take from 4 to 14 days. How individuals progress through the SATL process has great implications for healthcare providers and researchers. It is important to note that a major limitation to the SATL process is the lack of reference to health prevention and health promotion activities utilized by rural dwellers. This contrasts with both the SAP model proposed by O'Lynn (2006, 2010) and the HNAP model proposed by the authors of the present chapter, which accounts for health promotion and illness prevention and incorporates a holistic multitherapeutic approach.

SAP Model

In general, the SAP model supports the SATL process as described by Buehler et al. (1998, 2006, 2010, 2013), but with a few revisions. The authors described a symptom as a physical sign or sensation. SATL is focused on problem-solving and does not address activities to prevent illness and promote health. O'Lynn (2006, 2010) noted that the SATL definition of symptom was quite narrow and proposed that the concept of *symptom* be replaced with *health need*. A health need can be a biophysical need, as well as a spiritual, emotional, social, and psychological need. A health need is more holistic than a symptom and would provide a broader perspective of rural dwellers' response to perceived health and wellness needs (O'Lynn, 2006, 2010). The inclusion of psychological symptoms, such as those typically seen in depressive and anxiety disorders, is vital because mental health services are often unavailable or poorly implemented in rural communities (Rural Health Information Hub, 2018; Wilson et al., 2015).

Unlike the linear SATL process, the SAP model includes a circular process that allows for multiple actions—self-care, lay resources, and professional resources—to be incorporated in a sequential *or* concurrent fashion (Figure 13.2). This approach is different from the more linear SATL process, which details the process of resolving a single symptom or health problem, for example, fever or broken bone. The SAP can be used by individuals for multiple symptoms, an important consideration when responding to chronic illnesses. Chronic conditions, such as diabetes or congestive heart failure, are characterized by the recurrence of multiple symptoms with varying degrees of intensity and duration. Using the more circular SAP model, one can readily explain how an individual might use prayer, hot packs, support from friends, prescription drugs, and physical therapy concurrently to manage an illness or injury, and might vary use of these strategies over time as health needs wax and wane.

The SAP model also recognizes the act of ignoring a health need or symptom as a type of self-care action. This is often seen with rural men (Evans et al., 2011) and depressed

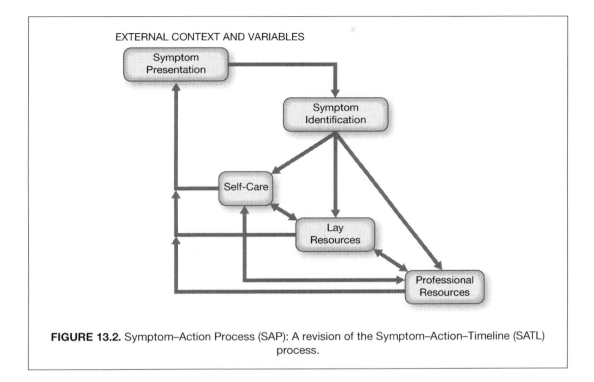

FIGURE 13.2. Symptom–Action Process (SAP): A revision of the Symptom–Action–Timeline (SATL) process.

persons seeking treatment for somatic health needs (such as fatigue, pain, or changes in appetite) while ignoring the depressive symptomatology (lack of interest in usual habits, sadness, etc.) that accompanies the somatic issues. Moreover, some cultural beliefs are rooted in traditions that perceive psychological health needs as conditions resulting from spiritual or magical causes or see the needs as a weakness (Garcia et al., 2011), highlighting the need to consider the context external to the decision-making process to understand rural persons' approach to health needs. In addition to culture and tradition, gender, race, ethnicity, educational achievement, socioeconomic status, family and social role, residential location, and barriers to resources, among others, provide the environment in which decisions are made.

Based on our initial and updated review of the literature, we propose renaming the SAP model as the HNAP model. By replacing the term *symptom* with *health need* we believe that the model more accurately reflects a broader spectrum of rural health demands, including psychological and physiological acute and chronic conditions.

METHOD USED FOR THE INITIAL LITERATURE REVIEW

Much of the literature pertaining to rural healthcare focuses on (a) disparities in health for rural dwellers as compared with nonrural dwellers, (b) description of the health of rural dwellers, (c) use of complementary alternative medicine (CAM) and treatments, (d) barriers to accessing healthcare services for rural dwellers, and (e) the experiences and demographics of healthcare providers in rural areas. None of these broad areas of literature directly addresses the SATL process or SAP model in identifying health needs and actions to resolve them, except for access barriers. Buehler et al. (1998, 2006,

2010, 2013) touched on access barriers in that additional effort is made to overcome the barriers if children were involved or symptoms were deemed emergent. Access barriers modulate the SATL process rather than serving as foundational antecedents in determining the components of the process itself. O'Lynn (2006, 2010) did not include access barriers in his literature review and as a result, barriers to care were not included in this review.

In March 2012, we conducted a search of peer-reviewed resources contained in the Cumulative Index to Nursing and Allied Health Literature (CINAHL), MedLine, Psych Info, PubMed, and Google Scholar, to locate research-based support for the SATL process and SAP model. Resources published from July 2004 through March 2012 were searched using the keyword *rural* and its associated keywords *rural health, rural environment, rural community, frontier,* and *rural populations.* Rural keywords were the primary sorting category to ensure that rural dwellers would be salient in the literature, although use of the SATL process and SAP model may be appropriate in nonrural populations as well. We then combined the rural keywords with other keywords, based on available keyword search options within each database that were suggestive of the SATL process and SAP model, including *self-care, health needs, health behaviors, illness behavior, attitudes and beliefs for self-care, decision-making, self-assessment, alternative therapies, complimentary medicine,* and *home remedies.* We excluded dissertation abstracts because of the difficulty of obtaining full texts of multiple dissertations. The search yielded a total of 583 journal articles.

From the 583 articles, we excluded review articles, case studies, and anecdotal reports, resulting in a new pool of 87 research-based journal articles. We then excluded all articles reporting studies occurring outside the United States, congruent with O'Lynn's (2006, 2010) review. This latter exclusion was reasonable because the study by Buehler et al. (1998, 2006, 2010, 2013) occurred in the United States. These steps resulted in 71 articles available for review.

Following a critical review of the 71 articles, we excluded studies that did not address components relevant to the SATL process or the SAP model and studies that focused only on healthcare providers. The final sample of articles for review included 21 research reports.

FINDINGS FROM THE INITIAL LITERATURE REVIEW 2004 TO 2012

The 21 studies included in this review were published between July 2004 and March 2012. Participants in these studies represented Arizona, Indiana, Louisiana, Michigan, Montana, New Mexico, North Carolina, North and South Dakota, Pennsylvania, Tennessee, Texas, West Virginia, and Wyoming. All studies included rural dwellers, although five studies (24%) included urban participants as a comparison group. The mean age of the rural dwellers in this literature review was 63.12 years. The Buehler et al. (1998, 2006, 2010, 2013) study did not include age ranges; therefore, this study was not included in the current review's mean age calculation. Table 13.1 shows the gender and racial or ethnic characteristics of the participants. Notably absent in the studies were participants identifying as Pacific Islander; few identified as Asian. Otherwise, non-Hispanic Caucasian, African American, Native American, and Hispanic participants were well represented.

Buehler et al. (1998, 2006, 2010, 2013) and O'Lynn (2006, 2010) noted a paucity in the literature of resources that describe the *process* rural individuals undertake in managing symptoms/health needs once they have been identified. We confirmed this paucity in the 2012 literature review. Of the 21 studies reviewed, 13 (62%) supported the tendency for adults to use self-care and lay resources before going to a health professional for nonemergent symptoms (Albert et al., 2008; Arcury et al., 2006, 2009; Buehler et al., 1998,

TABLE 13.1 Participants' Demographic Characteristics From the 2004 to 2012 Literature Review (*N* = 21 Studies)

Characteristic	*N*	%
Gender		
All female	6	29
Mixed	15	71
All male	0	0
Mean age	63.12 y (*N* = 20)	NA
Race Ethnicity		
All non-Hispanic White	3	14
Mixed	13	62
All minority	2	10
Unknown	3	14
Study location		
U.S. states represented	14	28

2006, 2010, 2013; Clark et al., 2008; Duran et al., 2005; Garcia et al., 2011; Harju et al., 2006; Ruggiero et al., 2011; Shreffler-Grant et al., 2005; Stoller et al., 2011; Vallerand et al., 2005; Zhang et al., 2009). However, none of these studies described or tested a comprehensive process of health needs identification and actions.

The majority of the studies we reviewed confirmed the *use of self-care strategies* to treat symptoms (Albert et al., 2008; Arcury et al., 2006, 2009; Brown & May, 2005; Buehler et al., 1998, 2006, 2010, 2013; Callaghan, 2005; Clark et al., 2008; Duran et al., 2005; Easom & Quinn, 2006; Garcia et al., 2011; Harju et al., 2006; Ruggiero et al., 2011; Shreffler-Grant et al., 2005; Stoller et al., 2011; Vallerand et al., 2005; Winters et al., 2006, 2010; Zhang et al., 2009). Many of these studies supported the self-care strategies described by Buehler, et al. (1998, 2006, 2010, 2013) and O'Lynn (2006, 2010), including taking over-the-counter medications, herbal remedies, CAM, and family remedies; referring to health information sources via the Internet, books, and television; and using physical treatments (e.g., heating pads, stretching, massage, or yoga). Several authors reported the value of prayer and spirituality as self-care strategies (Arcury et al., 2011; Duran et al., 2005; Easom & Quinn, 2006; Harju et al., 2006; Winters et al., 2010). Buehler et al. (1998, 2006, 2010, 2013) did not discuss these strategies. In some of the studies that compared rural and nonrural dwellers, researchers noted that rural dwellers were more likely than nonrural dwellers to use self-care strategies to treat symptoms (Garcia et al., 2011; Harju et al., 2006; Ruggiero et al., 2011; Winters et al., 2010).

We also found support for the *use of lay resources* in managing symptoms in the studies reviewed. Primarily, researchers reported the strategies of soliciting the assistance and support of friends and family in managing symptoms and in using formal support groups (Albert et al., 2008; Arcury et al., 2006, 2009, 2011; Buehler et al., 1998, 2006, 2010, 2013; Clark et al., 2008; Duran et al., 2005; Easom & Quinn, 2006; Garcia et al., 2011; Goins et al., 2010; Ruggiero et al., 2011; Shreffler-Grant et al., 2005; Stoller et al., 2011; Vallerand et al., 2005; Winters et al., 2006, 2010; Zhang et al., 2009). In addition, in nine (43%) of the studies that we reviewed, the researchers reported the progression to lay resource use after self-care had failed, or the use of lay resources prior to the use of professional resources (Arcury et al., 2006; Brown & May, 2005;

Buehler et al., 1998, 2006, 2010, 2013; Clark et al., 2008; Easom & Quinn, 2006; Harju et al., 2006; Shreffler-Grant et al., 2005; Vallerand et al., 2005; Winters et al., 2006).

In terms of gender, women were well represented in the sample of studies we reviewed, including six studies in which women were studied exclusively. In O'Lynn's review (2006, 2010) only one study (Sellers et al., 1999) was found that examined men or men's health exclusively; our literature review did not return any studies that focused exclusively on men. This limitation is significant because Sellers et al. noted that although both men and women may rely on self-care and lay resources before utilizing professional resources, men may interpret symptoms very differently and may delay the use of professional resources as long as possible (Levant & Habben, 2003; Sabo & Gordon, 1995; Sellers et al., 1999). Consequently, men may incorporate very different time frames for actions.

Generally, the results of the studies support the finding from Buehler et al. (1998, 2006, 2010, 2013) and O'Lynn (2006, 2010) that professional resources are utilized after self-care or lay resources are used. Some of the studies we reviewed included the use of complementary or alternative therapies to manage symptoms (Arcury et al., 2006, 2009, 2011; Buehler et al., 1998, 2006, 2010, 2013; Duran et al., 2005; Easom & Quinn, 2006; Harju et al., 2006; Shreffler-Grant et al., 2005; Winters et al., 2010). Complementary therapies included spiritual interventions, as noted earlier, but also included the use of professional resources such as those provided by a masseuse, acupuncturist, naturopath, chiropractor, and herbalist. Other results supported the finding that professional resources are utilized if symptoms persisted (Arcury et al., 2006; Brown & May, 2005; Buehler et al., 1998, 2006, 2010, 2013; Clark et al., 2008; Easom & Quinn, 2006; Harju et al., 2006; Shreffler-Grant et al., 2005; Vallerand et al., 2005; Winters et al., 2006, 2010).

Consistent with O'Lynn's review (2006, 2010), none of the investigators of the studies we reviewed provided specific time frames for utilizing resources as described by Buehler et al. (1998, 2006, 2010, 2013). However, research results did support the timeline tenets within the SATL process, particularly those referring to the use of professional resources. The results found that progression to and direct utilization of professional resources was quicker if (a) symptoms involved children (Buehler et al., 1998, 2006, 2010, 2013), (b) symptoms were perceived as emergent or crisis in nature (Arcury et al., 2006; Brown & May, 2005; Buehler et al., 1998; Clark et al., 2008; Easom & Quinn, 2006; Harju et al., 2006; Shreffler-Grant et al., 2005; Vallerand et al., 2005), (c) the individual perceived a need for a prescription to treat the symptom (Buehler et al., 1998, 2006, 2010, 2013; Harju et al., 2006; Winters et al., 2010), or (d) if the symptom would result in the individual missing work (Buehler et al., 1998, 2006, 2010, 2013; Winters et al., 2006; Harju et al., 2006).

Buehler et al. (1998, 2006, 2010, 2013) reported that if professional resources were not effective in relieving symptoms, participants continued to work with the professional, sought another professional (particularly a provider of alternative therapy), or accepted the symptom's nonresolution. As noted by O'Lynn (2006, 2010), we also found in the studies we reviewed that researchers did not address this specific decision point in the same fashion. However, a number of researchers reported the concurrent use of multiple strategies, including complementary or alternative therapies (Albert et al., 2008; Arcury et al., 2006, 2009, 2011; Brown & May, 2005; Buehler et al., 1998, 2006, 2010, 2013; Duran et al., 2005; Easom & Quinn, 2006; Garcia et al., 2011; Simmons et al., 2007; Stoller et al., 2011; Vallerand et al., 2005; Winters et al., 2006, 2010). A table of characteristic variables pulled from the literature review is displayed in Table 13.2.

TABLE 13.2 Characteristic Variables Found in the 2004 to 2012 Literature Review (*N* = 21 Studies)

Characteristic Variables	*n*	%
Self-care resources utilized	18	86
Lay resources	18	86
Decision-making process	17	81
Rural population only	16	76
Multiple strategies used	15	71
Self- and lay care used before professional services	13	62
Health promotion	11	52
Barriers to care	11	52
Lay resources to professional	9	43
Cultural beliefs	8	38
Symptom–Action Process discussed	7	33
Use of CAM therapies	7	33
Self-efficacy	5	24
Rural vs. nonrural population	5	24
Prayer/Spirituality self-care	4	19
Direct use of professional services when:		
Children are involved	1	5
Prescription is needed	3	14
Possible loss of employment	3	14

CAM, complementary alternative medicine.

FINDINGS FROM THE UPDATED LITERATURE REVIEW 2013-2020

In 2020, a search was conducted for articles published between January 2013 and December 2020 using the same databases used in the initial (2004–2012) review of literature. Rural and its associated keywords (*rural health, rural environment, rural community, frontier,* and *rural populations)* were the primary sorting category. The search yielded a total of 21,484 items; the majority were located using Google Scholar. The rural keywords were then combined with keywords suggested in the SATL and SAP models (*health needs, health seeking, symptom response, self-care, health behaviors, illness behavior, health and decision-making*); again the largest return came from Google Scholar when rural was combined with keywords *health behavior* (17,200) *and illness behavior* (1,460). To avoid duplication, and to ensure a manageable number of items to review, only the results from CINAHL, PsychInfo, and PubMed were used for this review (3,188). The articles were screened for items meeting the following parameters: research studies conducted with rural adults within the United States that were published in English in scholarly journals. Review articles, case studies, anecdotal reports, and studies that did not address components relevant to the SATL process or the SAP model were excluded. A total of 19 journal articles (Table 13.3) were appraised for this review.

Of the 19 studies appraised, nearly one-half focused on mental health needs ($n = 9$; 47%) and in all but two, the study samples included more women than men. No studies specifically addressed the process or timeline of seeking healthcare, however, they did provide insight into rural persons healthcare-seeking behaviors (see Table 13.4).

TABLE 13.3 Primary Focus for Studies in the 2013 to 2020 Literature Review ($N = 19$ Studies)

Primary focus	n	%
Meaning of health	1	5
Resources utilized	7	37
Decision-making process	1	5
Self-care	1	5
Complimentary medicine	1	5
Access to care	1	5
Health behaviors	3	15
Health seeking barriers	6	32
Rural vs. nonrural population	5	26
Population		
Rural population only	14	74
Rural and urban population	5	26

TABLE 13.4 Participants' Demographic Characteristics From the 2013 to 2020 Literature Review ($N = 19$ Studies)

Characteristics reported in study	n	%
Gender1		
All female	3	16
Mixed	16	84
All male	0	0
Age range	>18 ($n = 16$)	NA
Race/Ethnicity		
All non-Hispanic White	1	5
Mixed	16	84
All minority	0	0
Unknown	2	11
Study Location[1]		
U.S. states identified (Arkansas, Colorado, Iowa, Kentucky, Main, Minnesota, Montana, N. Carolina, North Dakota, Tennessee, New York, Virginia, Wisconsin, Wyoming	14	
U.S. regions identified	3	
Entire United States	4	

[1]Several studies were conducted in more than one state or were conducted in an area identified as a region within the U.S., or in the U.S. as a whole

Where one lives and a persons' rural values seem to matter when it comes to health-care behaviors. Lack of anonymity and privacy, recommendations to seek care from trusted insiders, distrust of outsiders, and social norms of self-reliance and independence affected healthcare seeking among rural persons with mental health needs (Alang, 2015; Andren et al., 2013; Cheesmond et al., 2019; Crumb et al., 2019; Fischer et al., 2016; Groh & Saunders, 2020; Saunders & Groh, 2019; Snell-Rood et al., 2017). A large study (N = 12,439) by Kirby et al. (2019) found that rural persons with mental health needs had fewer mental health visits and prescription drug fills compared to urban county residents. Although perceived stigma was identified by some investigators as a barrier to seeking mental healthcare for adults and children (Andren et al., 2013; Heflinger et al., 2014; Polaha et al., 2015; Snell-Rood et al., 2017), a child's age and a history of prior services were associated with greater willingness to seek mental health services for children (Polaha et al., 2015); health services were sought by depressed women when symptoms were severe (Snell-Rood et al., 2017); and men and women accessed mental healthcare following informal self-care and the recommendation of a trusted primary care provider (Andren et al., 2013).

Studies found that adults with physical health needs such as chronic illness and functional limitations, engaged in self-care, received informal care, and sought formal care when needed for health problems. In a study of 198 older African American and White rural adults (Bell et al., 2013), residents believed they understood their own health better than a physician and their behaviors best determined their health; one in five believed they could overcome illness with help and nearly 30% agreed that home remedies were better than drugs for treating illness. Prevention was not a priority for rural dwelling elders (Mize & Rose, 2019) who avoided preventative healthcare unless the situation was dire nor was prevention important to farmers (Earle-Richardson et al., 2015) who would see a provider for a problem, not preventative care. Although researchers agreed that many rural elders believe families should take care of their own (Savia et al., 2019) and are reluctant to accept formal care, their reliance on informal care and willingness to accept formal care was influenced by (a) filial beliefs, (b) the availability of and attitude toward community resources, (c) the availability of persons who could provide informal care, (d) finances, and (e) the degree of care required. Savia found (n = 503 adults >65 years) when services were available, and the need great, men and women would use the formal services either alone or in combination with informal care regardless of filial beliefs. However, older women living in poor counties were more likely than men to receive no care or use self-care or informal care only. Similarly, in a study of 33 women with symptoms of myocardial infarction (Jackson & McCulloch, 2014), women would seek formal healthcare if they correctly identified their symptoms; however, they were reluctant to do so if that disrupted their family, took too long, or invaded their privacy. Providing self-care can include taking responsibility to find a suitable healthcare provider. Tzeng et al. (2018) reported that rural residents were interested in using data to find a provider, hospital, or clinic (Tzeng et al., 2018). And in a study of 1,300 rural adults about their health concerns (Findling et al., 2020), residents were willing to accept outside government help for health issues facing the community.

DISCUSSION

The initial and updated literature reviews provide overall support for aspects of the SATL process and the SAP model used by rural dwellers. Although none of the researchers contradicted the model proposed by Buehler et al. (1998, 2006, 2010, 2013) or O'Lynn (2006, 2010), no researcher discussed or tested a comprehensive process for health needs identification and action. It should be noted, however, that the number of studies we reviewed was small. Most of the studies were cross-sectional and descriptive in design, limiting the ability to confirm the use of the SATL process or SAP model over time. We recommend studies be conducted that specifically focus on the process used in symptom and health need recognition and response using the SATL or SAP model.

Like O'Lynn's review (2006, 2010), although some studies appraised during the 2020 literature review included large sample sizes, most of the research we reviewed had small sample sizes and focused primarily on rural dwellers over 50 years of age. To be consistent with O'Lynn's review, we did not include participants residing outside the United States. We recommend studies be conducted with larger samples, younger participants, and with participants from outside of the United States, to further support the proposed change from the SAP to the HNAP model. Participants in the studies we reviewed were White, non-Hispanic with smaller numbers of persons identified as African American, Hispanic, American Indian/Alaskan Native, or Other. Very few studies included persons identifying Asian heritage; no study included those identifying as Pacific Islander. Women moderately outnumbered men in the studies we reviewed. We concur with O'Lynn (2006, 2010) that additional studies be conducted with a variety of racial and ethnic populations and with men in rural communities to further strengthen the recommended changes to the SAP model.

A limitation of the SATL process model is Buehler et al.'s (1998, 2006, 2010, 2013) lack of attention to symptoms that are recognized as problematic but ignored. For example, one may recognize a self-limiting symptom such as a strained muscle but choose no action to relieve the strain. An interesting finding in our review is that stigma and embarrassment influences health pattern behaviors in rural persons with mental health needs (Alang, 2015; Andren et al., 2013; Heflinger et al., 2014; Polaha et al., 2015; Simmons et al., 2007, Snell-Rood et al., 2017). Both the SAP (O'Lynn, 2006, 2010) and the current literature reviews found self-efficacy and health behavior patterns to be similar when comparing rural and nonrural dwellers' compliance with personal health needs management and both SAP and HNAP reviews allow for prevention and management of various health needs, including psychological needs (Andren et al., 2013; Crumb et al., 2019; Fischer et al., 2016; Garcia et al., 2011; Harju et al., 2006; Simmons et al., 2007; Snell-Rood et al., 2017; Winters et al., 2010; Harju et al., 2006). Additional research is needed to explore how embarrassment, stigma, stoicism, and other factors such as lack of anonymity, familiarity, isolation from lay resources, and attitudes of others (family members, community members, or primary care provider) influence individuals' recognition, interpretation, and response to health needs.

The emphasis on the timeline aspect of the SATL process model is problematic, in that, it suggests a rather linear progression through phases of symptom identification, and actions are taken while previous strategies may be abandoned because of unsatisfactory outcomes. We concur with O'Lynn (2006, 2010) that the literature we reviewed did not support this process and that instead, multiple modes of treatment are utilized singularly or concurrently. Our present review also supports O'Lynn in that as rural dwellers become more educated and familiar with interpreting and identifying recurring health symptoms, they may bypass self-care and lay care and go directly to professional resources. This is evident in those suffering from chronic conditions (Albert et al., 2008; Buehler et al., 1998, 2006, 2010, 2013; Easom & Quinn, 2006; Jackson & McCulloch, 2014; Snell-Rood et al., 2017; Stoller et al., 2011; Winters et al., 2006, 2010). A study done by Stoller et al. described the older rural adult who was managing both new symptoms and chronic diseases as a "bricoleur"—a kind of informal professional do-it-yourself person who blends information gathered from multiple sources. Managing the process of chronic symptoms and new health needs is well identified in the proposed HNAP model.

Buehler et al. (1998, 2006, 2010, 2013) and O'Lynn (2006, 2010) noted that time frames for action were influenced by whether the symptoms were associated with children (Polaha et al., 2015) or with emergent/dire conditions (Mize & Rose, 2019; Snell-Rood et al., 2017). Our present review provides support for this process. In addition, as noted previously, others have suggested that time frames for action are also influenced by whether symptoms (a) required a prescription, (b) caused one to miss work (Buehler et al., 1998, 2006, 2010, 2013; Harju et al., 2006; Winters et al., 2006, 2010), (c) interfered with family activities or invaded privacy (Jackson & McCulloch, 2014), and (d) were viewed worthy of professional help by family and community members (Andren et al., 2013; Fischer et al., 2016). It is reasonable to assume that barriers in accessing health resources for rural dwellers, as described widely in the literature, will influence how quickly or slowly one may adopt actions to address health need symptoms. As such, time frames are descriptive outcomes resulting from the contextual variables.

Perceived barriers such as stigma, pain, lack of information/knowledge, attitudes of family and friends, and community norms were noted in the studies in the current review (Callaghan, 2005; Crumb et al., 2019; Easom & Quinn, 2006; Fischer et al., 2016; Sriram et al., 2017; Snell-Rood et al., 2017; Vallerand et al., 2005). Lack of information and knowledge (coupled with pain) has been found to be related to health promotion activities (Easom & Quinn, 2006). Adding to that is psychological well-being and the ability of rural dwellers to self-identify their health needs (Callaghan, 2005; Duran et al., 2005; Garcia et al., 2011; Ruggiero et al., 2011; Simmons et al., 2007; Winters et al., 2010). O'Lynn (2006, 2010) recognized the importance of including psychological symptoms in the model and noted that mental health services are often unavailable or poorly implemented in rural communities. The HNAP model allows for psychological symptomatology to be identified and treated alongside physical symptoms (as would be the case in pain management, depression, and/or anxiety with new onset or chronic disease management). Depression in rural women is a growing public health concern, and many of the women underreport their symptoms due to stigma and/or a lack of knowledge regarding their symptoms (Simmons et al., 2007). Oftentimes with depression, anxiety, and other psychological disorders, symptoms present with somatic symptoms as well, making them difficult to identify. Our present review validated that multiple strategies are used (as depicted in the HNAP model) to address both psychological and physical health needs in rural populations.

RECOMMENDATIONS FOR THE NEW HNAP MODEL

Figure 13.3 shows a graphic depiction of the HNAP model. The action process of the HNAP is embedded in an external context identical to the SAP model. The two models are similar in all facets of identification, decision-making processes, and actions taken by rural dwellers. The only difference between the SAP and the HNAP model is the replacement of the term *symptom* with *health needs* to include physical and psychological health conditions and states. After health needs are identified in the HNAP model, individuals may incorporate various types of actions: (a) self-care, (b) lay resources, and (c) professional resources in a sequential or concurrent fashion. The contexts will influence which action, or combination of actions, is taken. The sloping nature of the action types reflects the propensity to progress from self-care to lay resource use to professional resource use. The double arrows between action types account for fluid movement among the aspects of the model and concurrent use of types of actions. More explicit in this model are the arrows leading from the action types back to the symptom occurrence aspect of

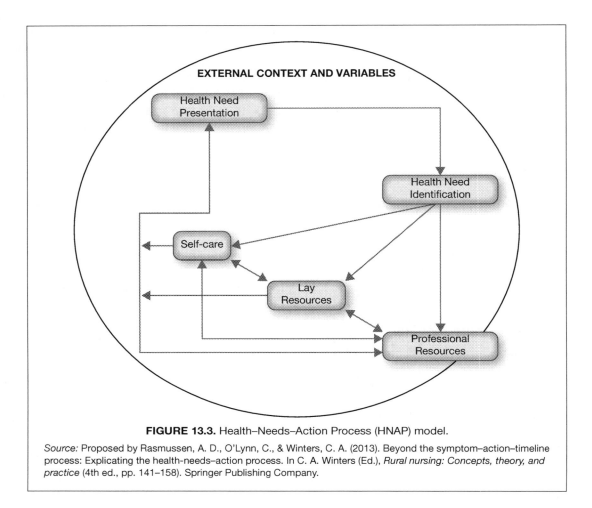

FIGURE 13.3. Health–Needs–Action Process (HNAP) model.

Source: Proposed by Rasmussen, A. D., O'Lynn, C., & Winters, C. A. (2013). Beyond the symptom–action–timeline process: Explicating the health-needs–action process. In C. A. Winters (Ed.), *Rural nursing: Concepts, theory, and practice* (4th ed., pp. 141–158). Springer Publishing Company.

the model. These arrows close the circle of the process and account for symptoms that might recur, new symptoms that develop, or new actions resulting from new information or previous actions taken by an individual.

Both the SATL process and HNAP model depict a process in which an individual identifies a problem or health need and takes action(s) to address it. As such, these models may describe the behaviors of all individuals, including nonrural dwellers, although individual and/or patterns of actions taken may differ across populations. To test and further strengthen the newly proposed HNAP model, we recommend that further research be conducted to:

1. Evaluate how well the revised HNAP model is empirically supported in diverse populations (particularly rural men, younger individuals, and minority populations) and diverse health contexts. If the revised model is well supported, then it may serve as an ideal framework for comparison studies examining health behaviors across participant demographic variables.

2. Explore evidence for international applicability of the HNAP model by updating the literature review with studies conducted outside the US.

3. Conduct studies to explore how various and multiple barriers, including structural and economic barriers, to health promotion, prevention, and treatment influence timelines, decisions, and processes within the HNAP model.

4. Conduct studies to explore how cultural, spiritual, and social practices; health beliefs, knowledge, and attitudes; and variable levels of health supports influence meaning-making and decision-making actions within the HNAP model.

CONCLUSION

Buehler et al. (1998, 2006, 2010, 2013) derived the SATL process model from a grounded theory study in which they described the process that a group of rural Montana women used to respond to health symptoms. O'Lynn (2006, 2010) completed a literature review to determine the level of support for the SATL process and proposed changes, resulting in a more circular model called SAP. In 2012 and again in 2020, literature reviews were conducted to determine the level of support for the SATL and SAP models and resulted in the HNAP model. The 2012 and 2020 reviews examined 40 research studies located in the CINAHL, MedLine, PsychInfo, PubMed, and Google Scholar databases that focused on the process rural dwellers use to respond to health needs. Those studies provide general support for the aspects of the SATL process, the SAP model, and the new HNAP model, although in only seven studies did researchers describe a sequential process of how rural dwellers respond to health symptoms (Albert et al., 2008; Arcury et al., 2009, 2011; Buehler et al., 1998, 2006, 2010, 2013; Stoller et al., 2011; Vallerand et al., 2005; Winters et al., 2010).

We recommend further research with younger participants, rural men, and racially and ethnically diverse populations to determine the support for the revised model. In addition, identifying whether cultural, physical, and/or psychological barriers inhibit rural populations (such as rural African American, American Indian/Alaskan Native, Hispanic, Pacific Islander, or those identifying as Asian heritage) from health promotion, prevention, and treatment would further support the revised SAP model, now renamed HNAP. Finally, we recommend an examination of studies completed outside the continental United States to determine whether the revised model has broad relevance to rural dwellers across the globe.

REFERENCES

Alang, S. M. (2015). Sociodemographic disparities associated with perceived causes of unmet need for mental health care. *Psychiatric Rehabilitation Journal, 38*(4), 293–299. http://dx.doi.org/10.1037/prj0000113

Albert, S. M., Musa, D., Kwoh, C. K., Hanlon, J. T., & Silverman, M. (2008). Self-care and professionally guided care in osteoarthritis—Racial differences in a population-based sample. *Journal of Aging and Health, 20*(2), 198–216. https://doi.org/10.1177/0898264307310464

Andren, K. A. K., McKibbin, C. L., Wykes, T. L., Lee, A. A., Carrico, C. P., & Bourassa, K. A. (2013). Depression treatment among rural older adults: Preferences and factors influencing future service use. *Clinical Gerontologist, 36*, 241–259. https://doi.org/10.1080/07317115.2013.767872

Arcury, T. A., Bell, R. A., Snively, B. M., Smith, S. L., Skelly, A. H., Wetmore, L. K., & Quandt, S. A. (2006). Complementary and alternative medicine use as health self-management: Rural older adults with diabetes. *Journal of Gerontology: Social Sciences, 61B*(2), S62–S70. https://doi.org/10.1093/geronb/61.2.s62

Arcury, T. A., Grzywacz, J. G., Neiberg, R. H., Lang, W., Nguyen, H. T., Altizer, K., A, Stoller, E. P., Bell, R. A., & Quandt, S. A. (2011). Daily use of complementary and other therapies for symptoms among older adults: Study design and illustrative results. *Journal of Aging and Health*, 23(1), 52–69. https://doi.org/10.1177/0898264310385115

Arcury, T. A., Grzywacz, J. G., Stoller, E. P., Bell, R. A., Altizer, K. P., Chapman, C., & Quandt, S A. (2009). Complementary therapy use and health self-management among rural older adults. *Journal of Gerontology: Social Sciences*, 64B(5), 635–643. https://doi.org/10.1093/geronb/gbp011

Bell, R. A., Grzywacz, J. G., Quandt, S. A., Neiberg, R., Lang, W., Nguyen, H., Altizer, K. P., & Arcury, T. A. (2013). Medical skepticism and complementary therapy use among older rural African Americans and Whites. *Journal of Health Care for the Poor and Underserved*, 24(2), 777–787. https://doi.org/10.1353/hpu.2013.0052

Brown, J. W., & May, B. A. (2005). Rural older Appalachian women's formal patterns of care. *Southern Online Journal of Nursing Research*, 2(6), 1–21. https://www.snrs.org/sites/default/files/SOJNR/iss02vol06.pdf

Buehler, J., Malone, M., & Majerus, J. (1998). Patterns of responses to symptoms in rural residents: The symptom-action-time-line process. In H. Lee (Ed.), *Conceptual basis for rural nursing* (pp. 153–162). Springer Publishing Company.

Buehler, J., Malone, M., & Majerus, J. (2006). Patterns of responses to symptoms in rural residents: The symptom-action-time-line process. In H. J. Lee & C. A. Winters (Eds.), *Rural nursing: Concepts, theory, and practice* (2nd ed., pp. 129–137). Springer Publishing Company.

Buehler, J., Malone, M., & Majerus, J. (2010). Patterns of responses to symptoms in rural residents: The symptom-action-time-line process. In C. A. Winters & H. J. Lee (Eds.), *Rural nursing: Concepts, theory, and practice* (3rd ed., pp. 153–162). Springer Publishing Company.

Buehler, J., Malone, M., & Majerus, J. (2013). Patterns of responses to symptoms in rural residents: The symptom-action-time-line process. In C. A. Winters (Ed.), *Rural nursing: Concepts, theory, and practice* (4th ed., pp. 131–140). Springer Publishing Company.

Callaghan, D. (2005). Healthy behaviors, self-efficacy, self-care, and basic conditioning factors in older adults. *Journal of Community Health Nursing*, 22(3), 169–178. https://doi.org/10.1207/s15327655jchn2203_4

Cheesmond, N. E., Davies, K., & Inder, K. J. (2019). Exploring the role of rurality and rural identity in mental health help-seeking behavior: A systematic qualitative review. *Journal of Rural Mental Health*, 43(1), 45–59. https://doi.org/10.1037/mh0000109

Clark, D. O., Frankel, R. M., Morgan, D. L., Ricketts, G., Bair, M. J., Nyland, K. A., & Callahan, C. M. (2008). The meaning and significance of self-management among socioeconomically vulnerable older adults. *Journal of Gerontology: Social Sciences*, 63B(5), S312–S319. https://dx.doi.org/10.1093%2Fgeronb%2F63.5.s312

Crumb, L., Mingo, T. M., & Crowe, A. (2019). "Get over it and move on:" The impact of mental illness stigma in rural, low income United States populations. *Mental Health and Prevention*, 13, 143–148. https://doi.org/10.1016/J.MHP.2019.01.010

Duran, B., Oetzel, J., Lucero, J., Jiang, Y., Novins, D. K., Manson, S., Beals, J., & American Indian Service Utilization and Psychiatric Epidemiology Risk and Protective Factors Project Team, University of Colorado Health Sciences Center. (2005). Obstacles for rural American Indians seeking alcohol, drug, or mental health treatment. *Journal of Consulting and Clinical Psychology*, 73(5), 819–829. https://psycnet.apa.org/doi/10.1037/0022-006X.73.5.819

Earle-Richardson, G., Scribani, M., Scott, E., May, J., & Jenkins, P. (2015). A comparison of health, health behavior, and access between farm and nonfarm populations in rural New York State. *The Journal of Rural Health*, 31, 157–164. https://doi.org/10.1111/jrh.12098

Easom, L. R., & Quinn, M. E. (2006). Rural elderly caregivers: Exploring folk home remedy use and health promotion activities. *Online Journal of Rural Nursing and Health Care*, 6(1), 32–46. https://doi.org/10.14574/ojrnhc.v6i1.164

Evans, J., Frank, B., Oliffe, J. L., & Gregory, D. (2011). Health, illness, men and masculinities (HIMM): a theoretical framework for understanding men and their health. *Journal of Men's Health*, 8(1), 7–15. https://doi.org/10.1016/j.jomh.2010.09.227

Findling, M. G., Blendon, R. J., Benson, J. M., Sayde, J. M., & Miller, C. E. (2020). Views of rural US adults about health and economic concerns. *JAMA Network Open*, 3(1), e1918755. https://doi.org/10.1001/jamanetworkopen.2019.18745

Fischer, E. P., McSweeney, J. C., Wright, P., Cheney, A., Curran G. M., Henderson, K., & Fortney, J. C. (2016). Overcoming barriers to sustained engagement iin mental health care: Perspectives of rural beterans and providers. *The Journal of Rural Health*, 32(4), 429–438. https://doi.org/10.1111/jrh.12203

Garcia, C. M., Gilchrist, L., Vazquez, G., Leite, A., & Raymond, N. (2011). Urban and rural immigrant Latino youths and adults' knowledge and beliefs about mental health resources. *Journal of Immigrant Minority Health*, 13, 500–509. https://doi.org/10.1007/s10903-010-9389-6

Goins, R. T., Spencer, S. M., & Williams, K. (2010). Lay meanings of health among rural older adults in Appalachia. *The Journal of Rural Health*, 27, 13–20. https://doi.org/10.1111/j.1748-0361.2010.00315.x

Groh, C. J., & Saunders, M. M. (2020). The transition from spousal caregiver to widowhood: Quantitative findings of a mixed-methods study. *Journal of the American Psychiatric Nurses Association*, 26(6), 527–541. https://doi.org/10.1177/1078390320917751

Harju, B. L., Wuensch, K. L., Kuhl, E. A., & Cross, N. J. (2006). Comparison of rural and urban residents' implicit and explicit attitudes related to seeking medical care. *The Journal of Rural Health*, 22(4), 359–363. https://psycnet.apa.org/doi/10.1111/j.1748-0361.2006.00058.x

Heflinger, C. A., Wallston, K. A., Mukolo, A., & Brannan, A. M. (2014). Perceived stigma toward children with emotional and behavioral problems and their families: The attitudes about child mental health questionnaire (ACMHQ). *Journal of Rural Mental Health*, 38(1), 9–19. https://doi.org/10.1037/rmh0000010

Jackson, M. N. G., & McCulloch, B. J. (2014). Heart attack symptoms and decision-making: The case of older rural women. *Rural and Remote Health*, 14, 2560. https://www.rrh.org.au

Kirby, J. B., Zuvekas, S. H., Borsky, A. E., & Ngo-Metzger, Q. (2019). Rural residents with mental health needs have fewer care visits than urban counterparts. *Health Affairs*, 38(12), 2057–2060. https://doi.org/10.1377/hlthaff.2019.00369

Levant, R., & Habben, C. (2003). The new psychology of men: Application to rural men. In B. Stamm (Ed.), *Rural behavioral health care: An interdisciplinary guide* (pp. 171–180). American Psychological Association. https://psycnet.apa.org/doi/10.1037/10489-013

Mize, D., & Rose, T. (2019). The meaning of health and health care for rural = dwelling adults age 75 and older in the Northwestern United States. *Journal of Gerontological Nursing*, 45(6), 23–31. https://doi.org/10.3928/00989134-20190509-03

O'Lynn, C. (2006). Updating the symptom-action-time-line process. In H. Lee & C. A. Winters (Eds.), *Rural nursing: Concepts, theory, and practice* (2nd ed., pp. 138–152). Springer Publishing Company.

O'Lynn, C. (2010). Updating the symptom-action-time-line process. In H. Lee, & C. A. Winters (Eds.), *Rural nursing: Concepts, theory, and practice* (3rd ed., pp. 163–178). Springer Publishing Company.

Polaha, J., Williams, S. L., Heflinger, C. A., & Studts, C. R. (2015). The perceived stigma of mental health services among rural parents of children with psychosocial concerns. *Journal of Pediatric Psychology*, 40(10), 1095–1104. https://doi.org/10.1093/jpepsy/jsv054

Rasmussen, A. D., O'Lynn, C., & Winters, C. A. (2013). Beyond the symptom–action–timeline process: Explicating the health-needs–action process. In C. A. Winters (Ed.), *Rural nursing: Concepts, theory, and practice* (4th ed., pp. 141–158. Springer Publishing Company.

Ruggiero, K. J., Gros, D. F., McCauley, J., de Arellano, M. A., & Danielson, C. K. (2011). Rural adults' use of health-related information online: Data from a 2006 national online health survey. *Telemedicine and e-Health*, 17(5), 329–334. https://psycnet.apa.org/doi/10.1089/tmj.2010.0195

Rural Health Information Hub. (2018). *Rural mental health*. https://www.ruralhealthinfo.org/topics/mental-health.

Sabo, D., & Gordon, D. F. (1995). Rethinking men's health and illness. In D. Sabo & D. F. Gordon (Eds.), *Men's health and illness: Gender, power, and the body* (pp. 1–22). Sage. https://doi.org/10.4135/9781452243757

Saunders, M. M., & Groh, C. J. (2019). Spousal dementia caregiving to widowhood: Perceptions of older urban and rural widows. *Western Journal of Nursing Research*, 42(8), 603–611. https://doi.org/10.1177/0193945919882727

Savia, J., Bivens, L. R., Roberto, K. A., & Blieszner, R. (2019). *Journal of Aging Health*, *31*(5), 837–860. https://doi.org/10.1177/0898264318761907

Sellers, S. C., Poduska, M. D., Propp, L. H., & White, S. I. (1999). The health care meanings, values, and practices of Anglo-American males in the rural Midwest. *Journal of Transcultural Nursing*, *10*, 320–330. https://doi.org/10.1177%2F104365969901000410

Shreffler-Grant, J., Weinert, C., Nicholls, E., & Ide, B. (2005). Complementary therapy use among older rural adults. *Public Health Nursing*, *22*(4), 323–331. https://dx.doi.org/10.1111%2Fj.0737-1209.2005.220407.x

Simmons, L. A., Huddleston-Casas, C., & Berry, A. A. (2007). Low-income rural women and depression: Factors associated with self-reporting. *American Journal of Health Behavior*, *31*(6), 657–666. https://psycnet.apa.org/doi/10.5993/AJHB.31.6.10

Snell-Rood, C., Hauenstein, E., Leukefeld, C., Feltner, F., Marcum, A., & Schoenberg, N. (2017). Mental health treatment seeking patterns and preferences of Appalachian women with depression. *American Journal of Orthopsychiatry*, *87*(3), 233–241. http://dx.doi.org/10.1037/ort0000193

Sriram, U., Morgan, E. H., Graham, M. L., Folta, S. C., & Seguin, R. A. (2017). Support and sabotage: A qualitative study of social influences on health behaviors among rural adults. *The Journal of Rural Health*, *34*(1), 88–97. https://doi.org/10.1111/jrh.12232

Stoller, E. P., Grzywacz, J. G., Quandt, S. A., Bell, R. A., Chapman, C., Altizer, K. P. Arcury, T. A. (2011). Calling the doctor: A qualitative study of patient-initiated physician consultation among rural older adults. *Journal of Aging and Health*, *23*(5), 782–805. https://doi.org/10.1177%2F0898264310397045

Tzeng, H. M., Okpalauwaekwe, U., Yin, C. Y., Jansen, S. L., Feng, C., & Barker, A. (2018). Do patients' demographic characteristics affect their perceptions of self-care actions to find safe and decent care? *Applied Nursing Research*, *43*, 24–29. https://doi.org/10.1016/j.apnr.2018.06.020

Vallerand, A. H., Fouladbakhsh, J. M., & Templin, T. (2005). Patients' choices for the self-treatment of pain. *Applied Nursing Research*, *18*, 90–96. https://doi.org/ doi: 10.1016/j.apnr.2004.07.003

Wilson, W., Bangs, A., & Hatting, T. (2015). *The future of rural behavioral health national rural health association policy brief*. National Rural Health Association. https://www.ruralhealthweb.org/NRHA/media/Emerge_NRHA/Advocacy/Policy%20documents/The-Future-of-Rural-Behavioral-Health_Feb-2015.pdf

Winters, C. A., Cudney, S., & Sullivan, T. (2010). Expressions of depression in rural women with chronic illness. *Rural and Remote Health*, *10*, 1–14. http:/www.rrh.org.au/journal/article/1533

Winters, C. A., Cudney, S., Sullivan, T., & Thuesen, A. (2006). The rural context and women's self-management of chronic health conditions. *Chronic Illness*, *2*, 273–289. https://doi.org/10.1177%2F17423953060020040801

Zhang, Y., Jones, B., Spalding, M., Young, R., & Ragain, M. (2009). Use of the Internet for health information among primary care patients in rural West Texas. *Southern Medical Journal*, *102*(6), 595–601. https://doi.org/10.1097/smj.0b013e3181a52117

CHAPTER 14

Acceptability: One Component in Choice of Healthcare Provider

Jean Shreffler-Grant

DISCUSSION TOPICS

- Discuss the aspects of local healthcare that affect the choices that rural dwellers make when deciding whether to use local care.
- How can the Acceptability Scale be utilized to improve local rural healthcare?
- Why do you think that the critical access hospital model of care has been implemented so widely across the United States?

INTRODUCTION

Since the early 1980s, access to healthcare has deteriorated in many rural areas in the United States as a result of the closure of rural hospitals and the associated loss of local providers and services that often accompany hospital closure. As one of the major employers in many rural communities, hospital closure can also have a negative impact on the economic situation of local businesses and individuals (Balasubramanian & Jones, 2016). In recent years, the rural hospital closure crisis has escalated with 2015 closure rates six times higher than in 2010 (Kaufman et al., 2016; National Rural Health Association [NRHA], 2020). During 2019, more U.S. rural hospitals (19) closed in 1 year than in the past 15 years and 11 additional hospitals have closed in the first 6 months of 2020 (Sheps Center for Health Services Research, 2020a). The NRHA (2020) reported that currently one in three rural hospitals may be at the risk of closure. Much of the blame for closures has long been attributed to factors external to rural communities, such as reduced Medicare reimbursement, a declining rural economy, provider shortages, and being located in states that did not expand Medicaid under the Affordable Care Act (Sheps Center for Health Services Research, 2020b). In contrast to external issues, a substantial volume of evidence has accumulated that indicates that the closures may, in part, be due to influences closer to home. Some rural hospitals are underutilized by local residents, who bypass them to seek care in larger towns

163

and cities (Allen et al., 2015; Amundson, 1993; DeFriese et al., 1992; Escarse & Kapur, 2009; Hall et al., 2010; Liu et al., 2007, 2008; Malone & Holmes, 2020; Radcliff et al., 2003; Weigel et al., 2017). Lee and McDonagh (2018) pointed out that decision-making and making choices about where and from whom to seek healthcare is relevant to the second theoretical statement originally proposed by Long and Weinert (1989). Rural dwellers are self-reliant and tend to seek help, including needed healthcare, from informal rather than formal sources. As discussed in this chapter, decision-making about healthcare involves making conscience choices about whether to access local healthcare resources or, alternately, to bypass local care to seek health services in a distant location.

Since the early 1990s, variations of critical access hospitals (CAHs) have been implemented as alternatives to rural hospitals that are at risk for closure. CAHs must be located in remote rural areas, are limited to short-stay lower-acuity services, and are allowed more flexibility in staffing and other licensure requirements. They are also reimbursed by Medicare based on reasonable cost instead of prospective payment, as compared with traditional rural hospitals. Cost-based Medicare reimbursement is considered advantageous for small hospitals that often serve a high proportion of older patients and are less likely to be able to average risk across large numbers of admissions, as may be necessary under prospective payment (Christianson et al., 1990). Following implementation of the Rural Hospital Flexibility Program, passed into law in 1997, CAHs have gained broad support in rural areas across the nation (Shreffler et al., 1999). By 2006, less than a decade after the CAH model was passed into law, a large majority (80%) of small rural hospitals and more than 60% of all rural hospitals had converted to CAHs (Pink et al., 2007). As of April 28, 2020, there were 1,352 CAHs nationwide (Flex Monitoring Team, 2020). Whether these new CAH models will be any more viable than traditional rural hospitals will likely be tied to how they are viewed and used by the rural residents they are intended to serve.

Improving equity in access to care has been an ongoing concern throughout most of the past half century (Aday et al., 1993; Patrick & Erickson, 1993), and rural access to care has been a particularly persistent problem (Gamm & Hutchison, 2003). Although equitable access to healthcare in and of itself may be intuitively desirable, it is through presumed links between access to quality health services, appropriate use, and resulting positive health outcomes that access becomes important (Millman, 1993). I conducted a study (1996) to examine rural residents' perspectives on access to healthcare in six communities in Montana with CAHs. The concept of "acceptability" is one dimension of access to care that can be used to explain why people do or do not use local rural healthcare services. As part of the larger study, a scale to measure acceptability was developed and validated. In this chapter, I focus on the Acceptability Scale (see Table 14.1).

ACCESS TO CARE

Conceptual Framework

Access to care was the conceptual framework guiding this study. I conceptualized access to care as having two dimensions. Potential access to care includes properties of the population and healthcare system that affect opportunities to enter into the healthcare system. Actual or realized access to care includes utilization and willingness to use the healthcare system and satisfaction with the care received (Aday & Andersen, 1975; Andersen et al., 1993).

TABLE 14.1. Individual Items Included in the "Acceptability Scale"

	Excellent	Good	Average	Fair	Poor	
Circle One Answer for Each Category						

1. How would you rate (facility name) in each of the following categories?

	Excellent	Good	Average	Fair	Poor	
a. Overall quality of care	5	4	3	2	1	Don't know
b. Medical care	5	4	3	2	1	Don't know
c. Nursing care	5	4	3	2	1	Don't know
d. Staff concern/ compassion	5	4	3	2	1	Don't know
e. "Personal" aspects of care	5	4	3	2	1	Don't know
f. Building cleanliness and condition	5	4	3	2	1	Don't know
g. Acceptability as source of care	5	4	3	2	1	Don't know

2. How would you rate each of the following aspects of overall medical care provided in your community? (Care provided by physicians, nurse practitioners, physician assistants, or other primary care providers at their office or local hospital)

	Excellent	Good	Average	Fair	Poor	
a. Competence of primary care providers	5	4	3	2	1	Don't know
b. Concern/ compassion for patient	5	4	3	2	1	Don't know
c. "Personal" aspects of care	5	4	3	2	1	Don't know
d. Competence of support staff	5	4	3	2	1	Don't know
e. Acceptability as source of care	5	4	3	2	1	Don't know

Source: Shreffler, M. J. (1996). Rural residents' views on access to care in frontier communities with medical assistance facilities. *Dissertation Abstracts International, 57,* 3131 (No. 9630109).

In several studies published in the 1980s on the relationship between access to care and utilization of care, Penchansky and Thomas (1981; Thomas & Penchansky, 1984) defined access as the fit between clients and the healthcare system. An adequate degree of fit was measured by objective utilization and subjective satisfaction. They identified five components of potential access that are referred to as "the 5 A's":

1. *Availability*—the supply of providers and services relative to clients' needs
2. *Accessibility*—where services are located relative to where clients are
3. *Accommodation*—how services are organized to accept clients
4. *Affordability*—costs of services relative to resources of clients
5. *Acceptability*—the clients' attitudes and opinions about the characteristics of providers and services

Discriminant validity of Penchansky and Thomas's (1981; Thomas & Penchansky, 1984) components of access to care was supported in their studies, and subsets of clients were found to differ significantly in the utilization of healthcare, based on how satisfied they were with the components that were salient for them. Although these investigators measured acceptability chiefly by consumers' attitudes and opinions about the physical environment in which care was delivered, they proposed that attitudes about personal and technical practice characteristics of providers and services were also relevant.

Methods

In the larger study to examine rural residents' perspectives on access to healthcare (Shreffler, 1996), I employed a descriptive survey design. Surveys were sent to a random sample of 100 households in each of six communities with CAHs, and I interviewed a subset of respondents by telephone. I obtained a 63.5% response rate on the mail survey ($N = 381$).

The principal aims in this study were to identify the predictors of use and willingness to use local healthcare, and respondents' satisfaction with care. In interpreting the term "predictors," it should be noted that I sought significant statistical relationships rather than cause and effect relationships. It was not possible to determine from the data whether people used local healthcare because they thought it was acceptable or whether they thought it was acceptable because they had used it.

There were four dependent variables in the analyses to address actual access to care. They were (a) use of the local CAH, (b) use of the local primary care provider, (c) willingness to use the local CAH, and (d) willingness to use the local provider. These "use" variables were dichotomous yes or no indicators of whether the respondents reported actual use of the CAH and the local provider in the recent past. The "willingness to use" variables were dichotomous yes or no indicators constructed from responses to a question about where respondents would first seek care for a variety of future health concerns. The future health concerns counted as "yes, willing to use" were concerns for which the local CAH and provider(s) offered healthcare services, rather than other services included in the question that were not available locally and for which patients would need to be referred elsewhere.

The major independent variables, or potential predictors, included potential access to care factors. All were measured by respondents' self-report and from their perspectives (vs. from the perspectives of the hospitals or providers). These included characteristics of the population (e.g., age, income, health insurance, and health status) and characteristics of the healthcare system that were operationalized according to "the 5 A's" from Penchansky and Thomas's work (1981; Thomas & Penchansky, 1984), that is, availability, accessibility, accommodation, affordability, and acceptability.

The Acceptability Scale comprised the summed values of responses to twelve 5-point Likert-type rating questions related to the concept of acceptability, included on the mail survey. I based my selection of the questions for inclusion in the scale on Penchansky and Thomas's work (1981; Thomas & Penchansky, 1984). The questions were then validated based on responses during telephone interviews to the question: "When you and your household members choose a medical care provider and a hospital to use, can you tell me what factors are important to you?" Responses were related to the technical quality of care, the "art" of care, and the appearance of the facility or office.

The Acceptability Scale items were components of two questions that asked respondents to rate a wide variety of aspects of healthcare in their local communities (see Table 14.1). Response options included excellent, good, average, fair, poor, and do not know. The scale had a possible point range of 12 to 60. The reliability coefficients for the Acceptability Scale were Cronbach's alpha = 0.97 and the Standardized item alpha = 0.97; the inter-item correlations analysis ranged from 0.54 to 0.88.

To identify the predictors of use and willingness to use local healthcare, I built four separate multivariate logistic regression models (one for each dependent variable) in which each dependent variable was regressed on a set of six community (dummy) variables to control for confounding by community. Then I added independent variables to the model together as a group (not stepwise). Next, I calculated odds ratios and 95% confidence intervals for the independent variables with $p \leq .05$.

I analyzed qualitative comments on several short-answer questions on the mail survey and open-ended questions from the telephone interview regarding access to care by using content analysis methods. I read all qualitative data multiple times and sorted them into similar categories based on the words used in the comments (manifest content) and the apparent meaning of the words (latent content; Catanzaro, 1988). I sought patterns and categories that might add to the understanding of rural residents' views on access to healthcare in their local communities. I then summarized these themes and categories and identified relevant themes using the actual phrases of the respondents.

Results

Table 14.2 shows the descriptive results of the "use of" and "willingness to use" dependent variables. As can be seen on the table, relatively few respondents ($n = 37$, 9.7%) reported that anyone in their household had used the local CAH for inpatient care in the prior 2 years, whereas roughly two-thirds of the respondents ($n = 260$, 68%) reported use of the local provider in the past year. Less than half of the respondents indicated willingness to use the CAH ($n = 162$, 43%) or local providers ($n = 182$, 48%) for future health concerns.

I computed Acceptability Scale scores for 261 of the total 381 households; the remaining households were excluded because of missing values or "don't know" answers. The mean Acceptability Scale score was 46.48 ($SD = 9.87$; range = 18–60 points [possible range = 12–60 points]).

On the basis of the logistic regression analysis (summarized in Table 14.3), respondents for households most likely to use the CAH for inpatient care were those who rated their knowledge of local healthcare highly, were older in age, and reported lower incomes. The odds ratio indicates the factor by which the odds of "use" or "willing to use" change when the corresponding variable is changed by one unit. Because in this chapter I focus on the Acceptability Scale, I do not discuss the other results at length, but just as illustration, for every unit increase in the knowledge rating category with an odds ratio of 2.308, the odds of use of the CAH increased by 130%. An odds ratio of 1 is equal odds, so

TABLE 14.2 Frequencies of Dependent Variables "Use of" and "Willingness to Use" Local Healthcare ($N = 381$)

Variable	N	%
"Used the CAHs" for inpatient care in prior 2 years	37	9.7
"Used local provider(s)" in the past year	260	68.0
"Willing to use the CAH" in the future	162	43.0
"Willing to use the local provider(s)" in the future	182	48.0

CAHs, critical access hospitals.

TABLE 14.3 Results of Multivariate Logistic Regression Models to Identify Predictors of "Use of" and "Willingness to Use" Local Healthcare

	B	SE	OR	95% CI
Use of CAHs and				
• Knowledge of local healthcare	0.836*	0.400	2.308	(5.05, 1.06)
• Respondent age	0.035*	0.017	1.036	(1.07, 1.01)
• Household income	−0.533*	0.221	0.587	(0.61, 0.56)
Use of local provider and				
• Acceptability scale score	0.096**	0.024	1.100	(1.15, 1.05)
Willing to use CAHs and				
• Acceptability scale score	0.065**	0.021	1.067	(1.11, 1.02)
• Use local provider	0.936*	0.452	2.549	(6.18, 1.05)
Willing to use local provider and				
• Acceptability scale score	0.088**	0.023	1.092	(1.14, 1.04)
• Used provider in the past	1.879**	0.504	6.546	(17.58, 2.44)
• Community affiliation	1.540**	0.549	4.664	(13.69, 1.59)

Data include significant independent variables only.
*$p \leq .05$
**$p \leq .01$
CAHs, critical access hospitals; CI, 95% confidence interval of the odds ratio; OR, odds ratio.

anything significantly over or less than 1 is considered. The Acceptability Scale as well as other variables in this model (distance from CAH, use of local provider, ease of transportation, and community affiliation) were not significant predictors of use of the CAH. I anticipated that few, if any, covariates would be significant in this model, with only 37 households that had reported the use of the CAH.

Households most likely to use the local provider(s) were those that had higher Acceptability Scale scores. For each additional point on the scale, the odds of use of the provider increased by 10%. Other variables in this model (knowledge of local healthcare, distance from CAH, respondent age, income, transportation, and community affiliation) were not significant predictors of use of the local provider.

Households most likely to be willing to use the CAH for future health problems were those with higher Acceptability Scale scores and those that had used the local provider(s) in the past year. Based on the odds ratios for each additional point on the Acceptability Scale, the odds of indicating willingness to use the CAH increased by 7%. Other variables in this model (knowledge, distance from CAH, age, income, transportation, and community affiliation) were not significant predictors of willingness to use the CAH.

Residents most likely to be willing to use the local provider(s) in the future were also those with higher acceptability scores, who used the local provider(s) in the past year, and reported that they were affiliated with the local community. Each point on the Acceptability Scale increased the odds of willingness to use the provider by 9%. Other variables in this model (knowledge, distance from CAH, age, income, and transportation) were not significant predictors of willingness to use the local provider.

Among those who used local healthcare, the Acceptability Scale score was also a significant predictor of satisfaction with care. Because I included only those households that had used both the CAH and local provider(s) in the recent past (n = 36) in this analysis, I used Mantel–Haenszel Chi-square tests to examine relationships between satisfaction and selected covariates. There was insufficient power to analyze this relationship using multivariate logistic regression models. The Acceptability Scale score was significantly associated with satisfaction with the local CAH, emergency care, local primary care provider(s), and the availability of night or weekend care ($p \leq .01$). Other variables examined were not significantly associated with satisfaction with care.

In the qualitative comments, the rural respondents offered many perspectives related to the relationship between acceptability and the use of local healthcare. "He knows what he's doing. He knows my son and my son knows him and that's comforting." "He's a country type doctor. I like that." "The way a hospital is equipped. I want a doctor who is top of the line." "For the doctor—that you have rapport with him, that he gives you accurate information, that you're comfortable that he knows what he's doing." "For the hospital—the nursing care, cleanliness. The doctor—personality. I go to see him the first time—did the medicines help, did the care help the problem?" "They don't have the services, the doctor's not as good, and it's not as good a hospital."

CONCLUSION

In this study, the Acceptability Scale was the most consistent predictor of "use of" and "willingness to use" local rural healthcare, as well as of satisfaction with care. Acceptability is that component of access to care that reflects potential clients' attitudes and opinions about the characteristics of providers and services. Unlike other aspects of access, acceptability reflects making a choice based on an opinion, judgment, and personal preferences on the part of consumers. The current rural reality for obtaining most goods and services including healthcare is that with access to vehicles, modern highways, and health insurance, rural residents are not as affected by distance in choosing healthcare as they once were. This study suggests that those who do not find local healthcare acceptable go elsewhere.

It is interesting to note that a large majority (95%) of the respondents in this study indicated that having local healthcare was very or somewhat important to their household members; "keeping" or maintaining the health services and providers they had was the predominant theme in the qualitative comments—yet only 9.7% of the households had a family member hospitalized in the CAH in the prior 2 years, and only 68.2% had used the local provider(s) in the prior year. A clarification of this discrepancy may be found by considering a second theme that emerged from the data—"just in case," as the following quotes show:

- "You always have certain people who are doubters … but they still want emergency care available in case they need it, even though they don't support it for everyday things."
- "I know that it's not paying its way in taxes, but we need it. It's like having an insurance policy. Insurance policies don't pay for themselves either, but you need it just in case."

Clearly there was support in these six communities for keeping their local healthcare, as evidenced by the large number of participants who reported that local healthcare was important to their household. The importance of local healthcare, however, was not associated with the use of it, whereas their perception of the acceptability of local healthcare was associated with use.

By improving researchers' understanding of what rural consumers deem acceptable in terms of services and providers, the Acceptability Scale can be used to improve healthcare access for rural residents. In the practice arena, attending to community residents' perceptions of competence, quality, the art of care, and appearance of facilities as well as developing strategies to strengthen and improve these perceptions may reduce outmigration from healthcare that is available locally. In the policy arena, as new models of care are developed or refined, paying substantial attention to features or characteristics that influence acceptability to consumers can make the difference between services that will be used and valued and services that will be bypassed by the residents they are intended to serve. When it comes to rural healthcare, Kinsella's (1982) old baseball adage, "If you build it, [they] will come," does not necessarily hold, unless what is built is acceptable to rural residents.

ACKNOWLEDGMENTS

This research was funded by Health Care Financing Administration Dissertation Grant 30-P-90510/0-01, Hester McLaws Award, Sigma Theta Tau Zeta Upsilon Research Award, and Montana State University College of Nursing.

REFERENCES

Aday, L. A., & Andersen, R. (1975). A framework for the study of access to medical care. In L. A. Aday & R. Andersen (Eds.), *Development of indices of access to medical care* (pp. 1–14). Health Administration Press.

Aday, L. A., Bagley, C. E., Lairson, D. R., & Slater, C. H. (1993). *Evaluating the medical care system: Effectiveness, efficiency, and equity*. Health Administration Press.

Allen, J. E., Davis, A. F., Hu, W., & Owusu-Amankwah, E. (2015). Residents' willingness-to-pay for attributes of rural healthcare facilities. *The Journal of Rural Health, 31*(1), 7–18. https://doi.org/10.1111/jrh.12080

Amundson, B. (1993). Myth and reality in the rural health service crisis: Facing up to community responsibilities. *The Journal of Rural Health, 9*, 176–187. https://doi.org/10.1111/j.1748-0361.1993.tb00512.x

Andersen, R. M., McCutcheon, A., Aday, L. A., Chiu, G. Y., & Bell, R. (1993). Exploring dimensions of access to medical care. *Health Services Research, 18*(1), 49–74. https://www.ncbi.nlm.nih.gov/pmc/articles/PMC1068709/

Balasubramanian, S. S., & Jones, E. C. (2016). Hospital closures and the current healthcare climate: The future of rural hospitals in the USA. *Rural and Remote Health, 16*, 1–5. http://www.rrh.org.au/articles/subviewnew.asp?ArticleID=3935

Catanzaro, M. (1988). Using qualitative analytical techniques. In N. F. Woods & M. Catanzaro (Eds.), *Nursing research: Theory and practice* (pp. 437–456). Mosby.

Christianson, J. B., Moscovice, I. S., Wellever, A. L., & Wingert, T. D. (1990). Institutional alternatives to the rural hospital. *Health Care Financing Review, 11*(3), 87–97. https://europepmc.org/article/pmc/pmc4193086

DeFriese, G. H., Wilson, G., Ricketts, T. C., & Whitener, L. (1992). Consumer choice and the national rural hospital crisis. In W. M. Gesler & T. C. Ricketts (Eds.), *Health in rural North America* (pp. 206–225). Rutgers University Press.

Escarse, J. J., & Kapur, K. (2009). Do patients bypass rural hospitals? Determinants of inpatient hospital choice in rural California. *Journal of Health Care for the Poor and Underserved, 20*(3), 625–644. https://doi.org/10.1353/hpu.0.0178

Flex Monitoring Team. (2020). *Critical access hospital locations.* http://www.flexmonitoring.org/data/critical-access-hospital-locations

Gamm, L., & Hutchison, L. (2003). Rural health priorities in America: Where you stand depends on where you sit. *The Journal of Rural Health, 19*(3), 209–213. https://doi.org/10.1111/j.1748-0361.2003.tb00563.x

Hall, M. J., Marsteller, J., & Owings, M. (2010). Factors influencing rural residents' utilization of urban hospitals. *National Health Statistical Report, 18*(31), 1–12. https://jhu.pure.elsevier.com/en/publications/factors-influencing-rural-residents-utilization-of-urban-hospital-8

Kaufman, B. G., Thomas, S. R., Randolph, R. K., Perry, J. R., Thompson, K. W., & Pink, G. H. (2016). The rising rate of rural hospital closures. *The Journal of Rural Health, 32*(1), 35–43. https://doi.org/10.1111/jrh.12128

Kinsella, W. P. (1982). *Shoeless Joe Jackson comes to Iowa.* Ballantine Books.

Lee, H. J., & McDonagh, M. K. (2018). Updating the rural nursing base. In C. A. Winters & H. J. Lee (Eds.), *Rural nursing: Concepts, theory, and practice* (5th ed., pp. 45–62). Springer Publishing Company.

Liu, J. J., Bellamy, G. R., Barnet, B., & Weng, S. (2008). Bypass of local primary care in rural counties: Effect of patient and community characteristics. *Annals of Family Medicine, 6*(2), 124–130. https://doi.org/10.1370/afm.794

Liu, J. J., Bellamy, G. R., & McCormick, M. (2007). Patient bypass behavior and critical access hospitals: Implications for patient retention. *The Journal of Rural Health, 23*(1), 17–24. https://doi.org/10.1111/j.1748-0361.2006.00063.x

Long, K. A., & Weinert, C. (1989). Rural nursing: Developing the theory base. *Scholarly Inquiry for Nursing Practice: An International Journal, 3*, 113–127.

Malone, T., & Holmes, M. (2020). Patterns of hospital bypass and inpatient care-seeking by rural residents. *Findings Brief. North Carolina Rural Health Research Program.* https://www.ruralhealthresearch.org/alerts/305

Millman, M. (Ed.). (1993). *Access to care in America.* National Academies Press.

National Rural Health Association. (2020). *NRHA save rural hospital action center.* https://www.ruralhealthweb.org/advocate/save-rural-hospitals

Patrick, D. L., & Erickson, P. (1993). *Health status and health policy: Quality of life in health evaluation and resource allocation.* Oxford University Press.

Penchansky, R., & Thomas, J. W. (1981). The concept of access: Definition and relationship to consumer satisfaction. *Medical Care, 19*, 127–140. https://doi.org/10.1097/00005650-198102000-00001

Pink, G. H., Holmes, G. M., Thompson, R. E., & Slifkin, R. T. (2007). Variations in financial performance among peer groups of Critical Access Hospitals. *The Journal of Rural Health, 23*(4), 299–305. https://doi.org/10.1111/j.1748-0361.2007.00107.x

Radcliff, T. A., Brasure, M., Moscovice, I. S., & Stensland, J. T. (2003). Understanding rural hospital bypass behavior. *The Journal of Rural Health, 19*(3), 252–259. https://doi.org/10.1111/j.1748-0361.2003.tb00571.x

Sheps Center for Health Services Research, University of North Carolina. (2020a). *170 rural hospital closures: 2005–present (128 since 2010).* https://www.shepscenter.unc.edu/programs-projects/rural-health/rural-hospital-closures/

Sheps Center for Health Services Research, University of North Carolina. (2020b). *Rural hospital closures: More information.* https://www.shepscenter.unc.edu/programs-projects/rural-health/rural-hospital-closures-archive/rural-hospital-closures/

Shreffler, M. J. (1996). Rural residents views on access to care in frontier communities with medical assistance facilities. *Dissertation Abstracts International, 57*, 3131 (No. 9630109).

Shreffler, M. J., Capalbo, S. M., Flaherty, R. J., & Heggam, C. (1999). Community decision-making about critical access hospitals: Lessons learned from Montana's Medical Assistance Facility program. *The Journal of Rural Health, 15*, 180–188. https://doi.org/10.1111/j.1748-0361.1999.tb00738.x

Thomas, J. W., & Penchansky, R. (1984). Relating satisfaction with access and utilization of services. *Medical Care, 22*, 553–568. https://doi.org/10.1097/00005650-198406000-00006

Weigel, P. A., Ullrich, F., Finegan, C. N., & Ward, M. M. (2017). Rural bypass for elective surgeries. *The Journal of Rural Health, 33*(2), 135–145. https://doi.org/10.1111/jrh.12163

CHAPTER 15

Telehealth in Rural Nursing Practice

K. M. Reeder, Victoria L. S. Britson,
and Mary Kay Nissen

DISCUSSION TOPICS

- What are the major influences of telehealth on rural and frontier nursing practice and healthcare?
- What are the advantages of using telehealth in rural and frontier environments?
- What is the role of the nurse in providing rural/frontier primary, urgent, and specialty care using telehealth modalities?
- How can nurses using telehealth help patients and families achieve desirable healthcare outcomes, avoid potentially preventable health concerns, and enhance quality of life?

INTRODUCTION

Telehealth nursing, also known as telenursing, involves the use of telecommunications and other technologies such as videoconferencing for sharing information and providing patient care, education, public health, and administrative services over distances (Fathi et al., 2017; Jones, 2017). Telehealth conceptually offers an approach to redesign and enhance nursing care outside of traditional healthcare settings, namely, hospitals and clinics (Fraiche et al., 2017; Totten et al., 2016). Changes in healthcare policy, including reimbursement structures, can create uncertainty and increase the risk for widening gaps in health among rural and frontier populations (Centers for Medicare & Medicaid Services [CMS], 2020; Kusmin, 2016). Telehealth programs have been designed to address these and other rural health disparities by increasing access and improving safety and quality of care, as well as reducing healthcare costs.

In 2020, the public health crisis created by the novel coronavirus (COVID-19) presented both opportunities and challenges in caring for persons living in rural and frontier communities. For example, Hong et al. (2020) found increased telehealth interest in the U.S. population as cases of the coronavirus increased; however, the number of U.S. hospitals providing telehealth services was not sufficient to meet the demand for telehealth. Although the rules on telehealth reimbursement were relaxed during the coronavirus pandemic by the CMS, the uptake of telehealth has been slow and fragmented (Smith et al., 2020). Nonetheless, telehealth programs are being designed and implemented to permanently address these and other rural health disparities by increasing access to care, improving the safety and quality of care, and reducing healthcare costs. This chapter includes discussion on the historic underpinnings of telehealth nursing, description of two telehealth patient care scenarios (institution-to-institution and direct-to-consumer) in nursing practice, and concludes with discussion on the implications of telehealth in nursing, including considerations for implementing telehealth patient care services programs and the current scope of telehealth nursing practice.

BACKGROUND

Extant literature on telehealth is vast and varied. Interchangeable terms, including eHealth (electronic health), mHealth (mobile health), and telemedicine (medical care at a distance via various telecommunication technologies) were used to operationalize telehealth, making comparisons between studies difficult. However, a recent systematic review and meta-analysis of 43 studies showed telehealth interventions may be as effective as face-to-face visits (Speyer et al., 2018). Evidence on cost and healthcare services use is also sparse (Snoswell et al., 2020). Thus, research is needed that further examines patient outcomes, including safety and quality of life outcomes and healthcare costs in rural and frontier populations with a variety of conditions and in a variety of contexts of care. Specifically, research is needed that examines patient and health services outcomes amenable to telehealth nursing interventions that will inform payers and policymakers on digital healthcare delivery and value-based models that accommodate continued technology innovation and expanded roles, while supporting current practices and translation of new evidence (Graves et al., 2013; Knapp, 2016; Smith et al., 2015).

Historically, the use of telehealth technologies by nurses was learned on-the-job, without formal training. Telehealth is increasingly being integrated into academic nursing curricula signifying the importance of telehealth in nursing practice. In the current healthcare milieu, training and experience in telehealth by RNs and APRNs in rural and frontier environments is critical to providing effective nursing care. Despite widespread efforts by the American Academy of Ambulatory Care Nursing (2011) and the American Telehealth Telemedicine Association (Gough et al., 2015) to provide evidence for telehealth use of standards of practice, there has been limited success in systematically implementing guideline-based telehealth care in clinical practice.

Providing healthcare using telehealth modalities differs from traditional nursing and advanced practice. Telehealth nursing requires collaboration and resourcefulness between on-site and distance site colleagues, as well as patients and families receiving telehealth care to achieve positive outcomes. In addition to traditional skills that underpin the nursing process and advanced practice, telehealth nurses must be skilled in the use of telehealth technologies, including the use of peripheral equipment and troubleshooting interruptions in telehealth interactions and assessments due to a variety of potential equipment and technology issues. Examples of technological equipment nurses use in conducting telehealth encounters include the electronic stethoscope for auscultation, otoscope and ophthalmoscope for ear and eye examinations, respectively, and handheld camera to visualize and assess wounds and other visible alterations.

During telehealth encounters, healthcare providers must be mindful of camera presence, extraneous noise, body language, and backgrounds visualized on the video screen by patients, families, and other members of the healthcare team. Like face-to-face encounters, telehealth patient encounters require adherence to professional and legal standards of confidentiality, ethics, communication, and cultural considerations. Communication during telehealth encounters often present additional challenges in that, there is frequently a slight delay in audiovisual transmission, resulting in an inadvertent talk-over audio effect during interactions, or pixelated or distorted visual effects. Thus, it is important to identify the need for repeated, or confirmatory, collection of history and physical assessment information to account for potential disruptions in telehealth technologies and asymmetries in interactions that might otherwise result in inaccuracies.

In a Delphi study, van Houwelingen et al. (2016) identified essential telehealth activities used by nurses who provide remote healthcare to Dutch community-dwelling patients. Consensus on 14 nursing telehealth entrustable professional activities (NT-EPAs) was formed for telehealth nursing practice. Specific competencies were then selected for each NT-EPA, which are needed to carry out each activity. For example, the activity pertaining to the coordination of care with the use of telehealth technology (NT-EPA #12) involves 14 competencies that address knowledge, communication, and clinical skills. Additional research is needed to validate the major nursing activities and their associated competencies in a variety of rural settings.

NEED FOR TELEHEALTH NURSING CARE IN RURAL POPULATIONS

Several factors specific to the needs of rural and frontier populations have contributed to the growth and expansion of telehealth in rural and frontier nursing practice. Residents of rural and frontier geographic areas are more likely to report lesser access to care, lower perceived quality of care, and poorer health outcomes when compared to metropolitan area residents (Agency for Healthcare Research and Quality, 2017). In 2016, an estimated 60 million (19%) Americans lived in rural counties (American Community Survey: 2011–2015). However, recruiting and retaining primary healthcare providers, specialists, and nurses in rural- and frontier-designated areas has been especially challenging.

HRSA has identified states and counties with medically underserved areas (MUAs)/medically underserved populations (MUPs). As illustrated in Figure 15.1, MUAs are specific geographic locations that lack sufficient primary healthcare, dental, and mental health providers; MUPs delineate population subgroups living in MUAs such as, the homeless, low-income individuals, and migrant populations (HRSA, 2020).

Higher rates of cigarette smoking, hypertension, obesity, leisure time physical inactivity, and lack of seatbelt use were found in rural populations compared to those in urban populations (Brooks, 2019; Garcia et al., 2019). In addition, social determinants of health such as education, income, poverty, and unemployment had a major influence on widening rural population health disparities (United States Department of Agriculture, 2020). Researchers have demonstrated that rural dwellers are more likely to have poorer health and live with more health risk factors and chronic conditions than their urban counterparts (Bolin et al., 2015; Moy et al., 2017). Moreover, nonmetropolitan area populations in the United States (Garcia et al., 2019; Moy et al., 2017) experience higher mortality from the top five leading causes of death (heart disease, cancer, unintentional injury, chronic lower respiratory disease, and stroke) and are trailing in the achievement of Healthy People 2020 objectives for the leading causes of death compared to metropolitan area populations (Callaghan et al., 2020).

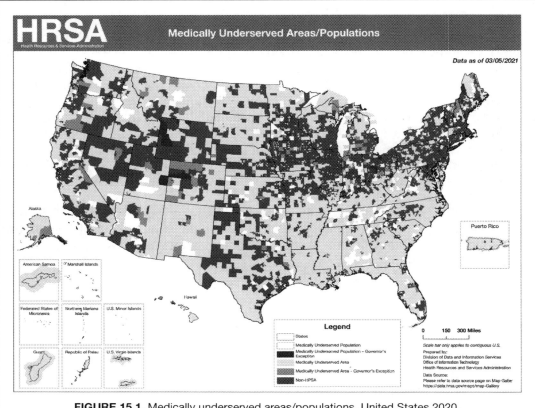

FIGURE 15.1. Medically underserved areas/populations, United States 2020.
Source: Health Resources & Services Administration. (2020). *HRSA data warehouse.* https://data.hrsa.gov/maps/map-gallery

Lack of health insurance and healthcare provider shortages for routine comprehensive care have contributed to widening gaps in primary care among rural and frontier populations. By 2015, there was an emerging trend whereby rural states had slightly lower uninsured rates than the general U.S. population and had similar primary care provider (PCP)-to-patient ratios as the general population (Kaiser Family Foundation, 2020). These findings, however, must be interpreted with caution, as improvements in insured rates and patient-to-provider ratios might be related to increases in health insurance realized with promulgation of the Affordable Care Act in 2010, and warrant further examination on the potential impact and sustainability of subsequent policy changes.

Telehealth nursing care can help to bridge the gaps in healthcare for persons in rural and frontier regions, and help patients gain local access to the necessary type and level of healthcare providers at distant sites to effectively address health concerns and optimize outcomes, including reducing mortality. When locally unavailable care or specialty consultations are needed, extensive travel to obtain these services may be required by patients and families. Transportation expense and time delays in care and specialized treatments, and road conditions, especially during inclement weather, can be significant barriers to accessing care. In these and other similar situations, audiovisual telehealth technologies can be used to connect rural and frontier populations with the needed healthcare services; thus, providing continuity of care for patients in their local communities and improving patient outcomes. Numerous published studies in a variety of settings and populations such as long-term, urgent, and emergency care showed patients who experienced a telehealth encounter had increased satisfaction with telehealth visits due to decreased travel time for specialty care, improved communication and continuity of care with PCPs, increased access to specialty providers, and prevention of unnecessary transfers to an ED or higher acuity level of care (Donelan et al., 2019; Hofmeyer et al., 2016; McLendon et al., 2019). To illustrate the potential impact of telehealth nursing on rural health outcomes, a commonly used method and a novel approach to telehealth care delivery are described below using hypothetical patient care scenarios: institution-to-institution for a long-term care (LTC) facility resident and direct-to-consumer approaches for a rural community-dwelling resident.

Institution-to-Institution Telehealth Scenario

Mrs. Smith, an 82-year-old widow with a history of diabetes, heart failure, and depression was assessed by her LTC nurse, and was noted to be disoriented, pale, coughing, and slightly short of breath. Vital signs were as follows: body temperature = 100.4°C, heart rate = 98/min, respiration rate = 22/min, and blood pressure = 114/78. Oxygen saturation via pulse oximetry was 91% on room air. The LTC nurse contacted the telehealth provider at the remote hospital approximately 300 miles from the LTC facility for a consultation. After establishing a secure Internet connection with the remote site, a telehealth consultation encounter was initiated by the remote site APRN who assessed Mrs. Smith with the on-site, in-person assistance of the LTC nurse.

After assessing Mrs. Smith, the APRN ordered lab work consisting of a complete blood count (CBC) with a differential, a basic metabolic panel (BMP), and a chest x-ray, which were performed at the LTC facility. Oxygen by nasal cannula was administered at 2 L/min, and albuterol nebulizer treatments were prescribed. After diagnostic test results were obtained, Mrs. Smith was diagnosed with a left lower lobe pneumonia and antibiotic therapy was initiated. An echocardiogram was performed. Mrs. Smith was monitored closely for signs and symptoms of worsening heart failure, which can be exacerbated by other conditions, such as pneumonia. With the appropriate and timely nursing interventions provided, Mrs. Smith's condition improved, and hospitalization was avoided. Mrs. Smith and her family were greatly relieved to have received appropriate medical care on site without having to be transferred to an acute care facility.

Direct-to-Consumer Primary Care Clinic Visit Telehealth Scenario

Tomar Lake, population 63, a small rural town on the border of two northern plains states, is the county seat for Fox County, a depressed region with fewer than 700 people. The town is known for harsh winter climate conditions and few community resources. The public school and grocery store recently closed, leaving the town with only local gas station convenience store food items. There is no healthcare available in Tomar Lake. With no viable jobs in town, most young people and families migrated to the nearest town, Coyote City (pop. 20,000), 70 miles west of town.

Mrs. Hutch is a 72-year-old widow, living alone on a fixed income in her small house in Tomar Lake. Most of her extended family migrated to Coyote City seeking employment. Mrs. Hutch's 23-year-old grandson, Ben, travels to Tomar Lake weekly to check on her and bring groceries. Mrs. Hutch does not drive and depends on Ben to take her to physician appointments in Coyote City. Feeling that she is a burden on her grandson and other family members, Mrs. Hutch often delays, and even avoids making and keeping needed follow-up blood pressure and diabetes care appointments with her PCP.

Mrs. Hutch's family recently voiced concerns about getting her to clinic visits, which have become increasingly more important as her healthcare needs have grown. Mrs. Hutch's family is asking her to sell her house in Tomar Lake and move into an assisted living facility in Coyote City. Mrs. Hutch does not want to leave her home of over 50 years, her church, and her friends in Tomar Lake. Mrs. Hutch is active in community and church activities and knows no one in the assisted living facility in Coyote City. She has become increasingly stressed over the pressure from family to relocate.

On April 11, 2020, Mrs. Hutch participated in choir practice, attended church services, and taught Sunday school. Later that week, Mrs. Hutch was notified by the health department that a local family had taken a cruise in late March and after their return home tested positive for COVID-19, the novel coronavirus that was rapidly becoming a worldwide pandemic. The family had attended the same activities that Mrs. Hutch had on Sunday and two of the children were in her Sunday school class.

Mrs. Hutch was alarmed and terrified that she may spread the virus to her grandson if he was required to drive her to the clinic. She called her PCP and explained her concerns. She was informed that the clinic was now providing virtual visits for patients and was able to add the app to her phone that was needed for the visit. After successfully logging on, Mrs. Hutch had an encounter with her PCP who completed an assessment, ordered labs, and also suggested that Mrs. Hutch use virtual visits for most of her future visits since she lived such a long distance from the clinic.

Mrs. Hutch was informed that the travel lab service would be in Tomar Lake in 2 days' time to perform testing for COVID-19 and could also draw needed blood work. Mrs. Hutch tested positive for COVID-19 but was able to remain at home and manage her symptoms with the help of her PCP and the use of virtual visits. As a result, Mrs. Hutch avoided exposing any family member or clinic staff to the coronavirus. Mrs. Hutch can now use the virtual clinic for many of her healthcare needs. Her family is pleased with the technology and feels that Mrs. Hutch may now stay in her home for many years to come.

The addition of telehealth services for primary care allowed Mrs. Hutch to access her PCP, clinic nurses, and pharmacist to discuss changes in health status and self-managed healthcare needs. With that, the direct-to-consumer telehealth services have given Mrs. Hutch the necessary human interaction with her nurse and other healthcare providers via the clinic's patient portal. With each virtual visit, Mrs. Hutch is more confident and comfortable in using the virtual system.

IMPLICATIONS OF TELEHEALTH FOR RURAL NURSING PRACTICE

Telehealth Program Implementation Considerations

The global pandemic caused by the novel coronavirus has brought to the forefront the limitations of face-to-face healthcare visits in America. Although telehealth technology has existed for several years, lack of reimbursement, tight regulations, and lack of provider education have limited the use of virtual care for consumers in the ambulatory care setting (Keesara et al., 2020).

Since promulgation of the Affordable Healthcare Act in 2010, proprietary and academic nurse-led clinics have increased in numbers due in part to increases in healthcare services demands. Telehealth services provided by nurse-led clinics are novel and growing methods of healthcare delivery systems, and provide opportunities for nurses, and other healthcare providers of multidisciplinary teams to render value-based care at reasonable cost (National University, 2016). Although the long-term impact of telehealth on healthcare costs and quality of care outcomes has yet to be realized, nurses are in a unique position to explore a variety of opportunities for delivering effective healthcare in ways that acknowledge the changing consumer landscape (Kaiser & Lee, 2015). With the development and expansion of sustainable technologies that support the delivery of tele-health primary care services, nursing practice can further expand nursing care services to rural dwellers and underserved populations.

Prior to purchasing equipment, training providers, and going live in program implementation, a precise vision for achieving strategic healthcare goals for specific rural populations must be articulated. A needs analysis can provide planners with a clear understanding of the nature and scope of unmet healthcare needs, provide a foundation for implementation, clarify objectives and shared expectations, improve coordination of services and resources, and provide support structures for program evaluation (Gough et al., 2015). Thus, the key to implementing a viable and sustainable telehealth care delivery program is thorough planning.

To deliver healthcare services using telehealth modalities, patient disclosures must be made, and mechanisms must be in place to assure adherence to regulatory and accreditation requirements, regardless of type of provider (e.g., nurse, physician). At a minimum, healthcare providers must disclose or provide (a) specific services provided; (b) provider contact information; (c) licensure and qualifications of providers and associates; (d) fees for services and how payment will be made; (e) financial interests, other than fees charged; (f) appropriate uses and limitations of the site, including emergency health situations; (g) uses and response times for emails, electronic messages, and other communications transmitted via telehealth technologies; (h) to whom patient health information may be disclosed and for what purpose; (i) rights of patients with respect to protected patient health information; and (j) information collected and any passive tracking mechanisms used (Federation of State Medical Boards, 2014).

Scope of Practice

In primary care practice settings, many conditions are amenable to telehealth intervention. Conditions most sensitive to telehealth intervention are those with a reasonable level of certainty for establishing a diagnosis and generating a treatment plan, especially when visual information coupled with access to a medical record containing diagnostic studies and imaging results is available (American Telemedicine Association, 2014). Thus, chronic disease management is commonly an integral aspect of telehealth care.

The American Academy of Ambulatory Care Nursing (AAACN) updated the scope and standards for telehealth nursing in 2018. Sixteen standards define the scope of practice for telehealth nursing incorporating current professional norms and practices and expectations of telehealth nursing. In the revised scope of practice standards, telehealth nursing is described as a practice, which is learned and requires the application of a core body of knowledge from biological, physical, and behavioral social sciences (AAACN, 2018).

Practice protocols and licensing requirements for telehealth nursing vary from state to state. In general, telehealth practice requires that nurse providers be licensed or under the jurisdiction of the state board of nursing of the state in which the patients receiving telehealth care are located. Thus, the practice of nursing occurs at the location of the patient at the time telehealth technologies are used in the delivery of healthcare services.

In 2020, telehealth practice in the United States was impacted by the global coronavirus pandemic. For example, reimbursement for telehealth services has been variable across states. As a result of the COVID-19 pandemic, however, CMS revised rules and regulations that provided parity in reimbursement for telehealth encounters; this meant that in-person and telehealth encounters would be reimbursed at the same rate, including ED, initial nursing facility and discharge, home, and therapy services. Thus, with these CMS changes, new, as well as established patients could stay at home and have a telehealth encounter with their PCP and other specialty providers (CMS, 2020).

As a result of the coronavirus pandemic, emergency protocols were enacted nationally to allow for the broader use of telehealth in providing ambulatory care. Expansions of telehealth in primary and specialty care will likely lead to continued and expanded use of telehealth as the pandemic eases and more providers and consumers become comfortable and confident in using telehealth modalities for providing and receiving healthcare services. With this, an expanded scope of practice for the provision of nursing care will be inevitable. Regardless of the type of nursing practice (e.g., clinic nurse, APRN, nurse leader, nurse educator), understanding and adhering to the scope of practice and federal and state regulations is critical to the success of implementing and sustaining telehealth nursing practice and documenting outcomes.

CONCLUSION

Telehealth nursing is one of the fastest growing areas of healthcare and has the potential to transform healthcare access, safety, and quality of healthcare for persons living in rural and frontier areas. Telehealth care trends currently shaping nursing practice include (a) transformation of the application of telehealth from increasing access to care to providing convenient sources of care, reducing unnecessary exposure to contagions, and reducing healthcare costs; (b) expansion of telehealth to address urgent care episodes and chronic conditions; and (c) migration of telehealth from hospitals to satellite clinics to homes with mobile devices (Dorsey & Topol, 2016).

Future telehealth applications are boundless. From remote primary care visits to precise monitoring and treatment of patients, nursing care via telehealth is key to serving people where they live. Chronic care management of diabetes and precise monitoring, with adjustments in the administration of insulin, for example, via electronic and virtual connections to patients' insulin pumps are possible. Telehealth technologies, including peripheral add-ons can be used to administer medications accurately and safely and to monitor untoward effects, reactions, therapeutic responses, toxicity, and incompatibilities (National Council of State Boards of Nursing, 2014). With vast and rapid changes in healthcare and healthcare technologies such as telehealth, it is imperative that nurses remain engaged and at the forefront of telehealth, as an ever-expanding care delivery system.

REFERENCES

Agency for Healthcare Research and Quality (2017). *National healthcare quality and disparities report chartbook on rural healthcare.* AHRQ Pub. No. 17(18)-0001-2-EF. https://www.ahrq.gov/sites/default/files/wysiwyg/research/findings/nhqrdr/chartbooks/qdr-ruralhealthchartbook-update.pdf

American Academy of Ambulatory Care Nursing. (2018). *Standards of practice for professional telehealth nursing.* https://www.aaacn.org/practice-resources/publications

American Telemedicine Association. (2014). *Practice guidelines & resources*. https://www.american-telemed.org/resource_categories/practice-guidelines/

Bolin, J., Bellamy, G., Ferdinand, A., Kash, B., & Helduser, J. (2015). *Rural healthy people 2020. Vol. 2.* Texas A&M Health Science Center School of Public Health, Southwest Rural Health Research Center. http://sph.tamhsc.edu/srhrc/docs/rhp2020-volume-2.pdf

Brooks, M. (2019). *Preventable deaths more common in rural America*. Medscape. https://www.medscape.com/viewarticle/920968

Callaghan, T. H., Ferdinand, A. O., Akinlotan, M., Primm, K., Lee, J. S., Macareno, B., & Bolin, J. (2020). *Healthy people 2020 progress for leading causes of death in rural and urban America: A chartbook*. https://srhrc.tamhsc.edu/docs/chartbook-march-2020.pdf

Centers for Medicare & Medicaid Services. (2020). *Medicare telemedicine health care provider fact sheet: Medicare coverage and payment of virtual services*. https://www.cms.gov/newsroom/fact-sheets/medicare-telemedicine-health-care-provider-fact-sheet

Donelin, K., Esteban, A. B., Sossong, S., Michael, C., Estrada, J. J., Cohen, A. B., Wozniak, J., & Schwamm, L. H. (2019). Patient and clinician experiences with telehealth for patient follow-up care. *American Journal of Managed Care, 25*(1), 40–44. https://www.ajmc.com/view/patient-and-clinician-experiences-with-telehealth-for-patient-followup-care

Dorsey, E. R., & Topol, E. J. (2016). State of telehealth. *New England Journal of Medicine, 375*(14), 154–161. https://doi.org/10.1056/NEJMra1601705

Fathi, J. T., Moden, H. E., & Scott, J. D. (2017). Nurses advancing telehealth services in the era of healthcare reform. *OJIN: The Online Journal of Issues in Nursing, 22*(2), Manuscript 2. https://doi.org/10.3912/OJIN.Vol22No02Man02

Federation of State Medical Boards. (2104). *Model policy for the appropriate use of telemedicine in the practice of medicine*. https://www.fsmb.org/siteassets/advocacy/policies/fsmb_telemedicine_policy.pdf

Fraiche, A. M., Eapen, Z. J., & McClellan, M. B. (2017). Moving beyond the walls of the clinic. *Journal of the American College of Cardiology: Heart Failure, 5*(4), 297–304. https://doi.org/10.1016/j.jchf.2016.11.013

Garcia, M. C., Rossen, L. M., Bastian, B., Faul, M., Dowling, N. F., Thomas, C. C., Schieb, L., Hong, Y., Yoon, P. W., & Iademarco, M. F. (2019). Potentially excess deaths from the five leading causes of death in metropolitan and nonmetropolitan counties-United States 2010–2017. *Morbidity and Mortality Weekly Report Surveillance Summaries, 68*(10), SS1–SS11. https://www.cdc.gov/mmwr/volumes/68/ss/ss6810a1.htm?s_cid=ss6810a1_w

Gough, F., Budhrani, S., Cohn, E., Dappen, A., Leenknecht, C., Lewis, B., Mulligan, D. A., Randall, D., Rheuban, K., Roberts, L., Shanahan, T. J., Webster, K., Krupinski, E. A., Bashshur, R., & Bernard, J. (2015). ATA practice guidelines for live on demand primary and urgent care. *Telehealth and e-Health, 21*(3), 233–241. https://doi.org/10.1089/tmj.2015.0008

Graves, B. A., Ford, C. D., & Mooney, K. D. (2013). Telehealth technologies for heart failure disease management in rural areas: An integrative research review. *Online Journal of Rural Nursing and Health Care, 13*(2), 56–83. https://doi.org/10.14574/ojrnhc.v13i2.282

Hofmeyer, J., Leider, J., Satorius, J., Tanenbaum, E., Basel, D., & Knudson, A. (2016). Implementation of telemedicine consultation to assess unplanned transfers in rural long-term care facilities, 2012–2015:) A pilot study. *The Journal of Post-Acute and Long-Term Care Medicine, 17*(11), 1006–1010. https://www.jamda.com/article/S1525-8610(16)30232-8/fulltext

Hong, Y., Lawrence, J., Williams, D., & Mainous, A. (2020). Population-level interest and telehealth capacity of US hospitals in response to COVID-19: Cross-sectional analysis of Google Search and National Hospital Survey Data. *JMIR Public Health Surveillance, 6*(2): e18961. https://doi.org/10.2196/18961

Jones, J. (2017). Telehealth. In J. J. Fitzpatrick & M. W. Kazer (Eds.), *Encyclopedia of nursing research eBook* (4th ed.). Springer Publishing Company.

Kaiser Family Foundation. (2020). *Health status indicators*. https://www.kff.org/state-category/health-status/?state=SD

Kaiser, L. S., & Lee, T. H. (2015). Turning value-based health care into a real business model. *Harvard Business Review*. https://www.medtronic.com/content/dam/medtronic-com/global/Corporate/Initiatives/harvard-business-review/downloads/turning-value-based-health-care-into-a-real-business-model-hbr.pdf

Keesara, S., Jonas, A., & Schulman, K. (2020). Covid-19 and health care's digital revolution. *New England Journal of Medicine, 2020, 382*: e82. https://doi.org/10.1056/NEJMp2005835

Knapp, T. R. (2016). *Legislative and policy recommendations for telehealth, telemedicine and digital healthcare delivery in the United States*. Unpublished paper. pp. 1–6.

Kusmin, L. D. (2016). Rural America at a glance. *Economic Information Bulletin No. (EIB-162)*. U.S. Department of Agriculture. https://www.ers.usda.gov/webdocs/publications/80894/eib-162.pdf?v=42684

McLendon, S. F., Wood, F. G., & Stanley, N. (2019). Enhancing diabetes care through care coordination, telemedicine, and education: Evaluation of a rural pilot program. *Public Health Nursing, 36*(17), 310–320. https://doi.org/10.1111/phn.12601

Moy, E., Garcia, M. C., Bastian, B., Rossen, L. M., Ingram, D. D., Faul, M., Massetti, G. M., Thomas, C. C., Hong, Y., Yoon, P. W., & Iademarco, M. F. (2017). Leading causes of death in nonmetropolitan and metropolitan areas—United States, 1999–2014. *Morbidity and Mortality Weekly Report Surveillance Summaries, 66*(1), SS1–SS8. http://dx.doi.org/10.15585/mmwr.ss6601a1

National Council of State Boards of Nursing. (2014). *The national council of state boards of nursing (NCSBN®) position paper on telehealth nursing practice*. https://www.ncsbn.org/3847.htm

National University. (2016). *National university nurse-managed clinic in Watts, Los Angeles collaborates with telehealth companies to expand access to virtual health care services*. https://www.nu.edu/News/Expand-Access-to-Virtual-Health-Care-Services.html

Smith, A. C., Thomas, E., Snoswell, C. E., Hayden, H., Ateev, M., Clemensen, J., & Caffery, L. J. (2020). Telehealth for global emergencies: Implications for coronavirus disease 2019) (COVID-19). *Journal of Telemedicine and Telecare, 26*(5), 309–313. https://doi.org/10.1177/1357633X20916567

Smith, C. E., Spaulding, R., Piamjariyakul, U., Werkowitch, M., Yadrich, D. M., Hooper, D., Moore, T. & Gilroy, R. (2015). mHealth clinic appointment PC tablet: Implementation, challenges and solutions. *Journal of Mobile Technology in Medicine, 4*(2), 21–32. doi:10.7309/jmtm.4.2.4. https://www.ncbi.nlm.nih.gov/pmc/articles/PMC4655176/pdf/nihms716959.pdf

Snoswell, C. L., Taylor, M. L., Comans, T. A., Smith, A. C., Gray, L. C., & Caffery, L. J. (2020). Determining if telehealth can reduce health system costs: Scoping review. *Journal of Medical Internet Research, 22*(10), e17298. https://doi.org/ 10.2196/17298: 10.2196/17298. https://www.ncbi.nlm.nih.gov/pmc/articles/PMC7605980/

Speyer, R., Denman, D., Wilkes-Gillan, S., Chen, Y., Bogaardt, H., Kim, J., Heckathorn, D., & Cordier, R. (2018). Effects of telehealth by allied health professionals and nurses in rural and remote areas: A systematic review and meta-analysis. *Journal of Rehabilitation Medicine, 50*(3), 225–235. https://doi.org/10.2340/16501977-2297

Totten, A. M., Womack, D. M., Eden, K. B., McDonagh, M. S., Griffin, J. C., Grusing, S., & Hersh, W. R. (2016). *Telehealth: Mapping the evidence for patient outcomes from systematic reviews*. Technical Brief No. 26. (Prepared by the Pacific Northwest Evidence-based Practice Center under Contract No. 290-2015-00009-I.) AHRQ Publication No.16-EHC034-EFAHRQ. https://www.ncbi.nlm.nih.gov/books/NBK379320/pdf/Bookshelf_NBK379320.pdf

United States Department of Agriculture. (2020). *State fact sheets: South Dakota*. http://www.ers.usda.gov/data-products/state-fact-sheets/state-data.aspx?StateFIPS=46&StateName=South%20Dakota#.VMk83GjF83l

van Houwelingen, C., Moerman, A., Ettema, R., Kort, H., & ten Cate, O. (2016). Competencies required for nursing telehealth activities: A Delphi study. *Nurse Education Today, 39*, 50–62. https://doi.org/10.1016/j.nedt.2015.12.025

CHAPTER 16

Emergency Medical Services on the Frontier

Lynn Jakobs

DISCUSSION TOPICS

- Think of a remote area in the United States that you have traveled to or would like to travel to. Then:
  - Locate the area's zip code utilizing an online zip code locator.
  - Access the following site www.ers.usda.gov/data-products/frontier-and-remote-area-codes/ and scroll to the 2010 EXCEL file containing zip-code level FAR codes and related data, and open it.
  - At the bottom of the page, click the tab labeled, FAR ZIP code data and you will see the list of FAR zip codes that you can group by state.
  - Try to locate the zip code for your chosen site. If your site is in a frontier designated area, it should be listed. If it is not there, it is not a frontier site. In that case, chose a zip code site that you might be interested in visiting.
  - You can also determine how remote your site is by noting the FAR level; level 4 is the most remote. You will note that there are four columns on the spreadsheet, labeled FAR 1 through FAR 4. If your site has a 1 in all columns, it qualifies as a FAR level 4. If it has a 1 in the first three columns, it qualifies as a FAR level 3, and so on. If there is a zero in one of the columns, your site does not quality for that level. For example, Nome, Alaska, is designated as a FAR level 3 site.
  - Once you have determined that your site is designated as frontier, use online resources to determine the closest hospital, and if the information is available, the type of EMS available.
  - Discuss how this information might:
    - Impact your decision to visit the area
    - Effect how you plan your trip, what you might need to bring, and so on
    - Effect who you might take with you: children, elderly parents, and so on

(continued)

(*continued*)

- Think of the circumstances surrounding your lifestyle; activities, work, family, and so on. If you lived in your chosen site (first activity), how likely would you be to volunteer for a local organization, and how much time could you commit to? What would factor into your decision?
- If were an RN, or an APRN living in a rural area, would you feel an ethical duty to help your local EMS system. If so, why?

INTRODUCTION

Imagine yourself, or a loved one, experiencing a life-threatening problem, such as severe chest pain or trauma; you dial 911, but no one answers. This is a situation that many frontier dwellers face (Jakobs, 2017, p. 73). It is also a situation that urban dwellers may face when they travel to frontier areas. Lack of access to timely and appropriate emergency medical services (EMS) was listed as the top priority by participants who responded to both the 2010 and 2020 Rural Healthy People survey (Schulze et al., 2015).

Several factors contribute to the lack of timely and appropriate rural emergency response: (a) distance, which equals time, (b) availability of EMS providers, and (c) level of training of responders and/or medical directors. Few studies that solely address EMS issues in frontier communities have been published; therefore, I included studies of rural EMS services with the knowledge that problems in rural areas are magnified in frontier areas. Due to this dearth of information regarding frontier healthcare, specifically EMS, I will include personal experiences from 17 years of nurse practitioner (NP) practice in a frontier community. In addition, this chapter addresses nursing's role regarding frontier EMS, technological advancements in EMS, and models that have been proposed to mitigate some of the problems related to provision of emergency services on the frontier.

BACKGROUND

The more rural the community, the higher the rate of injury-related hospitalizations, with rural residents 14% more likely to die from trauma-related incidents than urban residents (Jarman et al., 2016). Motor vehicle trauma (MVT) accounts for the highest number of these injuries (Coben et al., 2009; Meit et al., 2014). The fatality rate in 2016 was 2.5 times higher in rural areas than in urban areas (National Highway Traffic Safety Administration [NHTSA], 2018). This has been partly attributed to high rates of speed on country roads, as well as lower rates of seatbelt use (Garcia et al., 2017). Rural EMS intervention within 30 minutes of the MVT can improve outcomes; however, this response time may be unrealistic in frontier areas. Slow responses times may partly be responsible for a death rate of 42.6% within the first 4 hours of the crash in rural counties, compared to 21.1% in urban counties (Clark et al., 2013). A study that used the frontier and remote (FAR) taxonomy to determine the geographic setting of the MVT, found that approximately one in 15 EMS responses in the continental United States occur in FAR areas, and are more likely to involve advanced life support (ALS) care as well as on-scene death (Mueller et al., 2016).

Besides increased trauma injury rates, frontier dwellers have the same type of emergent medical problems as urban dwellers, but with more severe consequences. For example, heart disease (Singh & Siahpush, 2014), and stroke mortality (Georgakakos et al., 2020), is higher in rural areas than urban areas. The disparity in mortality has been partly related to delayed emergency response times and/or increased transport time, and the lack of an appropriate level of emergency response, that is, paramedic versus first responder (Institute of Medicine, 2007; D. Patterson et al., 2015). In the case of a life-threatening myocardial infarction, definitive treatment may be up to 2 hours away.

Urban dwellers who visit remote areas face the same disparity as frontier dwellers. Recreational activities tend to occur in frontier areas, and lead to seasonal population variations. For example, the average number of yearly visitors to Yellowstone National Park exceeds four million (National Park Service, 2020), and if you require ED services, the nearest hospital is almost 2 hours away. Besides tourism, other recreational activities in frontier areas include water sports, hiking, biking, off-highway vehicles, and camping. Urban residents who travel to remote areas for recreation may not foresee the possible need for medical care nor plan a strategy for emergent care. In my own frontier practice, I managed several toddlers who had fallen into fire pits. I also frequently managed patients with histories of controlled congestive heart failure who develop exacerbations after 36 hours or less of exposure to elevations of only 3,000 feet. I have also dealt with many vacationers who forgot to pack their medications, specifically hypertension and cardiac medications. They were surprised to learn that the closest pharmacy was 1 hour away.

TIME AND DISTANCE

Distance has been identified by providers and patients as one of the most significant barriers when seeking healthcare (Buzza et al., 2011). Longer distances, geographical obstacles, and adverse weather conditions can significantly affect EMS response or transport times (He et al., 2019). The mean EMS response times for rural ZIP codes are nearly double that of urban ZIP codes (Mell et al., 2017). In addition, EMS responders in remote areas face cellular and radio dead zones that limit communication for medical direction and provision of patient status updates (Larochelle et al., 2013).

Patients who sustain severe trauma are more likely to survive if they reach a trauma center in a timely manner (MacKenzie et al., 2006), and studies have shown that the odds of surviving a trauma-related incident are inversely related to time/distance to the nearest trauma center (Carr et al., 2017). A landmark study found that transport time to a trauma center is twice as long in rural areas compared to urban areas (Esposito et al., 1995), while a more recent study found that increased rurality was significantly related to lower access to trauma care (Carr et al., 2017). A unique variable in rural EMS situations is the potentially prolonged accident discovery and extrication time that increases with remoteness (Gonzalez et al., 2006; Peek-Asa et al., 2004). In a study of logging injuries, several reports described patients waiting hours until they were found, or EMS arriving on scene after a logger had died (Scott et al., 2019).

Distance is one of the main factors in deciding whether to use helicopter EMS (HEMS) or ground EMS to transport a trauma patient from the scene of injury to a trauma center (Stewart et al., 2011). Transport by HEMS can decrease the transport time to definitive care by greater than half (McCowan et al., 2007), and has been shown to decrease rural trauma mortality rates (Malekpour et al., 2017). In my own frontier practice, we routinely transferred patients by HEMS; this requires additional safety training for all providers involved, particularly in a *hot load* when the helicopter engines continue to run, and the blades continue to rotate.

Frontier areas also have high numbers of agriculture, forestry, and mining industries. The economies of 42% of frontier counties in the United States depend on farming, whereas another 8% depend on mining (National Center for Frontier Communities [NCFC], 2005). Along with forestry, fishing, and hunting, these industries account for the third highest rate of nonfatal occupational injuries and illnesses in private industry (Bureau of Labor Statistics, 2012). Farming injuries are predominately machine related (Kica & Rosenman, 2020), and surgical intervention is frequently required (Jawa et al., 2013). Farming and mining operations tend to cover large tracts of land, and for every 10% increase in the land area covered, EMS run times go up by an average of 0.62% (Lambert & Meyer, 2008).

Delayed transport times can adversely affect mortality related to medical problems as well. Myocardial infarction and stroke mortality increases with rurality (Singh & Siahpush, 2014). One study found that with acute myocardial infarction, a 1-minute increase in EMS response time causes an 8% decrease in survival (Wilde, 2013). Stroke mortality is 30% higher in the rural United States (Howard, 2013; Howard et al., 2017), which can partly be attributed to increased transport times. For example, one study of rural Idaho hospitals found transport delays of up to 66.7%, decreasing the time-treatment necessary for definitive stroke care (Gebhardt & Norris, 2006).

Critical access hospital (CAH) closures are affecting transport times as well. Approximately 6% of EMS agencies are hospital-based (NHTSA, 2014; D. Patterson et al., 2015), and all EMS agencies, when appropriate, transport patients to hospital EDs. Many frontier counties do not have a hospital; additionally, frontier counties without hospitals are often clustered together, compounding the distance EMS must travel from the scene to reach a hospital (Rural Health Information Hub, 2020). Hospitals in rural communities, often the closest emergency care for frontier residents, are closing at an alarming rate; 174 since 2005, and 132 since 2010 (Sheps Center for Health Services Research, n.d.). This has resulted in increased travel times for EMS, as 43% of closed hospitals are more than 15 miles to the next nearest hospital, and 15% are more than 20 miles away (Clawar et al., 2018).

RURAL AND FRONTIER EMS PROVIDERS

Availability

Seventy-five percent of rural emergency responders are volunteers, compared to just 7.5% of urban emergency responders (Williams et al., 2012). A study of 49 rural EMS agencies found that 69% face recruitment and retention problems (V. A. Freeman et al., 2009). In sparse frontier areas, recruitment efforts are further hampered due to fewer numbers of potential volunteers who are spread over wide geographic areas. Even frontier communities with an adequate number of volunteers can face problems with the availability of volunteer EMS providers due to lack of employer support for employee volunteers, and burnout (V. A. Freeman et al., 2009).

Availability of volunteer providers can vary depending on the economic structure of the frontier area. For example, in an agricultural area, volunteers may not be available during planting or harvest season (Jakobs, 2017, p. 73). The same may be true for mining or fishing areas. Workers in these industries may spend long hours on the job and have little time for volunteerism. When residents do volunteer, they may be unable to leave the job site to respond to an emergency call (V. Freeman et al., 2010).

Another issue is rural residents who commute to urban areas for work (Chandrasekhar, 2011). If these residents are also local EMS volunteers, the numbers of providers available to respond to an emergency is less during the work week. The CAH workforce is also effected as RNs are commuting out of rural areas in response to higher wages and more opportunities in urban hospitals (Johansen et al., 2018; Skillman et al., 2012), thus decreasing the potential of rural hospitals to recruit and retain a skilled nursing workforce.

For those rare frontier communities that have adequate providers to respond to a single call involving hospital transport, the community faces a possible 911 call with no one available to respond until they return. In some communities, this time of vulnerability can be as long as 6 hours (Jakobs, 2017, p. 74). The number of times a community is vulnerable increases in areas that see a population surge during tourist season (NCFC, 2006b).

The aging of frontier America not only affects the availability of frontier EMS providers, but also the number and nature of calls. Twenty-one of the 25 oldest counties in the nation are rural. Members of volunteer EMS agencies are aging too, with fewer young people to fill the gap. Since 2010, the increase in birth rate (natural change) has not matched the rate of out-migration (United States Department of Agriculture, 2015), leaving frontier communities with fewer young residents to replace older volunteers. In rural areas, the average age of volunteers tends to be older, with 45% over the age of 40 compared to 34% in urban areas (NCFC, 2006a). The aging of rural America also adds to the call volume of EMS agencies as health problems tend to increase with age, specifically falls (Coben et al., 2009). In some rural communities, 80% or more of the residents are over the age of 60 (Health Resources and Services Administration [HRSA], 2007).

LEVEL OF TRAINING

Volunteer EMS Providers

Frontier EMS agency providers may not be certified for *low-volume–high-risk* procedures, partly due to the insufficient amount of opportunities to practice them (D. Patterson et al., 2015). Disproportionate numbers of rural trauma injuries involving the central nervous system and airway have been reported (Esposito et al., 2003); these situations require advanced airway training that is beyond the scope of basic emergency medical technicians (EMTs) (NHTSA, 2019). There have been programs developed to provide EMTs with additional training to allow them to place endotracheal tubes (Pratt & Hirshberg, 2005); however, this skill takes practice to remain proficient. In my frontier community, a few of the EMTs have taken advanced training to allow them to place alternative airways, such as the Combitube, which require less practice.

Additional training takes time, and volunteer EMS providers have competing priorities for their time. Many have jobs, families, or other commitments and are reluctant to spend additional time training for situations that may rarely or never occur. EMS providers are required to recertify every 2 to 3 years, requiring many hours of instruction. Many rural volunteers have expressed concern that they cannot afford the cost of this process, both in time and dollars (HRSA, 2007). These two scenarios likely contribute to frontier EMS services having fewer providers qualified at the ALS level compared to more urban areas (Williams et al., 2012). The lack of providers with advanced certification leads to the *paramedic paradox*; paramedics are least available in frontier communities where they are most needed (Rowley, 2001).

Medical Directors

Medical direction in rural EMS has been identified as a major issue for a majority of U.S. states (Knott, 2003). With few rural and frontier EMS agencies staffed with ALS certified providers, it becomes more important to have adequate medical direction in the field. Small, isolated rural EMS agencies are twice as likely to rely on volunteer medical directors as compared to urban and large rural agencies. Additionally, nearly one in five small, isolated rural EMS agencies does not have access to medical consultation via radio, phone, or online (D. Patterson et al., 2015). Furthermore, volunteer rural EMS directors are less likely to be trained in emergency medicine, and are less likely to provide educational support functions such as continuing education (Slifkin et al., 2009). This can lead to poor patient outcomes, as agencies with paid medical directors are more likely to implement standard medical protocols for cardiac and stroke care (Greer et al., 2013).

NURSING INTEGRATION WITH RURAL AND FRONTIER EMS

Nurses play an important role in the provision of rural and frontier emergency services. One goal of the development of the CAH system was to improve EMS services in rural areas (Reif & Ricketts, 1999). The CAH workforce consists of both RNs and APRNs, such as NPs, who commonly assume the role of hospitalist and ED provider in a CAH. In the most rural hospitals, NPs may be the sole provider on-call when emergent patients present to the ED (Henderson, 2006; Nelson & Hooker, 2016; Ramirez & Cole, 2004).

The role of RNs in the provision of ED care in CAHs is a crucial one and has been expounded upon in the literature. Studies have demonstrated the *expert-generalist* nature of the role (Bushy & Bushy, 2001), the comfort level and training level of nurses who must perform advanced life-saving procedures (Broadley, 2014; Ross & Bell, 2009) and the stress associated with rural emergency nursing (Dekeseredy et al., 2019).

Without hospitals, frontier areas are more likely to have small medical clinics that utilize NPs to provide safety-net emergency treatment. There is a dearth of published information regarding the role of nursing in frontier EMS provision, most likely due the difficulty in accurately accessing this special population. Information regarding the role of NPs and their integration with frontier EMS systems, or directly with emergent patient situations, can be ferreted out of qualitative studies of frontier NP experience (Dean, 2012; Gorek, 2001; Jakobs, 2015; Lythgoe, 1999). These studies describe NPs taking x-rays of fractures, managing wounds, providing after-hours emergency care, and working with volunteer EMS agencies to provide ALS.

The isolation and lack of EMS resources causes many rural and frontier NPs to utilize their full scope of practice (Sharp, 2010). The extant evidence includes descriptions of isolated practices where NPs handle emergencies with patients of all ages (Bennett, 1981; Osborn, 1995; Rozier, 2000), as well as instances where the role requires NP to *take call* in case of emergency situations (Jakobs, 2017, pp. 82, 89, 110). Since all EMS in frontier areas is provided by volunteers, frontier NPs may rely on volunteers for manpower and backup during emergent patient situations (Jakobs, 2017, pp. 73, 104). In my own frontier experience, my partner and I were the only certified advanced cardiac life support (ACLS) responders within a 50-mile radius of the clinic, and during emergent situations would need the support of volunteer EMS providers.

The national EMS system does not recognize nurses or NPs in their taxonomy of responders (NHTSA, 2007); however, many EMS agencies do recognize mobile intensive care nurses (MICN) who function in a similar capacity to a paramedic (Nor Cal EMS, 2001; Shabazian, 1975). During my frontier NP experience, I became a certified MICN, which allowed me to integrate with the EMS system, give verbal and radio orders to the volunteers in the field, and stabilize patients at the clinic prior to transport for definitive care. EMS agencies could also benefit from the volunteerism of nurses, for example, the licensed vocational nurse at our clinic volunteered as an EMT, providing valuable assessment and intravenous access skills in the field.

TECHNOLOGICAL ADVANCEMENTS

Distance and expansive geographic EMS response areas are noted to have adverse effects on transport times. In one rural county, ambulances were outfitted with global positioning system navigation, with an increase in mean response times of 3.8 minutes (Gonzalez et al., 2009). This technology works in frontier areas as well, as it is not affected by geographic conditions (Garmin, n.d.); as long as you can see the sky, it will work.

Telemedicine is another technology that has also had an impact in the provision of EMS in rural areas. Its use in rural hospitals has improved the evaluation and management of trauma patients, allowing for more rapid transport to a tertiary center (Duchesne et al., 2008; Mohr et al., 2018). However, 46% of rural EDs do not use telemedicine and cost is the primary reason (Zachrison et al., 2020). This technology has also provided for physician assessment of potential stroke patients in the prehospital setting (Lippman et al., 2016). As promising as telemedicine appears to be, frontier areas often lack access (Jakobs, 2017, p. 75). Satellite technology has been proposed as a method to increase broadband connectivity in remote areas and may be the best option for telemedicine services in remote areas (Graziplene, 2009). The downside to this arrangement is that a frontier community must still have a broadband license, and the cost may be out of reach.

MODELS FOR RURAL/FRONTIER EMS

The increasing number of rural hospital closures has prompted an investigation into healthcare models that can preserve access to emergency care in rural and remote communities. Several models were suggested by the Medicare Payment Advisory Commission (MedPAC). One model, the Rural Free-Standing Emergency Department (RFSED) was proposed for use in the state of Georgia. This model allows hospitals that have closed, or face closure, to continue to function as rural safety nets by maintaining a fully staffed ED. However, the majority of FSEDs are found in larger, more affluent counties with just a handful in larger rural areas (Gutierrez et al., 2016). The low numbers of rural communities that have taken advantage of this program may be due to concerns over the financial viability of the model in rural areas (National Advisory Committee On Rural Health & Human Services, 2016).

A second model, the MedPAC Option 2, was targeted specifically for frontier communities (MedPAC Staff, 2015). The model was centered on the creation of a primary care clinic that would be open 8 to 12 hours a day with an adjacent ambulance service operating 24/7, creating a clinic by day and a stabilize-and-transfer model by night. Due to the need for a financial investment from the local community, as well as increased reimbursement rates from Medicare, it is unclear whether the proposal ever came to fruition.

A model for rural trauma care has also been proposed by some EMS agencies; it relies on the availability of emergency services at CAHs, many which have either closed or are in danger of closing. This model is based on the assumption that rural trauma care should not be an extension of urban trauma care, but rather rurality has unique features that preclude a one-size-fits-all approach (McSwain et al., 2012). Results of their study indicate greater than 90% of patients injured in rural communities could be treated at the local hospital, and they suggest the following: (a) local EMS systems should be taught triage criteria to determine whether or not patients can be treated locally, (b) hospital administrators should be educated as to the benefit of the model, (c) community members should be educated on the rationale for treating family and friends locally rather than transferring them to hospitals that could be hours away, and (d) trauma system registries should be utilized to ensure proper use of the trauma system.

The Centers for Medicare and Medicaid Services (CMS) is piloting a new model that was developed as a result of issues surrounding the transport of patients infected with the Coronavirus. The Emergency Triage, Treat, and Transport Model (ET3) is a 5-year payment model that will provide greater flexibility for EMS transfer or transport (CMS, 2019). Under the ET3 model, CMS will pay participating ambulance suppliers and providers to (a) transport an individual to a hospital ED, or other destinations covered under the regulations; (b) transport to an alternative destination partner, such as a primary care doctor's office or an urgent care clinic; or (c) provide treatment in place with a qualified healthcare partner, either on the scene or connected using telehealth. This model has promise for rural health clinics that, under current CMS reimbursement rules, would not be reimbursed for patients transported by ambulance from their homes to the clinic for treatment.

Paramedicine models have also been developed (O'Meara et al., 2018). Some paramedic services have invested heavily in FAR areas by establishing new ambulance stations, extending first responder programs, and employing additional clinical staff. There have been several designs proposed: (a) extended care paramedics, (b) community paramedics (CP), and (c) the Mobile Integrated Healthcare model. Of the three designs, the CP model more aptly fits the needs of FAR communities because it not only addresses emergency service needs but is flexible enough to provide other services to meet the needs of the community. These services may range from case management and home visits to vaccinations and wound care (Choi et al., 2016; D. G. Patterson et al., 2016). The major barriers to these proposed models are the scope of practice issues and reimbursement structures.

DISCUSSION

The results of Rural Healthy People 2010 and 2020 indicate that there is a significant disparity regarding access to the provision of safety-net emergency services in the frontier. Results of multiple studies demonstrate how distance, availability of appropriate EMS response, and adequate medical direction contribute to the problem. Additionally, the increasing number of CAH closures has an indirect negative effect on frontier EMS provision related to increased transport times.

Models to both improve and preserve access to EMS in rural and frontier areas have been proposed. Models that are more appropriate for frontier areas rely on an ongoing investment of funds from government agencies and local communities. Half of frontier communities have a higher poverty rate than the U.S. average (NCFC, 2012); therefore, it is unlikely that EMS models can be funded by residents. For this reason, paramedicine models are also unlikely to sustain themselves in frontier areas.

APRNs may provide the best overall solution for frontier communities. The Rural Health Clinic Services Act of 1977 authorized Medicare and Medicaid payment to qualified rural clinics for services provided by APRNs and promoted their use by mandating that at least 50% of the services in rural health clinics be provided by APRNs or physician assistants. This has since been revised to state that the rural health clinic must utilize the services of a physician's assistant, NP, or certified nurse midwife for at least 50% of the time the clinic is providing services (Rural Health Information Hub, 2021). The MedPAC option 2 model has similarities to a rural health clinic that, if staffed with an MICN, may provide ALS services and oversight for a local volunteer ambulance service. Financial viability of the clinic-by-day could be provided primarily by reimbursement for medical services, whereas viability of the stabilize-by-night would be supported by government funding, as proposed by MedPAC. Unlike the proposed paramedicine models, this model does not require a change in the scope of practice for NPs.

CONCLUSION

The provision of frontier EMS is complex and depends on many interrelated factors. Fostering the development of a culture of volunteerism and community service is important (HRSA, 2007); however, frontier areas often lack an adequate pool of potential volunteers. The federal government has proposed models that are flexible enough to meet the unique needs of remote communities.

It is important to note that frontier communities have unique characteristics that distinguish them from rural or urban communities; as well as from each other. Nurses embedded in these communities can play an integral part in the solution to EMS access in frontier areas.

REFERENCES

Bennett, M. (1981). *The rural family nurse practitioner: The quest for a role identity*. (Publication No. 303146652) [Doctoral dissertation, The University of New Mexico]. ProQuest Dissertations and Theses Global.

Broadley, A. (2014). *Evaluating nurses' comfort level with emergency situations in the critical access hospital setting: A partial replication study*. (Publication No. 1558183724) [Master's thesis, University of California, Davis]. ProQuest Dissertations and Theses Global.

Bureau of Labor Statistics. (2012). *Incidence rates and numbers of nonfatal occupational injuries and illnesses by private industry sector, 2010*. https://www.bls.gov/iif/oshwc/osh/os/osch0044.pdf

Bushy, A., & Bushy, A. (2001). Critical access hospitals: Rural nursing issues. *JONA: The Journal of Nursing Administration, 31*(6), 301–310. https://doi.org/10.1097/00005110-200106000-00008

Buzza, C., Ono, S. S., Turvey, C., Wittrock, S., Noble, M., Reddy, G., Kaboli, P., Reisinger, H. S. (2011). Distance is relative: Unpacking a principal barrier in rural healthcare. *Journal of General Internal Medicine, 26*(2), 648. https://doi.org/10.1007/s11606-011-1762-1

Carr, B., Bowman, A., Wolff, M., Mullen, M., Holena, D., Branas, C., & Wiebe, D. (2017). Disparities in access to trauma care in the United States: A population-based analysis. *Injury Prevention, 48*(2), 332–338. https://doi.org/:10.1016/j.injuiry.2017.01.008

Centers for Medicare & Medicaid Services. (2019). *Emergency triage, treat, and transport (ET3) model*. https://innovation.cms.gov/innovation-models/et3

Chandrasekhar, S. (2011). Workers commuting between the rural and urban: Estimates from NSSO data. *Economic and Political Weekly*, *46*, 22–25.

Choi, B. Y., Blumberg, C., & Williams, K. (2016). Mobile integrated health care and community paramedicine: an emerging emergency medical services concept. *Annals of Emergency Medicine*, *67*(3), 361–366. https://doi.org/10.1016/j.annemergmed.2015.06.005

Clark, D. E., Winchell, R. J., & Betensky, R. A. (2013). Estimating the effect of emergency care on early survival after traffic crashes. *Accident Analysis & Prevention*, *60*, 141–147. https://doi.org/10.1016/j.aap.2013.08.019

Clawar, M., Thompson, K., & Pink, G. (2018). *Range matters: Rural averages can conceal important information*. University of North Carolina at Chapel Hill, Sheps Center for Health Services Research.

Coben, J. H., Tiesman, H. M., Bossarte, R. M., & Furbee, P. M. (2009). Rural–urban differences in injury hospitalizations in the U.S., 2004. *American Journal of Preventive Medicine*, *36*(1), 49–55. http://dx.doi.org/10.1016/j.amepre.2008.10.001

Dean, E. (2012). In splendid isolation. *Nursing Standard*, *26*(46), 18–20. https://doi.org/10.1093/nq%2Fs11-v.123.348i

Dekeseredy, P., Kurtz Landy, C. M., & Sedney, C. L. (2019). An exploration of work related stressors experienced by rural emergency nurses. *Online Journal of Rural Nursing & Health Care*, *19*(2), 2–24. https://doi.org/10.14574/ojrnhc.v19i2.550

Duchesne, J. C., Kyle, A., Simmons, J., Islam, S., Schmieg Jr, R. E., Olivier, J., & McSwain Jr, N. E. (2008). Impact of telemedicine upon rural trauma care. *Journal of Trauma and Acute Care Surgery*, *64*(1), 92–98. https://doi.org/10.1097/ta.0b013e31815dd4c4

Esposito, T., Maier, R., Rivera, F., Griffith, J., Lazear, S., & Hogan, S. (1995). The impact of variation in trauma care times: urban versus rural. *Prehospital Disaster Medicine*, *10*(3), 161–166. https://doi.org/10.1017/S1049023X00041947

Esposito, T., Sanddal, T., Reynolds, S., & Sanddal, N. (2003). Effect of a voluntary trauma system on preventable death and inappropriate care in a rural state. *Journal of Trauma and Acute Care Surgery*, *54*(4), 663–670. https://doi.org10.1097/01.TA.0000058124.78958.6B

Freeman, V. A., Slifkin, R. T., & Patterson, P. D. (2009). Recruitment and retention in rural and urban EMS: results from a national survey of local EMS directors. *Journal of Public Health Management and Practice*, *15*(3), 246–252. https://doi.org/10.1097/phh.0b013e3181a117fc

Freeman, V., Rutledge, S., Hamon, M., & Slifkin, R. (2010). *Rural volunter EMS: Reports from the field* (N. R. H. R. a. P. A. Center, Trans.). Office of Rural Health Policy, Health Resources and Services Administration.

Garcia, M. C., Faul, M., Massetti, G., Thomas, C. C., Hong, Y., Bauer, U. E., & Iademarco, M. F. (2017). Reducing potentially excess deaths from the five leading causes of death in the rural United States. *MMWR Surveillance Summaries*, *66*(2), 1. https://www.cdc.gov/mmwr/volumes/66/ss/ss6602a1.htm

Garmin. (n.d.). *What is GPS?*. https://www.garmin.com/en-US/aboutGPS/

Gebhardt, J. G., & Norris, T. E. (2006). Acute stroke care at rural hospitals in Idaho: Challenges in expediting stroke care. *The Journal of Rural Health*, *22*(1), 88–91. https://doi.org/10.1111/j.1748-0361.2006.00004.x

Georgakakos, P., Swanson, M., Ahmed, A., & Mohr, N. M. (2020). Rural stroke patients have higher mortality: An improvement opportunity for rural emergency medical services systems. *The Journal of Rural Health*. https://doi.org/10.1111/jrh.12502

Gonzalez, R. P., Cummings, G. R., Mulekar, M. S., Harlan, S. M., & Rodning, C. B. (2009). Improving rural emergency medical service response time with global positioning system navigation. *Journal of Trauma and Acute Care Surgery*, *67*(5), 899–902. https://doi.org/10.1097/ta.0b013e3181bc781d

Gonzalez, R. P., Cummings, G. R., Mulekar, M. S., & Rodning, C. B. (2006). Increased mortality in rural vehicular trauma: Identifying contributing factors through data linkage. *Journal of Trauma*, *61*(2), 404–409. https://doi.org/10.1097/01.ta.0000229816.16305.94

Gorek, B. (2001). Nurse practitioners in rural settings. *Geriatric Nursing*, *22*(5), 263–264. https://doi-org.proxybz.lib.montana.edu/10.1067/mgn.2001.119478

Graziplene, L. R. (2009). *Creating telemedicine-based medical networks for rural and frontier areas*. http://businessofgovernment.org/sites/default/files/Creating%20telemedicine-based%20medicalpdf.pdf

Greer, S., Williams, I., Valderrama, A. L., Bolton, P., Patterson, D. G., & Zhang, Z. (2013). EMS medical direction and prehospital practices for acute cardiovascular events. *Prehospital Emergency Care*, *17*(1), 38–45. https://doi.org/10.3109/10903127.2012.710718

Gutierrez, C., Lindor, R. A., Baker, O., Cutler, D., & Schuur, J. D. (2016). State regulation of freestanding emergency departments varies widely, affecting location, growth, and services provided. *Health Affairs*, *35*(10), 1857–1866. https://doi.org/10.1377/hlthaff.2016.0412

He, Z., Qin, X., Renger, R., & Souvannasacd, E. (2019). Using spatial regression methods to evaluate rural emergency medical services (EMS). *The American Journal of Emergency Medicine*, *37*(9), 1633–1642. https://doi.org/10.1016/j.ajem.2018.11.029

Health Resources and Services Administration. (2007). *Rural and frontier EMS town hall meeting summary*. https://www.ruralhealthinfo.org/assets/277-537/rural-frontier-ems-town-hall.pdf

Henderson, K. (2006). TelEmergency: Distance emergency care in rural emergency departments using nurse practitioners. *Journal of Emergency Nursing*, *32*(5), 388–393. https://doi.org/10.1016/j.jen.2006.05.022

Howard, G. (2013). Ancel Keys lecture: Adventures (and misadventures) in understanding (and reducing) disparities in stroke mortality. *Stroke*, *44*(11), 3254–3259. https://doi.org/10.1161/strokeaha.113.002113

Howard, G., Kleindorfer, D. O., Cushman, M., Long, D. L., Jasne, A., Judd, S. E., Higginbotham, J. C., & Howard, V. J. (2017). Contributors to the excess stroke mortality in rural areas in the United States. *Stroke*, *48*(7), 1773–1778. https://doi.org/10.1161/STROKEAHA.117.017089

Institute of Medicine. (2007). *Emergency medical services: At the crossroads*. National Academies Press.

Jakobs, L. (2015). *Voices from the frontier: Stories of nurse practitioners working in remote settings*. (Publication No. 1700208880) [Doctorate Dissertation, University of North Dakota]. ProQuest Dissertations and Theses Global.

Jakobs, L. (2017). *The frontier nurse practitioner: A conceptual model for remote-rural practice*. Springer Publishing Company. http://doi.org/10.1891/9780826169129

Jarman, M. P., Castillo, R. C., Carlini, A. R., Kodadek, L. M., & Haider, A. H. (2016). Rural risk: geographic disparities in trauma mortality. *Surgery*, *160*(6), 1551–1559. https://doi.org/10.1016/j.surg.2016.06.020

Jawa, R. S., Young, D. H., Stothert, J. C., Yetter, D., Dumond, R., Shostrom, V. K., Cemaj, S., Rautiainen, R. H., & Mercer, D. W. (2013). Farm machinery injuries: The 15-year experience at an urban joint trauma center system in a rural state. *Journal of Agromedicine*, *18*(2), 98–106. https://doi.org/10.1080/1059924X.2013.766145

Johansen, L. J., Evanson, T. A., Ralph, J. L., Hunter, C., & Hart, G. (2018). Experiences of rural nurses who commute to larger communities. *Online Journal of Rural Nursing & Health Care*, *18*(2), 224–264. https://doi.org/10.14574/ojrnhc.v18i2.540

Kica, J., & Rosenman, K. D. (2020). Multisource surveillance for non-fatal work-related agricultural injuries. *Journal of agromedicine*, *25*(1), 86–95. https://doi.org/10.1080%2F1059924X.2019.1606746

Knott, A. (2003). Emergency medical services in rural areas: The supporting role of state EMS agencies. *The Journal of Rural Health*, *19*(4), 492–496. https://doi.org/10.1111/j.1748-0361.2003.tb00587.x

Lambert, T. E., & Meyer, P. B. (2008). New and fringe residential development and emergency medical services response times in the United States. *State and Local Government Review*, *40*(2), 115–124. https://doi.org/10.1177%2F0160323X0804000205

Larochelle, N., O'Keefe, M., Wolfson, D., & Freeman, K. (2013). Cellular technology improves transmission success of pre-hospital electrocardiograms. *The American Journal of Emergency Medicine*, *31*(11), 1564–1570. https://doi.org/10.1016/j.ajem.2013.07.032

Lippman, J. M., Smith, S. N. C., McMurry, T. L., Sutton, Z. G., Gunnell, B. S., Cote, J., Perina, D. G., Cattell-Gorden, D. C., Rheuban, K. S., Worrall, B. B., Southerland, A. M., & Solenski, N. J. (2016). Mobile telestroke during ambulance transport is feasible in a rural EMS setting: The iTREAT Study. *Telemedicine and e-Health*, *22*(6), 507–513. https://doi.org/10.1089/tmj.2015.0155

Lythgoe, A. M. (1999). *Transitions: The nurse practitioner as primary care provider in the frontier setting*. (Publication No. 304556127) [Master's thesis,] Gonzaga University]. ProQuest Dissertations and Theses Global.

MacKenzie, E., Rivara, F., Jurkovich, G., Nathens, A. F. K., Egleston, B., Salkever, D., & Scharfstein, D. (2006). A national evaluation of the effect of trauma-center care on Mortality. *New England Journal of Medicine*, *354*(4), 366–378. https://doi.org/10.1056/nejmsa052049

Malekpour, M., Younus, J. M., Jaap, K., Neuhaus, N., Widom, K., Rapp, M., Dove, J., Hunsinger, M., Blansfield, J., Shabahang, M., Torres, D., & Wild, J. (2017). Mode of transport and clinical outcome in rural trauma: A helicopter versus ambulance comparison. *The American Surgeon, 83*(12), 1413–1417.

McCowan, C. L., Swanson, E. R., Thomas, F., & Handrahan, D. L. (2007). Outcomes of blunt trauma victims transported by HEMS from rural and urban scenes. *Prehospital Emergency Care, 11*(4), 383–388. https://doi.org/10.1080/10903120701536867

McSwain, N., Totondo, M., Meade, P., & Duchesne, J. (2012). A model for rural trauma Care. *British Journal of Surgery, 99*(3), 309–314. https://doi.org/10.1002/bjs.7734

MedPA Staff. (2015). *Models for preserving access to emergency care in rural areas.* http://medpac.gov/-blog-/medpacblog/2015/11/24/models-for-preserving-access-to-emergency-care-in-rural-areas

Meit, M., Knudson, A., Gilbert, T., Yu, A. T.-C., Tanenbaum, E., Ormson, E., & Popat, S. (2014). The *2014 update of the rural-urban chartbook.* Rural Health Reform Policy Research Center. https://norc.org/PDFs/Walsh Center/Rural health US Report_Oct2014_dtp.pdf

Mell, H. K., Mumma, S. N., Hiestand, B., Carr, B. G., Holland, T., & Stopyra, J. (2017). Emergency medical services response times in rural, suburban, and urban areas. *JAMA Surgery, 152*(10), 983–984. https://doi.org/10.1001/jamasurg.2017.2230

Mohr, N. M., Young, T., Harland, K. K., Skow, B., Wittrock, A., Bell, A., & Ward, M. M. (2018). Emergency department telemedicine shortens rural time-to-provider and emergency department transfer times. *Telemedicine and e-Health, 24*(8), 582–593. https://doi.org/10.1089/tmj.2017.0262

Mueller, L., Donnelly, J., Jacobson, K., Carlson, J., Mann, C., & Wang, H. (2016). National characteristics of emergency medical services in frontier and remote areas. *Prehospital Emergency Care, 20*(2), 191–199. https://dx.doi.org/10.3109%2F10903127.2015.1086846

National Advisory Committee On Rural Health & Human Services. (2016). *Alternative models to preserving access to emergency care.* https://www.hrsa.gov/sites/default/files/hrsa/advisory-committees/rural/publications/2016-emergency-care.pdf

National Center for Frontier Communities. (2005). *Economic dependence2004 ERS county typology: Frontier education center.* http://frontierus.org/wp-content/uploads/2019/10/Economic-Dependence_Frontier-and-Remote-Map-2004.pdf

National Center for Frontier Communities. (2006a). *Emergency medical services in frontier areas: Volunteer community organizations: Rural Health Information Hub.* http://frontierus.org/wp-content/uploads/2019/10/EmergencyMedicalServicesFrontierAreas.pdf

National Center for Frontier Communities. (2006b). *Impact of seasonal population variations on frontier communities: Maintenance of the healthcare infrastructure: Rural health information hub.* http://frontierus.org/wp-content/uploads/2019/10/SeasonalPopVariations-FrontierCommunities2006.pdf

National Highway Traffic Safety Administration. (2014). *EMS system demographics.* US Department of Transportation. https://www.ems.gov/pdf/National_EMS_Assessment_Demographics_2011.pdf

National Highway Traffic Safety Administration. (2018). *Traffic safety facts: 2016 data.* Rural / urbancomparison of traffic fatalities. https://crashstats.nhtsa.dot.gov/Api/Public/ViewPublication/812521#:~:text=However%2C%20rural%20areas%20accounted%20for,all%20traffic%20fatalities%20in%202016.&text=Rural%20traffic%20fatalities%20decreased%20by,2007%20to%2017%2C656%20in%202016.

National Highway Traffic Safety Administration. (2019). *National EMS scope of practice model: Including change notices 1.0 and 2.0: National highway traffic safety administration.* US Department of Transportation. https://www.ems.gov/pdf/2017-National-EMS-Scope-Practice-Mode_Change-Notices-1-and-2.pdf

National Park Service. (2020). *Visitation statistics.* https://www.nps.gov/yell/planyourvisit/visitation-stats.htm

Nelson, S. C., & Hooker, R. S. (2016). Physician assistants and nurse practitioners in rural Washington emergency departments. *The Journal of Physician Assistant Education, 27*(2), 56–62. https://doi.org/10.1097/jpa.0000000000000074

Nor Cal EMS. (2001). *MICN scope of practice.* https://www.norcalems.org/pnp-manual/master-binder/04-ALS_PROTOCOLS/04-2000-MICN_Standardized_Procedures/04-2001-MICN_Scope_of_Practice.pdf

O'Meara, P., Wingrove, G., & Nolan, M. (2018). Frontier and remote paramedicine practitioner models. *Rural and Remote Health, 18*(3), 4550. https://doi.org/10.22605/RRH4550

Osborn M. (1995). Marie osborn: Rural health care nurse practitioner. *Interview by Maryann T Hardesty. Nurse practitioner Forum, 6*(3), 131–132.

Patterson, D. G., Coulthard, C., Garberson, L. A., Wingrove, G., & Larson, E. H. (2016). What is the potential of community paramedicine to fill rural health care gaps? *Journal of Health Care for the Poor and Underserved, 27*(4), 144–158. https://doi.org/10.1353/hpu.2016.0192

Patterson, D., Skillman, S., & Fordyce, M. (2015). *Prehospital emergency medical services personnel in rural areas: Results from a survey in nine states.* WWAMI Rural Health Research Center, University of Washington

Peek-Asa, C., Zwerling, C., & Stallones, L. (2004). Acute traumatic injuries in rural populations. *American Journal of Public Health, 94*(10), 1689–1693. https://dx.doi.org/10.2105%2Fajph.94.10.1689

Pratt, J. C., & Hirshberg, A. J. (2005). Endotracheal tube placement by EMT-Basics in a rural EMS system. *Prehospital Emergency Care, 9*(2), 172–175. https://doi.org/10.1080/10903120590924564

Ramirez, E. G., & Cole, F. L. (2004). Preparing for clinical NP practice in an emergency care setting. *Journal of Emergency Nursing, 30*(2), 176–178. https://doi.org/10.1016/j.jen.2004.02.006

Reif, S. S., & Ricketts, T. C. (1999). The Medicare critical access hospital program: The first year. *The Journal of Rural Health, 15*(1), 61–66. https://doi.org/10.1111/j.1748-0361.1999.tb00599.x

Ross, E. L., & Bell, S. E. (2009). Nurses' comfort level with emergency interventions in the rural hospital setting. *The Journal of Rural Health, 25*(3), 296–302. https://doi.org/10.1111/j.1748-0361.2009.00233.x

Rowley, T. (2001). Solving the paramedic paradox. *Rural Health News, 8*(3), 1–6.

Rozier, L. (2000). The rural nurse practitioner. In J. Hickey, R. Ouimette, & S. L. Venegoni (Ed.), *Advanced practice nursing: Changing roles and clinical applications* (2nd ed.). Lippincott.

Rural Health Information Hub. (2021). *Health and healthcare in frontier areas.* https://www.ruralhealth-info.org/topics/frontier

Schulze, A., Bolin, J., & Radcliff, T. (2015). Rural access to quality emergency services. In J. Bolin, G. Bellamy, A. Ferdinand, A. M. Vuong, B. A. Kash, A. Schulze, & J. W. Helduser (Eds.), *Rural healty people 2020.* (Vol. 1., pp. 25–32). The Texas A&M University Health Science Center, School of Public Health, Southwest Rural Health Research Center.

Scott, E., Hirabayashi, L., Krupa, N., & Jenkins, P. (2019). Emergency medical services pre-hospital care reports as a data source for logging injury surveillance. *Journal of Agromedicine, 24*(2), 133–137. https://doi.org/10.1080/1059924x.2019.1572558

Shabazian, D. (1975). Mobile intensive care unit nurse. *Journal of Emergency Nursing, 1*(4), 20.

Sharp, D. (2010). *Factors related to the recruitment and retention of nurse practitioners in rural areas.* Doctoral Dissertation, University of Texas at El Paso. ProQuest Dissertations & Theses Global: The Sciences and Engineering Collection database.

Sheps Center for Health Services Research. (n.d.). *174 rural hospital closures: January 2005–Present (132 since 2010).* https://www.shepscenter.unc.edu/programs-projects/rural-health/rural-hospital-closures/

Singh, G., & Siahpush, M. (2014). Widening rural–urban disparities in all-cause mortality and mortality from major causes of death in the USA, 1969–2009. *Journal of Urban Health, 91*(2), 272–292. https://doi.org/10.1007/s11524-013-9847-2

Skillman, S. M., Palazzo, L., Doescher, M., & Butterfield, P. (2012). Characteristics of rural RNs who live and work in different communities *WWAMI Rural Health Research Center, Final Report# 133.*

Slifkin, R. T., Freeman, V. A., & Patterson, P. D. (2009). Designated medical directors for emergency medical services: Recruitment and roles. *The Journal of Rural Health, 25*(4), 392–398. https://doi.org/10.1111/j.1748-0361.2009.00250.x

Stewart, K. E., Cowan, L. D., Thompson, D. M., & Sacra, J. C. (2011). Factors at the scene of injury associated with air versus ground transport to definitive care in a state with a large rural population. *Prehospital Emergency Care, 15*(2), 193–202. https://doi.org/10.3109/10903127.2010.541979

United States Department of Agriculture. (2015). *Rural America at a glance, 2015 edition.* (Economic Information Bulletin 145). United States Department of Agriculture. https://www.ers.usda.gov/publications/pub-details/?pubid=44016

Wilde, E. T. (2013). Do emergency medical system response times matter for health outcomes? *Health Economics*, 22(7), 790–806. https://doi.org/10.1002/hec.2851

Williams, I., Valderrama, A. L., Bolton, P., Greek, A., Greer, S., Patterson, D. G., & Zhang, Z. (2012). Factors associated with emergency medical services scope of practice for acute cardiovascular events. *Prehospital Emergency Care*, 16(2), 189–197. https://doi.org/10.3109/10903127.2011.615008

Zachrison, K. S., Boggs, K. M., Hayden, E. M., Espinola, J. A., & Camargo, C. A. Jr (2020). Understanding barriers to telemedicine implementation in rural emergency departments. *Annals of Emergency Medicine*, 75(3), 392–399. https://doi.org/10.1016/j.annemergmed.2019.06.026

CHAPTER 17

Palliative Care for the Rural Chronically Ill

JANE A. SCHANTZ

DISCUSSION TOPICS

- Many rural healthcare centers are staffed by generalists who do a wide variety of types of care in their daily work. Given this, what do you think is the best way for generalists to provide high-quality palliative care (PC) to their patients?
- Describe the differences and similarities between PC and hospice.
- Interdisciplinary teams (IDTs) typically consist of doctors, nurses, social workers, and chaplains. Why do you think this is important in PC? Where do these roles differ or overlap?

INTRODUCTION

Palliative care (PC; also known as palliative medicine) has come into its own as a medical specialty, primarily for adults with serious, life-threatening, and/or chronic illness. For many years, PC has been thought to be synonymous with end-of-life (EOL) care and hospice. But in the past decade, national organizations such as the Center to Advance Palliative Care (CAPC), the National Hospice and Palliative Care Organization, Hospice and Palliative Nurses Association, and American Academy of Hospice and Palliative Care have worked hard to distinguish and define palliative medicine in its own right, and to promote its establishment within the larger healthcare system. Although there remains a fair amount of misunderstanding among the general public and even the medical community as to what it is, "PC" is now a phrase with which many American adults are at least familiar, as it is a topic that is currently popular in the media. Typically, PC is described as being an umbrella specialty, within which EOL care and hospice reside. Both PC and hospice emphasize a palliative approach to symptom management and an interprofessional, team-based, holistic model of individualized care that focuses both on the patient and their loved ones. But increasingly there is an effort to separate the terms "PC" and "hospice," as PC matures as a field of medicine. This comes in part to dispel the common misunderstanding that "PC" is simply coded language for EOL care.

The purpose of this chapter is to report on the state of PC in rural settings, comparing it to what is assumed to be the standard, PC in urban/suburban settings. A case study will illustrate the need for home-based PC services for chronically but not yet terminally ill patients. We look at the most commonly identified challenges for rural PC, as well as strengths and recommendations for future programs.

PALLIATIVE CARE IN RURAL SETTINGS

In the United States, hospice services are regulated by Medicare, which defines eligibility as requiring a terminal diagnosis with a life expectancy of 6 months or fewer if the illness runs its expected course (Centers for Medicare & Medicaid Services, 2015, p. 3). In order to receive hospice, the patient must agree to forgo all curative treatment for the hospice diagnosis and any secondary diagnoses contributing to the patient's terminal prognosis. Conversely, PC is offered regardless of prognosis.

PC is defined as specialized medical and supportive care for people living with serious illness. As an interdisciplinary, holistic model of care, it focuses on relief of physical symptoms and the stresses associated with serious illness. Provided by a team of specially trained physicians, nurses, social workers, and others, the goal is to improve quality of life for the patient and the family. PC is offered at any stage in a serious illness, for persons of any age, and can be provided along with curative treatment.

PC is of special interest to nurses. Nurses have always played a key role in PC, as the patient-centered, holistic model is essentially the nursing model itself, and nurses are the central providers of hospice care.

Hospital-Based Palliative Care

Whether in urban, suburban, or rural settings, PC is most commonly practiced in the inpatient, acute care environment. Inpatient PC consultation is frequently sought amid an acute-on-chronic health crisis and usually focuses on one or more of the following: emotional support, symptom management, discussion of prognosis and goals of care, healthcare literacy and decision-making, advance directives, patient and family communication and coping, resource utilization, spiritual concerns, care coordination across levels of care, and/or EOL care and bereavement (Manfredi et al., 2000; Quill, 2015). These interventions have been repeatedly shown to increase patient and family satisfaction and well-being. They have also been shown to decrease healthcare costs at the EOL through improved symptom management, clarified goals of care, and shortened length of stay, as well as fewer hospital readmissions, ED visits, and emergent hospitalizations (Armstrong et al., 2013; Durie & Tanksley-Bowe, 2018; McGrath et al., 2013; Meier & Sieger, 2015; Wachterman et al., 2016). One landmark study showed cost savings of as much as $1,700 per admission for those who survived to discharge and $4,900 per admission for those who died while hospitalized (Morrison et al., 2008). These benefits have been demonstrated in both urban and rural hospitals. Durie and Tanksley-Bowe (2018) did a comparison of six hospitals within one rural region in Pennsylvania. Three hospitals had PC programs and three did not. The authors found that readmission rates were higher in the hospitals without PC programs than those that offered PC (71.6% vs. 55.1%, respectively).

At its 2015 national conference, CAPC declared, *mission accomplished* in reference to inpatient PC service penetration in hospitals across the United States. Indeed, between 2009 and 2015, the availability of hospital-based PC services increased by 78% nationally.

By 2019, 72% of U.S. hospitals with 50 or more beds reported having a PC team (Morrison & Meier, 2019). For rural hospitals, however, this declaration appears to be premature.

Approximately 51 million people live in the rural United States and depend on their community hospitals (American Hospital Association, 2015). In their state-by-state report card for 2019, CAPC reported that in sole community provider (SCP) hospitals only 40% reported PC programs. (SCP hospitals are by definition 35 miles or more from the nearest hospital and/or the sole providers of healthcare in a region.) In rural hospitals with 50 or more beds, the statistics are even worse—only 17% reported having a PC program. The availability of PC varied by state and by region. New England had the highest penetration at 92.3%, which is not surprising given the proximity to multiple major hospitals and academic medical centers. The east south central region had the poorest penetration, at 48.2% (Morrison & Meier, 2019). Critical access hospitals have fewer than 25 beds and a very small census mean of just over four patients per day. In these hospitals, which number more than 1,300 in the United States, PC programs are rare (Mayer & Winters, 2016). Issues such as low patient volumes and geographic isolation make it difficult to offer a variety of subspecialties (American Hospital Association, 2019).

In one study to assess rural PC needs, researchers surveyed 236 hospitals in seven Rocky Mountain states (Fink et al., 2013). The authors found significant barriers to providing PC, including lack of access to PC resources, lack of administrative support, lack of training and mentorship, and lack of basic knowledge about PC practice. They also found confusion as to the difference between PC and hospice. Although there was interest in professional development, distance, lack of time, and lack of coverage were all identified as additional barriers. These themes were repeated in studies of outpatient PC programs (Bakitas et al., 2015; Evans et al., 2003; Keim-Malpass et al., 2015; Leadbeater & Staton, 2014; Robinson et al., 2009, 2010).

Unfortunately, rural hospitals are closing at an increasing rate. According to the American Hospitals Association's *Rural Report* (2019), at least 95 rural hospitals closed in the past 10 years, and between 2005 and 2016 there were 380 mergers of rural hospitals. The impact of these closures on existing rural PC programs is unknown and requires further study. In the environment of ever-increasing budgetary pressures on small hospitals, the fact that PC programs are not income-generating but rather cost-saving makes them vulnerable to budget cuts.

Outpatient and Home-Based Palliative Care

Although successes in increased PC utilization in hospitals deserve celebration, many clinicians recognize that inpatient PC consultation, which is still too often employed only for EOL concerns, is akin to closing the barn door after the horses have escaped. Earlier intervention through outpatient and home-based PC services may prevent acute hospitalization. And for those patients who do receive early PC referral, the benefits of inpatient consultation may be amplified by ongoing outpatient support and home-based services to maintain effective symptom and chronic illness management, and to prevent unnecessary rehospitalization. The focus of national PC leaders has turned to applying the PC model to the management of chronic illness through outpatient and home-based PC services.

Rogers and Dumanovsky (2017) found that the majority of PC inpatients fell into one of four top diagnosis groups: 8% had neurologic disease, 12% had pulmonary disease, 13% had cardiac disease, and 26% had cancer. These categories represent diseases that often have a high degree of symptom burden over a prolonged period, well before the last 6 months of life. Pain, dyspnea, fatigue, weakness, dehydration, nausea, constipation, and other symptoms are common and can be disabling in advanced illness. Patient and family functional status can be significantly impaired without proper treatment and support. Outpatient and home-based PC services are aimed at effectively monitoring and treating patients with advanced chronic illness, reducing acute symptoms and exacerbations, supporting patient and family coping, facilitating access to resources, and smoothing transitions between care settings (Brumley, 2007; Davis et al., 2015; Twaddle & McCormick, 2016). The following case study illustrates the need for home-based PC services.

CASE STUDY

Horace (85) and Ida (83) Gregson (not their real names) had been married 65 years. He was a veteran and had worked in banking until his retirement and they had traveled the world together. Horace and Ida lived in their own modest split-level home. They had two adult children, both of whom lived several states away. Horace was admitted to hospice after an acute hospitalization for congestive heart failure (CHF). He had secondary diagnoses of cardiovascular disease with intermittent angina, chronic asthma, and macular degeneration, which had left him legally blind and unable to drive. Ida was able to care for him despite her moderately severe arthritis and her mild dementia. Horace was a proud man who did not like to be dependent on anyone, did not want to use oxygen, and insisted on continuing with certain routines such as fetching the mail and shoveling snow. He and Ida were resistant to home hospice at first but grew to be very fond of their hospice nurse, their home health aide, and the volunteer who drove them to get groceries and to the library for audiobooks.

The hospice nurse assessed Horace during weekly visits and worked with his physician to adjust medications for anginal pain, edema, hypertension, dyspnea, and a recurrent cellulitis on Horace's leg. The home health aide spent an hour a day for 5 days a week to assist Horace with showering and do some light housekeeping. Over time, Horace's symptoms of CHF stabilized, and it became increasingly clear he was not going to continue to qualify for hospice services. But Ida's dementia was worsening and her ability to care for Horace was inconsistent. The hospice team did not feel it was safe to discharge Horace from hospice services. Working within Medicare regulations, they found a way to recertify him for another benefit period, but at the end of that period, he had to be discharged. Horace and Ida hired some help with housecleaning twice a week but were unwilling to hire strangers for home healthcare. Within 6 weeks of discharge, Horace was taken to the ED after a fall at home. Following his hospital admission where he was given intravenous fluids, he was again referred to hospice in acute heart failure. Horace's hospice nurse found that he had been taking too much diuretic, as he could not see the labels on his pill bottles and Ida's dementia now made it difficult for her to manage his medications. Over the following 18 months, Horace was discharged from hospice, hospitalized, and readmitted to hospice two more times. In the 2 years since his initial hospice admission, the longest he went without hospice services was 2 months. By the time Horace died, Ivy's dementia was so severe, she was unable to care for him. Fortunately, Horace *was*

(continued)

(*continued*)

on hospice during his last 3 months of life, and the hospice team assisted the family in making plans for Ivy's care.

The issues represented in this case are all too common. Patients living with advanced chronic illness tend to be older, have multiple comorbidities, and may have family members who also carry a chronic disease burden. Medicare regulations stringently dictate that patients must be demonstrating a steady decline to continue to qualify for hospice; yet, this is not the usual illness trajectory for advanced cardiac or lung disease. Both of these illnesses are known for periods of fragile stability that may be prolonged but are easily disrupted by something like an overly salty meal or a common upper respiratory infection, which can quickly imperil these patients with symptoms such as severe dyspnea that require rapid, skilled intervention. Without access to PC services, these patients end up repeatedly hospitalized for acute symptoms that could often be managed at home with nursing support. Mr. Gregson was on and off hospice services for 2 years because there was no alternative care service available. He clearly deteriorated whenever services were removed, and he and his wife both suffered. Home-based PC is the solution to this problem.

Community or Home-Based Palliative Care

In a systematic review, Kirby et al. (2016) compared the needs of patients with life-limiting illness, and their families and caregivers, in rural versus urban settings. They found that rural EOL residents had higher rates of severe CHF, cancer, renal failure, and emphysema, with poorer symptom management, fewer physician visits, and poorer access to home care services, including PC. Patients and caregivers lacked information about PC and EOL care, and caregivers lacked support for practical skills that would allow patients to stay home longer (p. 291). Rural cancer patients were less likely to understand their prognosis, or to know that treatment intent was palliative rather than curative (p. 292). However, they also found that rural residents had resilience, greater acceptance of death, and good community support networks.

Ideally, community or home-based PC (CHBPC) is modeled on the interprofessional team used in both inpatient PC programs and home hospice services, represented by a physician and/or nurse practitioner (NP), RN, social worker, and chaplain; however, these services are not all reimbursable by Medicare and other forms of insurance (Meier et al., n.d.). Therefore, various program structures are being trialed around the country. The rural context brings additional barriers to reaching this ideal. There is still a lack of research on true PC in rural settings in the United States (Bakitas et al., 2015; Durie & Tanksley-Bowe, 2018; Kirby et al., 2016; Robinson et al., 2009). The literature on PC for patients at the EOL is somewhat more robust, especially when including research from other countries, as much of it originates in Canada and Australia. With the exception of financial analysis, much of this EOL research can be applied to the assessment of CHBPC, as the practice issues are closely related.

Certain themes stand out across the literature. There is wide general agreement that rural disparities in the availability of PC services, compared to urban and suburban communities, are common. Most also agree that outpatient and CHBPC programs in rural areas cannot be generically designed but must be tailored to the needs of the community being served (Bakitas et al., 2015; Caxaj et al., 2017; Kirby et al., 2016; Murphy, 2010; Pesut et al., 2013; Robinson et al., 2010; Temkin-Greener et al., 2012). Issues related to geographical distance and *windshield time*, lack of PC specialists, staff recruitment and retention, limited access to resources such as durable medical equipment and pharmacies, and financial constraints are common. Millions of people reside more than 60 minutes from a hospice agency, and many areas lack residential/inpatient hospice facilities as well as 24-hour (crisis) support. The idea of implementing telehealth technologies is frequently mentioned, with mixed reports on its feasibility and efficacy (Bakitas et al., 2015; Charlton et al., 2015; Evans et al., 2003; Holland et al., 2014; Lynch 2012; Paul et al., 2019; Robinson et al., 2010).

In looking at program development, additional topics unique to rural settings are being discussed and debated, including generalist versus specialist practice, rural–urban partnerships, and the role of the interdisciplinary team (IDT). Building capacity in communities was another strong theme. These aspects of PC practice encompass those areas that most urgently need to be tailored to fit the needs of the community being served. Across all models, nursing care is integral to PC and education for nurses and other providers is another major area of discussion.

A lack of providers educated in PC is creating a global workforce crisis in both urban and rural settings (Ernecoff et al., 2020; Kamal et al., 2017). Kamal et al. (2017) report an anticipated need for one PC physician for every 26,000 patients in the United States alone by 2030, with similar shortages apparent among the other professions within the IDT. In rural healthcare generally, the aforementioned hospital closures have been shown to result in a decrease in the number of primary care physicians but an increase in the number of advanced practice providers such as NPs (Mobley et al., 2020). These trends imply an increasing opportunity for APRNs to fill this void, whether as generalists or as PC specialists, in both urban and rural environments.

Within the community of PC providers, there is much discussion of whether and how primary care providers can help to meet the increasing need for PC services. Many rural and remote settings rely on generalists to cover the wide variety of healthcare needs for these communities. Any model of CHBPC necessarily relies on these local providers, whether for direct treatment or referral, and building and maintaining good relationships with them is crucial. In fact, utilizing existing professionals is repeatedly reported as an element of program successes. Because PC is only a small portion of what they do, however, it is more difficult for these professionals to obtain and maintain sufficient training and skills to meet the variety of needs presenting within PC. In a systematic review of randomly controlled trials of PC interventions, Ernecoff et al. (2020) looked at the characteristics and outcomes of interventions, comparing primary care providers to PC specialists. They concluded that interventions by specialists were more comprehensive and demonstrated better outcomes regarding improved physical symptoms. Various solutions to this discrepancy are being tried, many focusing on specialist support being made available to the generalists.

Hospice organizations are one source of specialist support. Traveling teams of PC specialists may visit patients directly or be available via tele or videoconferencing. Mobile health clinics are another potential solution (Bakitas et al., 2015; Lynch 2012; Robinson et al., 2009; Spice et al., 2012). Howell et al. (2011) reported on a shared care model that involves primary care patients in need of PC, an advanced practice nurse who acted as care coordinator, input on symptom assessment and management by an IDT, and involvement of home care services. The results were improved patient quality of life and reduction of symptoms. Mitchell et al. (2016) evaluated another pilot program that also involved a specialist NP coordinating care with support of the patient's generalist primary care provider and a one-time IDT case conference for each patient. The results included prompt initiation of treatment with good follow-up and coordinated, integrated care. Patients reported being satisfied with the service. Financial viability was not established.

NP-led, home-based PC consultation services are becoming more common in rural areas, as evidenced by programs in the Lehigh Valley of Pennsylvania, Southern Tier region of New York state, and counties surrounding Madison, Wisconsin. These programs have been implemented by hospice agencies and hospital-based healthcare systems. Typically, the services consist of an initial home consultation by the specialist NP lasting 1 to 2 hours, and periodic follow-up visits. The consultation includes a special focus on any symptoms requiring palliation, discussion of healthcare goals and advance directives, and an assessment of patient and family coping, caregiver burnout, and other needs associated with living with chronic illness. Recommendations are made to the patient's primary care provider with regard to symptom management and/or referrals for family support. This is a cost-effective approach to home-based PC as NPs can bill for their visits; however, reimbursement rates may not cover the cost and programs are often subsidized. Additionally, these programs often lack direct involvement of an IDT. The increasing incidence of such programs will provide an excellent opportunity for further research.

Telephone and videoconferencing may seem like an obvious answer to the geographical challenges of rural care. In some programs, these have been successfully utilized, whereas in others, results were more mixed. Watanabe et al. (2013) describe a virtual clinic where patients traveled to a facility, received an in-person assessment by a nurse including physical assessment and completion of a variety of assessment tools, and then participated in an IDT videoconference that resulted in recommendations for care. The nurse provided the follow-up. Although this method was determined to be feasible and patients reported satisfaction, problems identified included patient travel time, increased time needed for scheduling, and limited awareness of the clinic despite promotional efforts. Leadbeater and Staton (2014) found that often the necessary technology was not available in rural areas. In a small proof-of-concept study, Paul et al. (2019) found that web-based videoconferencing could be used effectively for PC consultation with rural elders. They had a clinical nurse specialist and home care nurse assist with facilitating the visit by being present in the patients' homes while meeting with a PC physician via Skype. The authors found that all participants (providers, patients, and family) felt the visits were effective and expressed satisfaction with the care delivered. This method saved time for the PC physician as well as the patient/family. The authors cautioned however that web-based videoconference visits should not replace all in-person visits, might be best used for follow-ups, and should not replace investment in local healthcare resources and facilities. An important part of any PC program is after-hours telephone support, which has been shown to increase a sense of security and reduce feelings of isolation experienced by families caring for a PC patient (Wilkes et al., 2004). Many existing programs do not yet offer this component, usually due to lack of funding and/or staffing.

Ceronsky et al. (2013) studied the effects of the Minnesota Rural Palliative Care Initiative, which sought to build PC capacity over 18 months using 10 community teams in a variety of service areas ranging in population from 9,000 to 200,000. All communities had existing hospice programs and four participating hospitals were critical access hospitals. The teams involved the collaboration of a wide variety of existing agencies and institutions, comprising an interdisciplinary approach. Only one community had a previously existing PC program. Based on their analysis, the authors proposed five recommendations:

- Community development of PC services requires external resources and support.
- Sustainability and continued progress are reliant on ongoing networking.
- Community-based metrics must be defined to assess the impact on cost, quality, and readmissions as well as patient and family satisfaction.
- Sustainability of programs in rural communities would be supported by reimbursement for PC services as a covered benefit.
- Program development for PC should occur within larger healthcare system redesign to maximize efficiency.

Currently, research is focusing on a variety of aspects of rural PC, inclusion of which is beyond the scope of this chapter. Barriers to home-based PC is one important area of study (Bowman et al., 2019; Brant et al., 2019; Pugh et al., 2019; Tedder et al., 2017.) There are efforts underway in Canada to develop culturally appropriate PC programs that meet the unique needs of rural Indigenous people (Caxaj et al., 2017; Kelley et al., 2018). PC for reducing unnecessary hospital admissions in rural populations is being more widely studied (Durie & Tanksley-Bowe, 2018; van de Mortel et al., 2017). PC for rural people with cancer is another focus (Dionne-Odom et al., 2018; Orsak et al., 2019). More research such as this is needed to guide PC program development in rural areas.

CONCLUSION

As our nation's population ages in the next two decades, there will be mounting pressure to find effective ways to care for burgeoning numbers of chronically ill adults. Palliative medicine offers a sound solution by providing holistic patient- and family-centered care with an emphasis on quality of life. Much work needs to be done to develop models of home-based care that are tailored to the communities they serve and covered by Medicare and other insurers. Nurses will undoubtedly play key roles in delivering this specialized care and are well suited to do so.

REFERENCES

American Hospital Association. (2015). *Rural and small hospitals fact sheet*. http://www.aha.org/content/13/fs-rural-small.pdf

American Hospital Association. (2019). *Rural report: Challenges facing rural communities and the roadmap to ensure local access to high-quality, affordable care*. https://www.aha.org/system/files/2019-02/rural-report-2019.pdf

Armstrong, B., Jenigiri, B., Hutson, S. P., Wachs, P. M., & Lambe, C. E. (2013). The impact of a palliative care program in a rural Appalachian community hospital. *American Journal of Hospice and Palliative Medicine, 30*(4), 380–387. https://doi.org/10.1177/1049909112458720

Bakitas, M. A., Elk, R., Astin, M., Ceronsky, L., Clifford, K. N., Dionne-Odom, N., Emanuel, L. L., Fink, R. M, Kvale, E., Levkoff, S., Ritchie, C., Smith, T. (2015). Systematic review of palliative care in the rural setting. *Cancer Control, 22*(4), 450–464. https://doi.org/10.1177/107327481502200411

Bowman, B. A., Twohig, J. S., Meier, D. E. (2019). Overcoming barriers to growth in home-based palliative care. *Journal of Palliative Medicine, 22*(4), 408–412. https://doi.org/10.1089/jpm.2018.0478

Brant, J. M., Fink, R. M., Thompson, C., Li, Y. H., Rassouli, M., Majima, T., Osuka, T., Gafer, N., Ayden, A., Khader, K., Lascar, E., Tang, L., Nestoros, S., Abdullah, M., Michael, N., Cerruti, J., Ngaho, E.,

Kadig, Y., Hablas, M., … Silberman, M. (2019). Global survey of the roles, satisfaction, and barriers of home health care nurses on the provision of palliative care. *Journal of Palliative Medicine, 22*(8), 945–960. https://doi.org/10.1089/jpm.2018.0566

Brumley, R. (2007). Increased satisfaction with care and lower costs: Results of a randomized trial of in-home palliative care. *Journal of the American Geriatrics Society, 55*(7), 993–1000. https://doi .org/10.1111/j.1532-5415.2007.01234.x

Caxaj, C. S., Schill, K., & Janke, R. (2017). Priorities and challenges for a palliative approach to care for rural indigenous populations: A scoping review. *Health Social Care Community, 26*, e329–e336. https://doi.org/10.1111/hsc.12469

Centers for Medicare & Medicaid Services. (2015). *Medicare benefit policy manual.* https://www.cms .gov/Regulations-and-Guidance/Guidance/Manuals/downloads/bp102c09.pdf

Ceronsky, L., Shearer, J., Weng, K., Hopkins, M., & McKinley, D. (2013). Minnesota rural palliative care initiative: Building palliative care capacity in rural Minnesota. *Journal of Palliative Medicine, 16*(3), 310–313. https://doi.org/10.1089/jpm.2012.0324

Charlton, M., Schlichting, J., Chioreso, C., Ward, M., & Vikas, P. (2015). Challenges of rural cancer care in the United States. *Oncology (Williston Park, N.Y.), 29*(9), 633–640. http://www.ncbi.nlm.nih.gov/ pubmed/26384798

Davis, M., Temel, J., Balboni, T., & Glare, P. (2015). A review of the trials which examine early integration of outpatient and home palliative care for patients with serious illnesses. *Annals of Palliative Medicine, 4*(3), 99–121. https://doi.org/10.3978/j.issn.2224-5820.2015.04.04

Dionne-Odom, J. N., Taylor, R., Rocque, G., Chambless, C., Ramsey, T., Azuero, A., Ivankova, N., Martin, M. Y., & Bakitas, M. A. (2018). Adapting an early palliative care intervention to family caregivers of persons with advanced cancer in the rural deep south: A qualitative formative evaluation. *Journal of Pain and Symptom Management, 55*(6), 1519–1530. https://doi.org/10.1016/ j.jpainsymman.2018.02.009

Durie, C., & Tanksley-Bowe, C. (2018). Rural readmissions in the palliative care vacuum. *Journal of Hospice & Palliative Nursing, 20*(2), 160–165. https://doi.org/10.1097/NJH.0000000000000421

Ernecoff, N. C., Check, D., Bannon, M., Hanson, L. C., Dionne-Odom, J. N., Corbelli, J., Klein-Fedyshin, M., Schenker, Y., Zimmermann, C., Arnold, R. M., & Kavalieratos, D. (2020). Comparing specialty and primary palliative care interventions: Analysis of a systematic review. *Journal of Palliative Medicine, 23*(3), 389–396. https://doi.org/10.1089/jpm.2019.0349

Evans, R., Stone, D., & Elwyn, G. (2003). Organizing palliative care for rural populations: A systematic review of the evidence. *Family Practice, 20*(3), 304–310. https://doi.org/10.1093/fampra/cmg312

Fink, R. M., Oman, K. S., Youngwerth, J., & Bryant, L. L. (2013). A palliative care needs assessment of rural hospitals. *Journal of Palliative Medicine, 16*(6), 638–644. https://doi.org/10.1089/jpm.2012.0574

Holland, D. E., Vanderboom, C. E., Ingram, C. J., Dose, A. M., Borkenhagen, L. S., Skadahl, P., Pacyna, J. E., Austin, C. M., & Bowles, K. H. (2014). The feasibility of using technology to enhance the transition of palliative care for rural patients. *CIN: Computers, Informatics, Nursing, 32*(6), 257–266. https://doi.org/10.1097/CIN.0000000000000066

Howell, D., Marshall, D., Brazil, K., Taniguchi, A., Howard, M., Foster, G., & Thabane, L. (2011). A shared care model pilot for palliative home care in a rural area: Impact on symptoms, distress, and place of death. *Journal of Pain and Symptom Management, 42*(1), 60–75. https://doi.org/10.1016/ j.jpainsymman.2010.09.022

Kamal, A. H., Bull, J. H., Swetz, K. M., Wolf, S. P., Shanafelt, T. D., & Myers, E. R. (2017). Future of the palliative care workforce: Preview to an impending crisis. *The American Journal of Medicine, 130*(2), 113–114. https://doi.org/10.1016/j.amjmed.2016.08.046

Keim-Malpass, J., Mitchell, E. M., Blackhall, L., & De Guzman, P. B. (2015). Evaluating stakeholder-identified barriers in accessing palliative care at an NCI-designated cancer center with a rural catchment area. *Journal of Palliative Medicine, 18*(7), 634–637. https://doi.org/10.1089/jpm.2015.0032

Kelley, M. L., Prince, H., Nadin, S., Brazil, K., Crow, M., Hanson, G., Maki, L., Monture, L., Mushquash, C. J., O'Brien, V., & Smith, J. (2018). Developing palliative care programs in Indigenous communities using participatory action research: A Canadian application of the public health approach to palliative care. *Annals of Palliative Medicine, 7*(Suppl. 2), S52–S72. https://doi.org/10.21037/ apm.2018.03.06

Kirby, S., Barlow, V., Saurman, E., Lyle, D., Passey, M., & Currow, D. (2016). Are rural and remote patients, families and caregivers needs in life-limiting illness different from those of urban dwellers? A narrative synthesis of the evidence. *Australian Journal of Rural Health*, 24(5), 289–299. https://doi.org/10.1111/ajr.12312

Leadbeater, M., & Staton, W. (2014). The role and organisation of community palliative specialist nursing teams in rural England. *British Journal of Community Nursing*, 19(11), 551–555. https://doi.org/10.12968/bjcn.2014.19.11.551

Lynch, S. (2012). Hospice and palliative care access issues in rural areas. *American Journal of Hospice and Palliative Medicine*, 30(2), 172–177. https://doi.org/10.1177/1049909112444592

Manfredi, P. L., Morrison, R. S., Morris, J., Goldhirsch, S. L., Carter, J. M., & Meier, D. E. (2000). Palliative care consultations: How do they impact the care of hospitalized patients? *Journal of Pain and Symptom Management*, 20(3), 166–173. http://www.ncbi.nlm.nih.gov/pubmed/11018334

Mayer, D. D. M., & Winters, C. A. (2016). Palliative care in critical access hospitals. *Critical Care Nurse*, 36(1), 72–78. https://doi.org/10.4037/ccn2016732

McGrath, L. S., Foote, D. G., Frith, K. H., & Hall, W. M. (2013). Cost effectiveness of a palliative care program in a rural community hospital. *Nursing Economics*, 31(4), 176–183. http://www.ncbi.nlm.nih.gov/pubmed/24069717

Meier, D. E., Bowman, B., Collins, K. B., Dahlin, C., & Twohig, J. S. (n.d.). *Palliative care in the home: A guide to program design*. Center to Advance Palliative Care.

Meier, D. E., & Sieger, C. E. (2015). *A guide to building a hospital-based palliative care program*. Center to Advance Palliative Care.

Mitchell, G. K., Senior, H. E., Bibo, M. P., Makoni, B., Young, S. N., Rosenberg, J. P., & Yates, P. (2016). Evaluation of a pilot of nurse practitioner led, GP supported rural palliative care provision. *BMC Palliative Care*, 15(1), 93. https://doi.org/10.1186/s12904-016-0163-y

Mobley, E., Ullrich, F., Baten, R. B. A., Shrestha, M., & Mueller, K. (2020). *RUPRI center for rural health policy analysis rural policy brief: Health care professional workforce composition before and after rural hospital closure*. https://rupri.public-health.uiowa.edu/publications/policybriefs/2020/hospital%20closure%20workforce.pdf

Morrison, R. S., & Meier, D. E. (2019). *America's care of serious illness: 2019 state-by-state report card on access to palliative care in our nation's hospitals*. Center to Advance Palliative Care and the National Palliative Care Research Center.

Morrison, R. S., Penrod, J. D., Cassel, J. B., Caust-Ellenbogen, M., Litke, A., Spragens, L., & Meier, D. E. (2008). Cost savings associated with U.S hospital palliative care consultation programs. *Archives of Internal Medicine*, 168(16), 1783–1790. https://doi.org/10.1001/archinte.168.16.1783

Murphy, S. (2010). Territory palliative care: A model for remote area palliative care provision. *Progress in Palliative Care*, 18(1), 27–30. https://doi.org/10.1179/096992610X12624290276304

Orsak, G., McGaha, P., Brandon, P., Swan, A., & Singh, K. P. (2019). A longitudinal pilot study for examining symptom reduction in patients with cancer in a palliative care program: A primarily rural northeast Texas population. *Hospital Topics*, 97(2), 54–59. https://doi.org/10.1080/00185868.2019.1605322

Paul, L. R., Salmon, C., Sinnarajah, A., & Spice, R. (2019). Web-based videoconferencing for rural palliative care consultation with elderly patients at home. *Supportive Care in Cancer*, 27, 3321–3330. https://doi.org/10.1007/s00520-018-4580-8

Pesut, B., Hooper, B., Sawatsky, R., Robinson, C. A., Bottorf, J. L., & Dalhuisen, M. (2013). Program assessment framework for a rural palliative supportive service. *Palliative Care: Research and Treatment*, 7, 7–17. https://doi.org/10.4137/pcrt.s11908

Pugh, A., Castleden, H., Giesbrecht, M., Davison, C., & Crooks, V. (2019). Awareness as a dimension of health care access: Exploring the case of rural palliative care provision in Canada. *Journal of Health Services and Research Policy*, 24(2), 108–115. https://doi.org/10.1177/1355819619929782

Quill, T. (2015). The initial interview in palliative care consultation. In R. M. Arnold (Ed.), *UpToDate*. https://www-uptodate-com

Robinson, C. A., Pesut, B., & Bottorff, J. L. (2010). Issues in rural palliative care: Views from the countryside. *Journal of Rural Health*, 26, 78–84. https://doi.org/10.1111/j.1748-0361.2009.00268.x

Robinson, C. A., Pesut, B., Bottorff, J. L., Mowry, A., Broughton, S., & Fyles, G. (2009). Rural pallia-
    tive care: A comprehensive review. *Journal of Palliative Medicine*, *12*(3), 253–258. https://doi
    .org/10.1089/jpm.2008.0228

Rogers, M., & Dumanovsky, T. (2017). *How we work*. Center to Advance Palliative Care.

Spice, R., Paul, L. R., & Biondo, P. D. (2012). Development of a rural palliative care program in the
    Calgary Zone of Alberta Health Services. *Journal of Pain and Symptom Management*, *43*(5), 911–924.
    https://doi.org/10.1016/j.jpainsymman.2011.05.019

Tedder, T., Elliot, L., & Lewis, K. (2017). Analysis of common barriers to rural patients utilizing hospice
    and palliative care services: An integrated literature review. *Journal of the American Association of
    Nurse Practitioners*, *29*, 356–362. https://doi.org/ 0.1002/2327-6924.12475

Temkin-Greener, H., Zheng, N. T., & Mukamel, D. B. (2012). Rural-urban differences in end-of-life
    nursing home care: Facility and environmental factors. *Gerontologist*, *52*(3), 335–344. https://doi
    .org/10.1093/geront/gnr143

Twaddle, M. L., & McCormick, E. (2016). Palliative care delivery in the home. In C. Ritchie & M. Silveira
    (Eds.), *UpToDate*. https://www.uptodate.com/contents/palliative-care-delivery-in-the-home

Van de Mortel, T. F., Marr, K., Brumeister, E., Koppe, H., Ahern, C., Walsh, R., Tyler-Freer, S., & Ewald,
    D. (2017). Reducing avoidable admissions in rural community palliative care: A pilot study of care
    coordination by General Practice registrars. *Australian Journal of Rural Health*, *25*, 141–147. https://
    doi.org/10.1111/ajr.12309

Wachterman, M. W., Pilver, C., Smith, D., Ersek, M., Lipsitz, S. R., & Keating, N. L. (2016). Quality of
    end-of-life care provided to patients with different serious illnesses. *JAMA Internal Medicine*, *176*(8),
    1095–1102. https://doi.org/10.1001/jamainternmed.2016.1200

Watanabe, S., Fairchild, A., Pituskin, E., Borgersen, P., Hanson, J., & Fassbender, K. (2013). Improving
    access to specialist multidisciplinary palliative care consultation for rural cancer patients by vid-
    eoconferencing: Report of a pilot project. *Supportive Care in Cancer*, *21*(4), 1201–1207. https://doi
    .org/10.1007/s00520-012-1649-7

Wilkes, L., Mohan, S., White, K., & Smith, H. (2004). Evaluation of an after-hours telephone support
    service for rural palliative care patients and their families: A pilot study. *Australian Journal of Rural
    Health*, *12*(3), 95–98. https://doi.org/10.1111/j.1440-1854.2004.00568.x

CHAPTER 18

Challenges and Opportunities to Palliative Care for Rural Veterans

TAMARA L. TASSEFF

Disclaimer

The views expressed in this book chapter are those of the author and do not necessarily reflect the position or policy of the Department of Veterans Affairs or the U.S. Government.

DISCUSSION TOPICS

Select one rural community to:

- Compare and contrast nonveteran rural populations with rural Veteran populations.
- Explore the strategies the rural community could implement to provide culturally sensitive care to military Veterans.
- Explain how palliative care and hospice care are similar or dissimilar.
- Describe the barriers to implementing concurrent palliative care. Identify specific strategies to address those barriers.

INTRODUCTION

Rural Veterans are an important subset of both the Veteran and the rural population with differing healthcare needs that are sometimes misunderstood. Concurrent palliative care, when delivered as a critical component of comprehensive primary care in rural areas, may offer the best opportunity for rural Veterans to remain productive amid the increasing incidence of multiple chronic conditions (MCCs). In this chapter, we describe the rural Veteran culture, outline the current research on the barriers to palliative care in the rural setting, and provide direction in the opportunities that exist addressing the concerns of the rural Veteran population.

WHO ARE RURAL VETERANS?

Only 4% of people living in the United States are Veterans (National Center for Veterans Analysis and Statistics, 2017). Rural Veterans are a unique subset of the larger rural-dwelling population. Similar to their rural counterparts, rural Veterans are older, on average, and experience higher rates of poverty, poorer health, and have fewer healthcare options than those living in urban areas. Geographic barriers, limited broadband Internet, and decreased availability of healthcare and support services add to the challenges of living and safely aging in place in many rural areas.

Approximately 5 million Veterans, 25% of the total Veteran population, live in rural or highly rural areas. Of these, 57% are enrolled in the Veterans Administration (VA) and 55% have one or more service-connected disabilities. Minorities (25%), women (7%), those making less than $35,000 a year (55%), and those without home Internet access (35%) provide a snapshot of rural Veterans who receive some form of benefits or healthcare from VA. When compared with Veterans living in urban areas, the percentage of rural Veterans enrolled in VA is 20% higher (37% urban, 57% rural), and nearly half are age 65 or older (U.S. Department of Veterans Affairs Office of Rural Health, n.d.).

Men and women who served during the Vietnam era represent nearly 28% of all rural Veterans (Holder, 2017). America's rural Veterans represent serving in World War II (5%), the Korean War (9%), the Vietnam Era (39%), pre-9/11 (11%), and post-9/11 (10%) with the largest group of Veterans serving in peacetime only (Holder, 2017). Although Vietnam-era Veterans constitute the largest segment of rural Veterans, post-9/11 Veterans who served in Iraq and Afghanistan account for 460,000 rural Veterans (Office of Rural Health, n.d.). Thirty-one percent of rural Veterans report some form of disability; those who served from September 2001 to present day, account for the highest number of service-connected disabilities (Holder, 2017). The majority of rural Veterans have multiple, complex, physical, and mental health needs that require ongoing care throughout their lives (Farmer et al., 2016).

The Influence of Veteran Culture

Kuehner (2013), a Navy nurse practitioner and Veteran, describes the diverse nature of Veterans as individuals who are united by national service and are influenced by a collective military culture. Yet, each has a unique story and perspective without any one story revealing the complexity of care needs faced by the Veterans after their military service has ended. Similar to Kuehner's assessment of the larger Veteran population, rural Veterans are diverse and may associate characteristics of both Veteran and rural cultural attributes.

Duty, honor, respect, self-sacrifice, integrity, loyalty, and courage are an inseparable part of many rural Veterans and the larger Veteran population, regardless of the military era or length of their military service (Kuehner, 2013; Meyer, 2015). The military culture is one in which personal privacy is relinquished (Meyer, 2015). Because of this cultural attribute, Veterans may distrust healthcare providers based on their experiences with military providers who are compelled to disclose information that may influence the goals of the Department of Defense (Kuehner, 2013).

The military cultural attribute of self-sacrifice for the good of the larger population devalues personal well-being. This leads to a perception that health-seeking behaviors are selfish (Meyer, 2015). This perception is further promoted by the military culture that promotes a "hypermasculine paradigm" (Ashley & Brown, 2015, p. 535) in which help seeking is viewed as weakness. Seeking help for mental health–related issues is often viewed as taboo by many Veterans; however, the newest generation of Veterans, those who served in Iraq and Afghanistan, may be more open to seeking mental health assistance than older Veterans. In a survey of 1,501 Iraq and Afghanistan Veterans, 58% reported sustaining a mental health injury and 82% reported seeking mental health assistance (Maffucci & Frazier, 2015).

Other studies of Veterans reported that rural Veterans may utilize EDs more than urban Veterans to seek mental health treatment rather than seek assistance from available VA or community counseling centers (Johnson et al., 2015). Differences related to the military ethos or warfighter mentality led to recent changes in the *Diagnostic and Statistical Manual of Mental Disorders (DSM)* criteria for posttraumatic stress disorder (PTSD). The original wording in the diagnostic criteria for PTSD used the language related to the patient's endorsement of helplessness, yet military members are trained to confront self-doubt and helplessness as an enemy to be engaged, the opposite of helplessness (Meyer, 2015).

Rural Veterans, many of whom joined the military in late adolescence between the ages of 17 and 19 years, internalized the military culture and core values into their personal identities (Kuehner, 2013; Meyer, 2015). Just over 20% of 1,501 Veterans of Iraq and Afghanistan believe that civilians understand the sacrifices that Veterans have made despite the majority believing they are supported by the public (Maffucci & Frazier, 2015).

Influence of Rural Culture on Rural-Dwelling Veterans

Autonomy, self-reliance, and defining health as the ability to be productive, rather than as the absence of disease (Long & Weinert, 2018), are the attributes of rural culture. Similar to nonveteran rural dwellers, rural Veterans frequently encounter transportation challenges, tend to travel farther to receive care, have poorer physical and mental health, poorer quality of life, higher rates of disability, and smaller incomes than urban dwellers and urban Veterans; however, rural Veterans are more likely than rural nonveterans to have healthcare insurance (National Center for Veterans Analysis and Statistics, 2016). A large majority of Iraq and Afghanistan Veterans (71%) surveyed reported service-connected disabilities and chronic pain (64%) and/or PTSD (77%) connected to their military service (Maffucci & Frazier, 2015). Many of these Veterans receive care from the VA and within their local communities.

An estimated 30% to 75% of rural Veterans receive care from local community providers in addition to VA healthcare (U.S. Department of Veterans Affairs, 2016a). Despite access to multiple sources of care, often referred to as "dual care," rural Veterans face additional disparities that are different than those encountered by urban Veterans and rural dwellers. In earlier studies, for example, rural Veterans with dementia have a greater likelihood of not receiving timely and effective ambulatory care and were more likely than nonveteran rural dwellers and urban Veterans to experience an avoidable hospitalization (Thorpe et al., 2010).

Many health professionals and the public perceive Veterans to have abundant access to care from the VA, and within the community through TRICARE (www.tricare.mil). Yet, only active duty military members and Veterans who have retired from the military or are Congressional Medal of Honor recipients are eligible for TRICARE, the military equivalent of insurance (Department of Defense, 2016). Further complicating coordination of care and payment for services rendered, many Veterans and healthcare providers were confused by the Veterans Choice Program (Maffucci & Frazier, 2015). In efforts to simplify and improve care coordination and access to care in the community, the Veterans Choice Act was allowed to sunset and was replaced by the MISSION Act in 2019. Improvements include the establishment of a new VA Community Care Program, the ability of providers to provide telehealth across state lines to Veterans located anywhere in the United States, and streamlined eligibility criteria that includes when the Veteran and referring provider agree that community care is within the Veteran's "medical best interest" (U.S. Department of Veterans Affairs, 2019).

Many rural Veterans face undue health burdens related to higher rates of chronic disease and disability. Gale and Heady (2013) reported a lack of military/Veteran cultural competence and understanding of service-connected health issues and mental health needs of rural Veterans. Only one-third of Americans under the age of 30 are directly related to a military service member, which could widen the gap of understanding related to Veteran cultural competence (Meyer, 2015). Johnson et al. (2015) noted rural Veterans with psychiatric diagnoses, including PTSD, were at higher risk of not receiving appropriate medical services, yet this was not observed in the urban Veteran population. In earlier studies, Thorpe et al. (2010) examined rural–urban access to ambulatory care for Veterans with dementia and found preventable admissions were four times higher for rural Veterans than urban Veterans. They also found that the association between rurality and preventable hospital admissions was not attributable to overall higher preventable hospital admissions in rural areas. Nayar et al. (2013) found that 74% of rural providers, compared with 59% of urban providers, believed non-VA physicians had enough experience to treat war-related PTSD. The complexities of experiences unique to rural Veterans create additional challenges to providing culturally competent palliative care and hospice care in rural areas.

RESEARCH ON THE BARRIERS, CHALLENGES, AND OPPORTUNITIES FOR PALLIATIVE CARE IN THE RURAL SETTING

Understanding the barriers to palliative care begins with embracing the broad definition of palliative care—preventing and alleviating suffering at any stage in a serious illness, with the goal of improving the quality of life of patients and families facing physical, psychological, or spiritual problems associated with a serious illness (World Health Organization [WHO], 2015). Despite the broad definition of palliative care and the appropriateness of delivering palliative care at any age and at any stage of a serious illness, 86% of the people who could benefit from palliative care never receive it (WHO, 2015). Basic palliative care can be delivered by primary care providers as a component of comprehensive primary care. Specialized palliative care is often delivered by providers with advanced training in palliative medicine. Palliative care is not hospice care. Hospice care is a special subset of palliative care focused on the end-of-life period. Palliative care focuses on the individual with the serious illness, their goals, how they would prefer to live, what they value, and what matters most.

Research related to the perceptions of palliative care held by physicians, nurses, and patients shows these misperceptions exist throughout the world and are not isolated to the United States. Very little published current research exists related to the barriers to palliative care in rural areas. A significant gap exists related to rural Veterans' perceptions of palliative care and barriers to rural Veterans' experiences of receiving palliative care.

Concurrent palliative care, to improve the quality of life, may be offered simultaneously with traditional treatment. Rural Veterans suffering from diabetes, heart disease,

Parkinson's, Alzheimer's or other dementias, multiple sclerosis, cancer, kidney disease, and rheumatoid arthritis may be candidates for concurrent palliative care. However, even when physicians and nurses recognize the value of palliative care, they may associate palliative care with a cancer diagnosis and not within the broader context as appropriate to multiple serious chronic conditions (Golla et al., 2014; Kavalieratos et al., 2014). Nurses and physicians more familiar with end-of-life or hospice care may be proponents of palliative care yet may believe that palliative care is appropriate only at the point traditional medical treatments have stopped (Verschuur et al., 2014). This limits a broader application of palliative care to a wide range of serious, chronic illnesses appropriate at any point within the disease trajectory.

Despite the expanded definition and practice of expanded palliative care services over the past 20 years, little has changed related to the public's, nurses', and providers' largely held misperceptions that palliative care is synonymous with hospice or end-of-life care. However, in a public opinion research study, 8 out of 10 consumers stated they would want palliative care for themselves or a loved one after hearing the definition (Morgan, 2019). Defining palliative care prior to discussing it may provide hope for many earlier in the illness process, such as aging rural Veterans suffering from MCCs and serious illness.

Current world events, specifically the global pandemic related to COVID-19, are reshaping how healthcare providers and the public perceive palliative care. Primary healthcare providers are consulting virtually with palliative care specialists about how to provide supportive care for their patients, some of whom are recovering and returning home to their families (Powell & Silveira, 2020). Similarly, palliative care teams, including those within VA, are conducting an increasing number of e-Palliative Care or Veteran virtual care visits to address the needs of more Veterans outside of traditional face-to-face visits. This global pandemic may have done more to correct misperceptions and increase the utilization of palliative care than any targeted efforts over the past 20 years. A Public Broadcasting Service (PBS) News Hour interview of Dr. Diane Meier of the Center to Advance Palliative Care noted that the current global pandemic has elevated the value of palliative care and the importance of having important conversations about what people value (Woodruff, 2020). The unintended, yet positive, consequence of the COVID-19 pandemic may advance the understanding and utilization of palliative care, especially in rural areas where access has traditionally been limited. This understanding and advancement of palliative care may be especially beneficial for rural Veterans and nonveterans, who may be at an increased risk of serious complications, on average, based on older age and poorer health status when compared to those living in urban areas.

Challenges—The Increasing Incidence of Chronic Conditions and the Aging Population

Rural Veterans, similar to the aging, rural-dwelling population, are experiencing an increasing incidence of chronic disease that further challenges rural healthcare. Developing MCCs increases with aging, and nearly 50% of 45- to 64-year-olds have MCCs and 80% of people older than 65 have MCCs (Gerteis et al., 2014). The rapidly aging population in the United States, increased life expectancy, and the rise in MCCs will increase demands on the U.S. healthcare system, especially in rural areas already burdened by health professional shortages. Increased economic burdens, bothersome symptoms, and stress will likely decrease the quality of life for those living with MCCs and their families (Goodman et al., 2013). This is especially true in rural areas where only 10% of physicians and 16% of nurses practice (Bolin et al., 2015).

The majority of rural Veterans are currently over the age of 65 (Office of Rural Health, n.d.); the vast majority will be living with MCCs. Aging rural Veterans and rural non-veterans will be competing for limited healthcare resources, such as available skilled nursing, hospital, and home care in rural areas. Suboptimal symptom management reduces quality of life for rural Veterans and rural-dwelling people suffering from serious chronic illnesses or MCCs (Centers for Disease Control and Prevention, 2013; Institute of Medicine [IOM], 2015). Aging rural Veterans and their families may face additional challenges related to dementia in addition to increases in the incidence of MCCs.

Challenges—Rural Veterans and Early Onset Dementia

Recent studies find rural dwellers and rural Veterans who have sustained head trauma, including concussions, have a higher risk of developing dementia or Alzheimer's disease (Alzheimer's Association, 2015). Veterans diagnosed with PTSD, or who have sustained moderate traumatic brain injuries (TBIs), have double the risk of developing Alzheimer's disease and the risk quadruples for rural Veterans who have experienced severe TBIs, such as injuries sustained from roadside bomb blasts in Iraq and Afghanistan (Qureshi et al., 2010). Although more research is needed, it is conceivable that rural Veterans may develop Alzheimer's years earlier than the traditional Alzheimer's patient (Sibener et al., 2014). An aging rural population of Veterans and nonveterans, increases in MCCs, and limited availability of skilled nursing beds, healthcare and community support resources, and healthcare professionals require proactive planning now. Palliative care may provide additional options for Veterans in rural areas; however, more palliative care options are needed in many rural areas.

Challenges—Confidence and Competence Providing Palliative Care Services

Many physicians and nurses lack experience, confidence, or comfort providing palliative care, especially on an outpatient or ambulatory care basis (Raphael et al., 2014; Schroedl et al., 2014). Managing referrals (Smith et al., 2013), funding and staffing issues (Raphael et al., 2014; Smith et al., 2013), and difficulties with estimating survival or disease trajectory of nonmalignant diagnoses (Schroedl et al., 2014) remain challenging. Physicians and nurses who practice in rural areas may already experience geographical and professional isolation and may believe concurrent palliative care should be reserved solely for palliative medicine specialists. Additionally, it is posited that certain professional vulnerabilities may exist for healthcare professionals who believe palliative care is more than end-of-life care when many of their colleagues and patients may perceive that palliative care is solely end-of-life care and reimbursement models lag behind best practices. Although growing evidence supports the cost-effectiveness of palliative care services (WHO, 2015), convincing rural healthcare administrators and community boards that palliative care is responsible, efficient, and cost-effective care can be challenging and time consuming. However, opportunities exist to proactively screen, explore, and implement alternate healthcare delivery models, and change perceptions through mentoring and education.

Opportunities—Screenings and Creative Alternate Healthcare Delivery Models

Routine screening interventions may assist rural providers with providing higher quality, culturally sensitive care while identifying rural Veterans at risk of developing dementia or who may be experiencing a reduced quality of life related to a serious chronic condition and suboptimal symptom management. Less than 40% of non-VA providers screen patients for military service (Meyer, 2015). The VA maintains a website that contains a Military Service Toolkit that provides a screening tool and helpful ideas on how to approach screening patients for military service and questions that may be used to help identify Veterans and their specific healthcare needs (VA/U.S. Department of Veterans Affairs, n.d.). Other screening tools may help with early identification of Veterans who could benefit from early palliative care. One such validated screening tool is the 40-item Care Assessment Need (CAN) score used by VA primary care providers to assess frailty and predict patients at greatest risk of hospitalization and mortality as evidenced by CAN scores greater than 95 (Ruiz et al., 2018). Additionally, the VA is currently implementing multiple technological options to enhance healthcare delivery in rural areas, including the delivery of palliative care using telemedicine and electronic tablet-based virtual healthcare visits. The 2020 COVID-19 global pandemic has spurred rapid advancement to deliver more care to Veterans using telemedicine virtual visits to avoid exposing Veterans to more serious health complications.

Routine screening of rural Veterans with serious chronic conditions may help to identify suboptimal symptom management and reduced the quality of life earlier in the disease trajectory. Earlier identification can assist with addressing and managing stress, suboptimal symptoms, and decreased quality of life associated with a serious illness. Many rural healthcare providers have implemented routine depression screening, and this screening is extremely important to rural Veterans. Only 6% of Iraq and Afghanistan Veterans considered taking their own lives prior to entering military service and the majority, 53% to 73%, reported excellent premilitary health; however, 40% of these same Veterans have considered taking their own lives since joining the military and less than 10% reported excellent current overall health (Maffucci & Frazier, 2015). Screening of information provides information helpful to considering and designing alternate healthcare delivery models for rural areas.

The VA has shifted focus to community-based outpatient clinics and medical home models of care and is increasing the use of telemedicine virtual visits. Veterans who are home-bound may receive home-based primary care visits or virtual visits. Researchers continue to explore innovative ways to provide palliative care to rural Veterans who are isolated by geography, lack of technology, transportation, or lack of needed services close to home. VA research and development efforts are underway to improve access to care for rural Veterans through field-based pilot projects, telemedicine/telehealth, and virtual consults to better support Veterans and their caregivers located in rural and remote areas (U.S. Department of Veterans Affairs, 2016b). The VA offers multiple continuing education opportunities for community-based non-VA providers and nurses in addition to research collaboration.

Opportunities—Changing Perceptions Through Education and Mentoring

Military culture and palliative care education for health professionals, administrators, and the community are two of the best investments in redesigning rural healthcare delivery models. In 2011, a White House initiative, *Joining Forces*, was launched to promote a greater understanding of the military culture and improve support for Veterans. Despite ending in January 2017, over 660 nursing schools in all 50 states (Rossiter, 2015) and more than 100 medical schools across the United States (Association of American Medical Colleges, n.d.) committed to greater support of Veterans' health and culturally sensitive care. Although the vast majority of medical schools reported curriculum on PTSD and TBIs, roughly 25% reported addressing the military culture within their curriculum (Meyer, 2015; Ross et al., 2015).

Physician and nurse perceptions of palliative care likely affect medical and nursing practice. Palliative care perceptions affect when, how, and whether palliative care is initiated; impact referral practices; and determine whether concurrent palliative care or only end-of-life care is offered. The IOM (2015) called for better education, communication, policies, payment, and planning related to quality of care through the end of life. The American Association of Colleges of Nursing (AACN) has also studied and adopted 17 updated palliative care competencies for undergraduate nursing students utilizing a panel of palliative care experts and key nursing academic representatives (Ferrell et al., 2016).

The intent of nursing and medical schools is promising; however, more educational and palliative care mentoring opportunities are needed to support rural providers and nurses. For the past 18 years, the VA has offered interprofessional fellowships in palliative care at a number of VA medical centers (Weller et al., 2019). Additional mentoring opportunities with health professionals who possess expertise in treating Veterans, and with palliative medicine specialists, are needed for rural providers and nurses. Additional mentorship opportunities, especially virtual opportunities, could significantly advance concurrent palliative care availability for rural Veterans and rural-dwelling people. More creative solutions and ideas are needed to support and increase the practice of palliative care in rural areas. Telemedicine and virtual consults, also called e-palliative care, similar to successful e-ICU collaboratives operating in some rural areas, are starting to break down palliative care access barriers for Veterans living in rural areas. Educating community healthcare providers, Veterans, and their families about the multiple options available through VA and their community will be critical to expanding and providing palliative care services in rural areas.

Although palliative care can be delivered concurrently at any point in the disease trajectory, hospice care requires a certification of a terminal illness with a life expectancy of 6 months or less. Veterans who qualify for hospice care may continue to receive both curative treatment and hospice care through VA or VA and community hospice partnerships. One of the most significant advances in end-of-life palliative care is concurrent hospice care. Sometimes referred to as *concurrent care*, this type of care allows Veterans who qualify for hospice benefits to avoid the terrible choice of deciding between curative treatment and hospice; something unavailable to most nonveterans living in the United States. However, there is still more work to do to improve understanding of palliative care, how it differs from hospice care, and what options may be available to help Veterans living in rural areas.

Community education, delivered in collaboration with the VA, Veterans, and palliative care experts, is an important step in advancing the understanding of the military culture and the benefits of concurrent palliative care and concurrent hospice care within rural communities. A broadened understanding of the rural Veteran culture and concurrent palliative care may allow rural communities to dialogue and discuss proactive solutions to limited healthcare and community resources. Enlisting the help of rural Veterans, who may be looking for a renewed purpose and mission, may provide insight into how to partner on rural models of healthcare delivery that incorporate concurrent palliative care and utilize rural Veterans to identify and assist other rural Veterans in need of concurrent palliative care while providing real-time insight into the rural Veteran culture. The VA Office of Rural Health is currently supporting research related to removing access barriers and improving identification, communication, and treatment of rural Veterans diagnosed with serious illnesses.

Opportunities—Research, Legislative Reform, and Application of the Evidence to Practice

Improving the access and availability of concurrent palliative care for rural Veterans is a complex mission in need of a collaborative multifaceted approach. Palliative care, delivered as a complement to primary care for rural Veterans with serious chronic conditions, may provide increased quality of life while promoting ethical, efficient, individualized, cost-effective, and resource-conscious care. Controlling symptoms may reduce the stress and symptom burden for both rural Veterans and their families. Rural Veterans of working age may perceive symptom management related to chronic conditions, or permanent disabling injuries as aligning with rural values such as remaining productive and regaining self-reliance, thus supporting an improved quality of life.

Legislators are also recognizing that palliative care offers affordable, efficient, high-quality care beyond end-of-life care. A bill introduced in the U.S. House of Representatives, H.R. 1676—Palliative Care and Hospice Education and Training Act, is aimed at improving palliative care and hospice education in medical and nursing schools, increasing research, and supporting the development of faculty careers in palliative medicine (Engel, 2017). Although the bill passed the House on July 23, 2018, the Senate failed to pass it (govtrack.us).

More research related to rural Veterans, support for faculty, mentors, and education of healthcare professionals in rural communities is needed to promote an understanding of rural Veterans and to correct palliative care misperceptions. Research, education, and application of the evidence to improve concurrent palliative care delivery will be needed to improve the quality of life for rural Veterans and their families living with serious chronic conditions.

CONCLUSION

In a time of healthcare professional shortages, decreasing reimbursements, and limited resources, current healthcare models are insufficient to address the needs of Veterans living with serious illnesses in rural areas. Current economic situations and global health crisis, such as the COVID-19 pandemic, are showing the gaps in the U.S. healthcare delivery system. Current healthcare delivery models are unsustainable and require transformation. Collaborations between rural providers and the VA not only serve to assist rural Veterans, but may also be the best opportunity to develop a national healthcare model that improves the access and availability of concurrent palliative care for rural-dwelling people throughout the United States.

REFERENCES

Alzheimer's Association. (2015). 2015 Alzheimer's disease facts and figures. *Alzheimer's & Dementia*, *11*(3), 88. https://www.alz.org/facts/downloads/facts_figures_2015.pdf

Ashley, W., & Brown, J. C. (2015). The impact of combat status on Veterans' attitudes toward help seeking: The hierarchy of combat elitism. *Journal of Evidence-Informed Social Work*, *12*(5), 534–542. doi:10.1080/15433714.992695

Association of American Medical Colleges. (n.d.). *AAMC supports joining forces*. https://www.aamc.org/advocacy/campaigns_and_coalitions/258074/joiningforces.html

Bolin, J. N., Bellamy, G. R., Ferdinand, A. O., Vuong, A. M., Kash, B. A., Schulze, A., & Helduser, J. W. (2015). Rural Healthy People 2020: New decade, same challenges. *The Journal of Rural Health, 31*(3), 326–333. doi:10.1111/jrh.12116

Centers for Disease Control and Prevention. (2013). *The state of aging and health in America 2013* (p. 60). U.S. Department of Health and Human Services. http://www.cdc.gov/aging/help/dph-aging/state-aging-health.html

Department of Defense. (2016). *Eligibility*. http://www.tricare.mil/Plans/Eligibility

Engel, E. (2017, March 24). Text—H.R.1676—115th Congress (2017-2018): Palliative Care and Hospice Education and Training Act [webpage]. https://www.congress.gov/bill/115th-congress/house-bill/1676/text

Farmer, C. M., Hosek, S. D., & Adamson, D. M. (2016). Balancing demand and supply for Veterans' health care: A summary of three RAND assessments conducted under the Veterans Choice Act. *Rand Health Quarterly, 6*(1), 12. https://www.ncbi.nlm.nih.gov/pmc/articles/PMC5158276/

Ferrell, B., Malloy, P., Mazanec, P., & Virani, R. (2016). CARES: AACN's new competencies and recommendations for educating undergraduate nursing students to improve palliative care. *Journal of Professional Nursing, 32*(5), 327–333. doi:10.1016/ j.profnurs.2016.07.002

Gale, J., & Heady, H. (2013). Rural vets: Their barriers, problems, needs. *Health Progress, 94*(3), 49–52. http://digitalcommons.usm.maine.edu/insurance/5

Gerteis, J., Izrael, D., Deitz, D., LeRoy, L., Ricciardi, R., Miller, T., & Basu, J. (2014). *Multiple chronic conditions chartbook* (No. AHRQ Q14-0038) (p. 52). Agency for Healthcare Research and Quality. http://www.cdc.gov/chronicdisease/overview/

Golla, H., Galushko, M., Pfaff, H., & Voltz, R. (2014). Multiple sclerosis and palliative care: Perceptions of severely affected multiple sclerosis patients and their health professionals: A qualitative study. *BMC Palliative Care, 13*(1), 1–23. doi:10.1186/1472-684X-13-11

Goodman, R. A., Posner, S. F., Huang, E. S., Parekh, A. K., & Koh, H. K. (2013). Defining and measuring chronic conditions: Imperatives for research, policy, program, and practice. *Preventing Chronic Disease, 10*, E66. doi:10.5888/pcd10.120239

Holder, K. A. (2017). Veterans in rural America (American Community Survey Reports ACS-36; p. 22). Census Bureau. https://www.census.gov/content/dam/Census/library/publications/2017/acs/acs-36.pdf

Institute of Medicine. (2015). *Dying in America: Improving quality and honoring individual preferences near the end of life*. National Academy of Sciences. http://publications.amsus.org/doi/full/10.7205/MILMED-D-15-00005

Johnson, C. E., Bush, R. L., Harman, J., Bolin, J., Evans Hudnall, G., & Nguyen, A. M. (2015). Variation in utilization of health care services for rural VA enrollees with mental health-related diagnoses. *The Journal of Rural Health, 31*(3), 244–253. doi:10.1111/jrh.12105

Kavalieratos, D., Mitchell, E. M., Carey, T. S., Dev, S., Biddle, A. K., Reeve, B. B., Abernethy, A. P., & Weinberger, M. (2014). "Not the 'Grim Reaper Service'": An assessment of provider knowledge, attitudes, and perceptions regarding palliative care referral barriers in heart failure. *Journal of the American Heart Association, 3*(1), 1–11. doi:10.1161/JAHA.113.000544

Kuehner, C. A. (2013). My military: A navy nurse practitioner's perspective on military culture and joining forces for Veteran health. *Journal of the American Association of Nurse Practitioners, 25*, 77–83. doi:10.1111/j.1745-7599.2012.00810.x

Long, K. A., & Weinert, C. (2018). Rural nursing: Developing the theory. In C. A. Winters (Ed.), *Rural nursing concepts, theory, and practice* (5th ed., pp. 17–30). Springer Publishing Company.

Maffucci, J., & Frazier, C. (2015). *7th annual member survey: The most comprehensive look into the lives of post-9/11 Veterans*. Iraq and Afghanistan Veterans of America. https://iava.org/wp-content/uploads/2016/05/IAVA_MemberSurvey_Final_single_pgs.pdf

Meyer, E. G. (2015). The importance of understanding military culture. *Academic Psychiatry, 39*, 416–418. doi:10.1007/s40596-015-0285-1

Morgan, L. (2019, December 17). Public opinion research on palliative care | Get palliative care. https://get-palliativecare.org/public-opinion-research-on-palliative-care-and-living-with-a-serious-illness/

National Center for Veterans Analysis and Statistics. (2016, August). *Characteristics of rural Veterans: 2014 data from the American Community Survey*. U.S. Department of Veterans Affairs. https://www.va.gov/vetdata/docs/SpecialReports/Rural_Veterans_ACS2014_FINAL.pdf

National Center for Veterans Analysis and Statistics. (2017). *Profile of Veterans: 2017* [PowerPoint]. https://www.va.gov/vetdata/docs/SpecialReports/Profile_of_Veterans_2017.pdf

Nayar, P., Apenteng, B., Yu, F., Woodbridge, P., & Fetrick, A. (2013). Rural Veterans' perspectives of dual care. *Journal of Community Health*, 38(1), 70–77. doi:10.1007/s10900-012-9583-7

Powell, V. D., & Silveira, M. J. (2020). What should palliative care's response be to the COVID-19 pandemic? *Journal of Pain and Symptom Management*, 60(1), e1–e3. https://dx.doi.org/10.1016%2Fj.jpainsymman.2020.03.013

Qureshi, S. U., Kimbrell, T., Pyne, J. M., Magruder, K. M., Hudson, T. J., Petersen, N. J., Yu, H.-J., Schulz, P. E., & Kunik, M. E. (2010). Greater prevalence and incidence of dementia in older Veterans with posttraumatic stress disorder. *Journal of the American Geriatrics Society*, 58(9), 1627–1633. doi:10.1111/j.1532-5415.2010.02977.x

Raphael, D., Waterworth, S., & Gott, M. (2014). The role of practice nurses in providing palliative and end-of-life care to older patients with long-term conditions. *International Journal of Palliative Nursing*, 20(8), 373–379. doi:10.12968/ijpn.2014.20.8.373

Rossiter, R. (2015, November 10). AACN supports Joining Forces Wellness Week. *Press Release*. American Association of Colleges of Nursing.

Ross, P. T., Ravindranath, D., Clay, M., & Lypson, M. L. (2015). A greater mission: Understanding military culture as a tool for serving those who have served. *Journal of Graduate Medical Education*, 7(4), 519–522. doi:10.4300/JGME-D-14-00568.1

Ruiz, J. G., Priyadarshni, S., Rahaman, Z., Cabrera, K., Dang, S., Valencia, W. M., & Mintzer, M. J. (2018). Validation of an automatically generated screening score for frailty: the care assessment need (CAN) score. *BMC Geriatrics*, 18, 106. https://doi.org/10.1186/s12877-018-0802-7

Schroedl, C., Yount, S., Szmuilowicz, E., Rosenberg, S. R., & Kalhan, R. (2014). Outpatient palliative care for chronic obstructive pulmonary disease: A case series. *Journal of Palliative Medicine*, 17(11), 1256–1261. doi:10.1089/jpm.2013.0669

Sibener, L., Zaganjor, I., Snyder, H. M., Bain, L. J., Egge, R., & Carrillo, M. C. (2014). Alzheimer's disease prevalence, costs, and prevention for military personnel and Veterans. *Alzheimer's & Dementia: The Journal of the Alzheimer's Association*, 10(3), S105–S110. doi:10.1016/j.jalz.2014.04.011

Smith, A. K., Thai, J. N., Bakitas, M. A., Meier, D. E., Spragens, L. H., Temel, J. S., Weissman, D. E., & Rabow, M. W. (2013). The diverse landscape of palliative care clinics. *Journal of Palliative Medicine*, 16(6), 661–668. doi:10.1089/jpm.2012.0469

Thorpe, J. M., Houtven, C. H., Sleath, V., & Thorpe, C. T. (2010). Rural-urban differences in preventable hospitalizations among community-dwelling Veterans with dementia. *Journal of Rural Health*, 26(2), 146–155. doi:10.1111/j.1748-0361.2010.00276.x

U.S. Department of Veterans Affairs. (n.d.). VA community provider toolkit: Serving Veterans through partnership. https://www.mentalhealth.va.gov/communityproviders/screening_howto.asp

U.S. Department of Veterans Affairs Office of Rural Health. (n.d.). *Rural Veterans*. http://www.rural-health.va.gov/aboutus/ruralvets.asp

U.S. Department of Veterans Affairs. (2016a). *Dual health system users: Strategies to implement optimal care coordination*. Health Services Research & Development. https://www.hsrd.research.va.gov/news/feature/dual_use.cfm

U.S. Department of Veterans Affairs. (2016b). Health services research & development. https://www.hsrd.research.va.gov/for_researchers/sig/default.cfm#rural

U.S. Department of Veterans Affairs. (2019, June 6). *VA launches new health care options under MISSION Act* [Press release]. https://www.va.gov/opa/pressrel/pressrelease.cfm?id=5264

Verschuur, E. M., Groot, M. M., & van der Sande, R. (2014). Nurses' perceptions of proactive palliative care: A Dutch focus group study. *International Journal of Palliative Nursing*, 20(5), 241–245. doi:10.12968/ijpn.2014.20.5.241

Weller, R., Healy, J., Hettler, D. L., Howe, J. L., Smith, H. M., Steckart, M. J., & Periyakoil, V. S. (2019). VA Interprofessional fellowship in palliative care: 15 years of training excellence. *Journal of Social Work in End-of-Life & Palliative Care*, 15(2–3), 85–98. https://doi.org/10.1080/15524256.2019.1645797

Woodruff, J. (2020, June 30). *A brief but spectacular take on compassionate care during COVID-19*. https://www.youtube.com/watch?v=49P7D--AF3g

World Health Organization. (2015, July). *Palliative care*. http://www.who.int/mediacentre/factsheets/fs402/en

Rural Youth Suicide Risk Assessment and Intervention for Rural Healthcare Providers and Families

STACY M. STELLFLUG AND KEE A. DUNNING

DISCUSSION TOPICS

- Discuss a time you did not feel validated in a conversation. Describe what happened? How did you feel? What could have been done differently?
- Do you ever find yourself in a power struggle with another person (parent, child, spouse, coworker, etc.)? Pair up with another student and do a role-play of your situation. Try to incorporate the Kee Concepts in your interaction.
- Role-play a scenario in which one of your colleagues is a suicidal youth and has just told you they are thinking about taking their life tonight. Discuss what you would do in this situation.

INTRODUCTION

Suicide is a significant cause of mortality in the United States. According to the Centers for Disease Control and Prevention (CDC) Web-Based Injury Statistic Query and Reporting System, suicide was the 10th leading cause of death overall in the United States. Suicide claimed the lives of 48,344 people in 2018 (CDC, 2018). Suicide was the second leading cause of death for people ages 10 to 24 years in 2018, second only to unintentional injury (CDC, 2018). Although suicide knows no boundaries, suicide has made itself at home in rural areas across the United States. Increased rates of suicide in rural dwellers was first observed and described in the early 1990s and has continued to increase annually (Singh et al., 2002). As counties become less urbanized, suicide rates have increased (Chen & Ingram, 2015). No single age group or population has seen a more dramatic increase in suicide rates than rural youth. In this chapter, we review the suicide risk factors at both the macro and micro levels. We briefly discuss the suicide risk assessment and intervention. The primary focus will be the presentation of pragmatic communication techniques to augment rural youth suicide risk assessment and intervention for both rural healthcare providers and families. The communication techniques described in this chapter are lessons learned by the chapter authors after many years of experience working with suicidal youth.

Suicide Risk Factors

Who is at risk for suicide? Suicide does not discriminate; every one of us is at risk. Common factors have been identified in individuals who have attempted and/or completed suicide. Factors such as prior suicide attempt, depression or other mental health disorders, substance abuse disorders, family history of mental health disorders or substance abuse, family history of suicide, family violence, and access to firearms have been hypothesized to increase an individual's risk for suicide (CDC, 2018). Additional risk factors have been identified and include lack of social support, feelings of hopelessness, and stressful life events (Singh et al., 2002).

Individuals in rural settings face many of the factors identified earlier coupled with additional obstacles related to geographic and environmental variations. Rural dwellers do not readily have access to specialty care like mental healthcare. Many rural dwellers do not have access to basics such as primary care provided by family nurse practitioners, physicians, or physician assistants. If a primary care provider is available, rural dwellers may have geographic barriers to cross to reach care. Geographic barriers can include mountain passes, gravel roads, and two-lane highways traversing hundreds of miles across open prairie with more cows than humans visible. In states where the motto "pull yourself up by your bootstraps" is both figurative and literal, a reticence to access mental healthcare services may also play a role. This is especially true in small towns where everyone seems to know your business, sometimes before you do.

Suicide Risk in a Rural State

You would be hard pressed to find a resident in the state of Montana who has not been touched by suicide in one way or another. A bit about the State of Montana. Montana is the fourth largest state in the United States and one of the most sparsely populated states with an average of 6.86 people per square mile (U.S. Census Bureau, 2018b). There are 56 counties in the State of Montana. Of those counties, 53 are considered to be rural based on definitions from multiple federal agencies (Office of Management and Budget, 2012; U.S. Census Bureau, 2018a; U.S. Department of Agriculture, 2019). Of Montana's 53 rural counties, 45 meet criteria for frontier counties (National Institutes of Health National Network of Libraries of Medicine, 2019). The term frontier is used to describe an area characterized by some combination of low population size and high geographic remoteness. It is the most remote end of the urban, suburban, and rural continuum (National Center for Frontier Communities, 2019).

Frontier and rural areas have historically experienced difficulties with access to healthcare. Long travel distances to essential services are common in Montana. Of the 56 Montana counties, 54 are designated as Health Professional Shortage Ares (HPSA), 55 are designated as Mental Health HPSA, and 41 as Dental HPSA (Montana DPHHS, 2019). Frontier and rural dwellers in Montana comprise a population with unique issues related to accessing healthcare and unique healthcare needs. Montanans are more likely to die prematurely as a result of cancer and unintentional injury deaths (CDC, 2018). Motor vehicle accidents are the primary cause of unintentional injury deaths in Montana. Motor vehicle accidents disproportionally take the lives of American Indians (AI) and residents living in rural counties (Montana Department of Transportation, 2011–2015; Montana DPHHS, 2019). Montana's suicide rate has continued to be one of the highest in the nation, with an average 240 completed suicides annually and 990 ED visits annually for suicide attempts (CDC National Center for Health Statistics, 2019). Suicide in Montana disproportionately affects youth.

Suicide Risk in Rural Montana Youth

For all age groups, Montana has had the dubious distinction of being in the top five states for highest suicide rates for more than 30 years. Montana youth suicide rates for persons aged 11 to 17 is 12.6 per 100,000 (CDC, 2018). Determining the risk factors associated with increased suicide risk for Montana youth has been difficult. Common factors previously associated with increased risk for death by suicide have been studied, reviewed, and acted upon with various initiatives. Despite targeted interventions and education, high youth suicide rates have persisted in Montana. Approximately 9% of Montana residents lack health insurance (Goe, 2019). The poverty rate in rural Montana tends to be higher at 13.4%, compared to 12.1% in urban areas (Kaiser Family Foundation, 2018). Rural Montanans tend to be undereducated and have higher levels of unemployment. The aforementioned factors may play a role in the higher number of youth suicide in Montana; however, it has been difficult to make a direct link to the risk factors and the increased rate of suicide.

Demographics of Montana youth dying by suicide tend to follow those exhibited by other states. Males are more likely than females to die by suicide in Montana. AIs in Montana are more likely to die by suicide with a rate of 28 per 100,000 population. This number is especially disconcerting considering AIs comprise only 6% of the general Montana population. Also, of great concern is the decreasing age of youth dying by suicide in Montana. Montana youth in the age range of 10 to 14 had a suicide rate of 12.6 per 100,000 people in 2018; this rate is almost triple the national rate for the same age group of 4.5 per 100,000 people (CDC, 2018). Over the past 10 years, 65% of Montana youth suicides were completed with a firearm (CDC, 2018).

Comparing Youth Risk Behavior Nationally and in Montana

Increasing rates of youth suicide across the United States led the CDC to develop the Youth Risk Behavior Surveillance System (YRBSS) in 1990. The YRBSS was initiated to monitor health risk behaviors that could contribute to the leading causes of death, disability, and social problems among all youth in the United States. A component of the YRBSS has included assessment of suicidal thoughts and behaviors. Since 1991 students at the national, state, and local levels have completed the YRBSS on a biannual basis (Kann et al., 2018). In 2017, the CDC released the first YRBSS Data Summary and Trends Report analyzing data and trends from the previous 10 years (Kann et al., 2018). An identified area of priority in the 2017 report was mental health. Table 19.1 outlines several factors in which Montana youth scored poorly compared to national percentages.

Montana youth are more likely to carry a weapon and carry a weapon while on school property. Montana youth also reported feeling sad/hopeless, considering suicide, planning how to die by suicide, and attempting suicide more frequently than their national counterparts. Nationally, males outnumber females in all age ranges for completed suicides. Although the same holds true for Montana youth, the number of females completing suicide in Montana is six times higher than the national average (Kann et al., 2018).

TABLE 19.1 Youth Risk Behavior Surveillance Data for Montana Youth

Percentage of High School Students Who:	National % (CI)	Montana % (CI)
Drove when they had been drinking alcohol	5.5 (4.9–6.3)	7.6 (6.6–8.8)
Drove when they had been using marijuana	13.0 (11.7–14.6)	54.2 (51.4–57.0)
Carried a weapon	15.7 (13.3–18.4)	25.2 (23.6–26.9)
Carried a weapon on school property	3.8 (2.9–4.8)	8.5 (7.4–9.8)
Carried a gun	4.8 (4.1–5.7)	7.7 (6.8–8.9)
Were electronically bullied	14.9 (13.7–16.2)	17.6 (16.3–19.0)
Felt sad or hopeless	31.5 (29.6–33.4)	31.0 (29.2–32.9)
Seriously considered attempting suicide	17.2 (16.2–18.3)	20.8 (19.2–22.6)
Made a plan about how they would attempt suicide	13.6 (12.4–14.8)	16.6 (15.5–17.9)
Actually, attempted suicide	7.4 (6.5–8.4)	9.5 (8.3–10.9)
Suicide attempt resulted in an injury, poisoning, or overdose that had to be treated by a doctor or nurse	2.4 (2.1–2.9)	3.1 (2.6–3.7)

Suicide Risk Assessment and Intervention

There are multiple depression screening tools, suicide risk assessment tools, suicidal ideation scales, and intervention trainings available to assess and intervene with individuals who are or may be suicidal. Unfortunately, many of the available tools have not been tested and validated in patients 18 years of age and younger. That being said, both the American Academy of Child and Adolescent Psychiatry (AACAP) and the American Academy of Pediatrics (AAP) recommend all pediatric patients be screened annually starting as early as 10 to 12 years of age (Sisler et al., 2020). Neither organization identifies a preferred screening or risk assessment tool, but they do offer suggested tools. Examples of tools suggested by AACAP and AAP include the SSHADESS assessment (Strengths, School, Home, Activities, Drug/Substance Use, Emotions/Eating/Depression, Sexuality and Safety), the Patient Health Questionnaire (PHQ-9), the more specific PHQ-9 Adolescent version, and the Columbia-Suicide Severity Rating Scale (C-SSRS). We will briefly review these tools below. It is important to note, no one tool, has been deemed the Gold Standard for assessment of suicide in youth. Lack of consensus on a single tool may point to a multifactorial picture of the "cause" of suicide.

Regardless of the tool or scale used to assess youth, the goal is to gather enough information to formulate a plan to prevent suicide attempts and/or intervene before an attempt becomes a completed suicide. Suicide prevention and intervention strategies must be multifaceted and tailored to the individual to address their risk factors and potential protective factors. Authors Cramer and Kapusta (2017) assessed and described major suicide risk and protective factors as informed by a social–ecological model to better understand the dynamic interrelations among personal and environmental factors. A social–ecological model starts with the individual, moves next to their interpersonal relationships, followed by community relationships, and finally societal relationships. Each level of a social–ecological model is influenced by factors at another level (Cramer & Kapusta, 2017).

In Cramer and Kapusta's (2017) model, identification of biological and personal factors that may contribute to increased suicide risk is necessary to implement interventions specific to the youth. Arming a youth with tools for conflict resolution, life skill training, and communication skills can bolster the youth's ability to address potential risk factors and augment the next level of social–ecological interaction, relationships (Cramer & Kapusta, 2017). The second level, relationship, is an assessment of the youth's social circle of peers, partners, and family members. Through assessment of relationships, identification of a strong support network and promotion of healthy relationships, can add to the youth's toolbox of skills necessary to work through difficult situations.

The third level of social–ecological interaction is the community. Specifically, identifying where social relationships occur for the youth is helpful in determining interventions aimed to reduce social isolation and decrease potential barriers. Finally, the fourth level examines the societal factors that may affect the youth including social and cultural norms. Interventions at the fourth level may require a more global approach targeted at processes and policies. Identification and mitigation of risk factors along with augmentation of protective factors across the continuum may serve for effective and lasting changes for the youth. All of the aforementioned factors are essential for a comprehensive approach to working with suicidal youth.

In years of clinical experience and direct work with suicidal rural youth, the authors of this chapter share their experience assessing suicidal rural youth. We have asked rural youth who have considered suicide in the past about the scales/tools/interventions used to assess them when they presented to healthcare systems as a suicidal youth. The rural youth frequently report they know "how" to answer the assessment tool questions. The rural youth are acutely aware of adults/healthcare providers asking questions about suicide risk because it is part of their job or a box that has to be checked. Rural youth are also aware when adults/healthcare providers are asking about suicide risk because they genuinely respect and care about the youth.

Conceptual Framework

Two concepts from Rural Nursing Theory as described by Long and Weinert (1989) germane to the discussion of rural youth suicide risk and assessment are self-reliance and outsider/insider. Youth are reluctant to accept help from people they do not trust or know. The rural nursing concept of self-reliance and its relationship to outsider/insider are essential components in understanding youth behavior, communication, and planning intervention (Long & Weinert, 1989).

Rural dwellers have been noted to delay seeking treatment until they are in crisis. Similarly, rural youth will act in a way that has been modeled by adults in their lives by not disclosing mental struggles and trying to manage things on their own. When they are willing to disclose, rural youth prefer to disclose to someone they trust or someone they believe can be trusted. Building rapport with rural youth quickly is not only desirable but is essential to begin the process of assessment and continue on to intervention. Trust and respect are critical components of communication, especially with rural youth.

Gatekeeper Training

Gatekeeper training has been touted as an essential assessment and intervention tool to identify and reduce suicide risk (Bell, 2016). Gatekeepers are individuals in a community who have regular contact with other members of a community and may be able to identify persons at risk for suicide and refer them to support services (Bell, 2016). A specific example of gatekeeper training is the Question, Persuade, Refer (QPR) training. QPR training is modeled after cardiopulmonary resuscitation (CPR) training concepts with the overall goal to improve survival (Bell, 2016). The Chain of Survival as described in

CPR training is based on the notion of an increased likelihood of survival if cardiac arrest symptoms are recognized early and interventions are implemented as soon as possible (American Heart Association & International Liaison Committee on Resuscitation, 2015). QPR is also based on early recognition and intervention in an effort to improve survival and decrease suicide-related injury and death. Knowledge learned by adults/healthcare providers in gatekeeper training has been shown to degrade with time after the initial completion of the training. Typically, a decrease to baseline knowledge levels has been shown within 6 months of completing gatekeeper training (Bell, 2016; Cross et al., 2011; Holmes et al., 2019). The same findings have also been found in other lifesaving skills/knowledge courses such as cardiopulmonary resuscitation.

Assessment Tools

Identification of factors that have been suggested to increase risk of suicide in youth is an important facet of care. As previously mentioned, several tools such as SSHADESS, PHQ-9/PHQ-9 Adolescent version, and the C-SSRS, have been suggested for use in patients 18 years of age and younger. The SSHADESS screen is based on a social–ecological model and explores risk and protective factors that may be present across eight domains or aspects of the youth's life. The SSHADESS tool provides a more detailed assessment by implementing a strength-based interviewing approach and requires the practitioner to have time to explore answers provided. The PHQ-9 and the PHQ-9 Adolescent consist of nine items based on the diagnostic criteria for depression. Each question is answered by rating with zero being not at all and three being nearly every day (Johnson et al., 2002). The PHQ-9 and PHQ-9 Adolescent version are most often used in primary care settings as a screening tool to identify the presence and severity of depression and as an assessment tool to monitor treatment response (Kroenke et al., 2001). The C-SSRS uses simple questions and algorithms to gauge severity of suicidal ideation, intensity of ideation, behavior and lethality (Posner et al., 2011). The C-SSRS is most often used in acute care settings and serve as a guide for interventions. Regardless of the tool used, establishing quick rapport and effective communication are essential.

Most often multiple risk factors interact at different levels to lead a youth from suicide risk to suicide action. A key factor in early identification and risk reduction is less about a tool or scale and more about how we as adults and healthcare providers communicate with youth. Suicidal youth have identified interpersonal conflict with family and peers as well as invalidation of thoughts and feelings by others as tipping points for suicide action (McManara-O'Brien et al., 2019). The authors of this chapter see great value in the augmentation of the current tools, scales, and training with techniques targeted to develop rapport and an authentic relationship quickly with all people, but especially with one of our most valuable resources, youth. In the next section, chapter author Kee Dunning, a licensed clinical social worker, will describe tools she has found invaluable in her psychotherapy practice and in life.

Kee Concepts of Communication

The following concepts are the themes of 40 plus years of practice in mental health, working primarily with children and their families. As a psychotherapist in private practice, I noticed recurring themes regardless of who I was seeing in my office. From these themes, I developed a list of communication concepts and called them *Kee Concepts*. Fortunately, my name allowed for a clever play on words in branding the concepts. I use the concepts with all of my clients regardless of age, and I teach the concepts across multiple professional disciplines including nursing. The coalescing of the themes into Kee Concepts of Communication is in many ways an informal ethnographic study of the many youth (and their families) I have had the honor to sit with and learn from. While therapy with me can occur within the confines of four walls, most often it occurs "in the wild" walking, talking, and experiencing the lives of my clients in their words. My work and the Kee Concepts of Communication will also be featured in a forthcoming Ken Burn's documentary on mental health. For clarity, I will refer to Kee Concepts of Communication simply as Kee Concepts from this point forward. I could continue to espouse the benefits of the concepts in both professional and personal life; however, I encourage you to read on and decide for yourselves the utility of these communication pearls Figure 19.1.

RESPECT

The foundation of Kee Concepts is respect. The word respect comes from the Latin word, respectus, which means attention, regard, and consideration (Meissner & Auden, 1894). The concept of respect can refer to our ability to value and honor another individual. We honor and value the other person's thoughts, words, and actions, even if we do not approve of or believe in the individual's thoughts, words, or actions. Respect is a cornerstone of human interaction and of life itself. Respect is the foundation upon which all conversation should be based. Being respectful is always possible, as it is a choice we make.

Children in therapy will often say grown-ups do not respect them. These young people say, "Nobody cares what I think, they don't really listen to me." Instead, youth will say adults want to "tell me what to do, how to think, and what I am thinking because they know best, because they are the grown up." The number one statement heard in therapy with children is "I just want them to listen to me!" Whether it be parents, teachers, coaches, or any adult youth encounter in their day-to-day life, they want to be heard. Respect means being heard, and we are not listening to our youth.

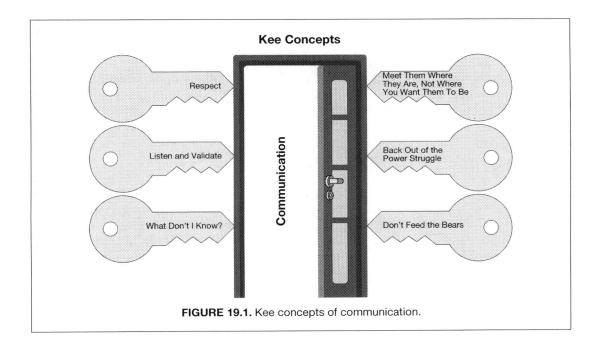

FIGURE 19.1. Kee concepts of communication.

Paramount to communicating with all people, especially youth, is a need to reframe the way we interact and communicate with others. How many times have you asked a patient a question, but in your mind, you have already answered the question for them? How many times have you asked a question and not really paid attention to the answer? How do we reframe our interactions to convey respect? We need to "Stop. Think. Plan."

Before each interaction, pause for a moment and ask yourself the following questions:

- What choices do I have for a response?
- What am I thinking and feeling about my interaction?
- Is what I am about to say respectful?
- Is what I am saying kind and loving?
- What about my tone of voice?
- What about my posture?
- Is what I am about to say necessary?
- If after I have said it, will I need to apologize?
- Would I be proud if I heard my own child use the same words and tone I am about to use?

Once you have answered these questions, make a plan, then act! Remember, it is always possible to be impeccable with your words, it is a choice you consciously make, so choose wisely.

LISTEN AND VALIDATE

Pay attention! Listen up! Are you really listening to me and what I have to say? Are you sure? Very few things strike fear in the heart of healthcare providers across all professions like these five words … "I feel like killing myself." Youth will often say the first reaction of adults when they hear those words is to say, "No, you don't?" or "Why would you want to take your life when your life is so good?" As adults, we often feel a need to fix the problem for our youth or talk them out of what they are thinking and/or feeling. Ask yourself, why is it so hard for adults to listen and support a youth in crisis? Youth are not asking us to fix anything. Youth really just want us to pay attention to what they are saying, acknowledge we have heard their words, and what they are trying to tell us. Youth do not want adults to talk them out of what they are feeling or thinking.

As healthcare providers (and adults) thinking about what listen and validate means you may be asking yourself several questions: How do I know whether I am actually listening? What in the world does it mean to validate? Do I just repeat what I heard back to the person? Will the person know I am trying to validate them? These are excellent questions to ask ourselves when we consider how we communicate and in case you were not aware, you were just validated!

Validation is actually hearing what the other person said and recognizing the emotion that may be a part of what they are communicating. Back to our suicidal youth, instead of telling the youth what they do not want to do or questioning why they would even be considering suicide, try approaching the youth by listening and validating. "I hear you saying you want to take your life and you sound scared (or whatever emotion you see/feel). Can you tell me more?" You are not agreeing with what the youth said, instead you are opening the door for more dialogue and allowing the youth a safe place to say what is on their mind at that moment. You may even be surprised how well this technique works in a variety of milieus. Listening and validating is about being genuine in your interactions and allowing yourself the opportunity to be open and authentic.

WHAT DO NOT I NOT KNOW?

Think about the word judgment. What does judgment mean to you? The word judgment has its roots in Latin, deriving from the root *ius*, meaning law or right paired with the root *dico* which, means to indicate or point out (Meissner & Auden, 1894). Have you ever passed judgment on another? What happened when you judged another human being and then took the time to actually listen to what they had to say? Did you find yourself thinking afterward, "I had no idea you [fill in the blank]?" The blank can be filled with any situation such as, not sleeping well, having to put a pet to sleep, just finding out your best friend died, or any number of situations too wide and broad to list here.

As human beings, we all pass judgment on others many times a day, sometimes without consciously recognizing we are judging until after the fact. Imagine, if instead of passing judgment we stopped ourselves and asked, "What don't I know about this person I am interacting with?" We all have a story and experiences that will influence the way we approach our lives. As previously mentioned, youth do not always feel as though we as adults respect or actually listen to them. What if I approached the young person in my examination room with respect, kindness, and a willingness to actually hear what they say, before passing judgment? As a practitioner, I might learn far more about this youth than if I made up my mind about what was going on before even walking in the exam room door. I might learn that this young person experienced the tragic loss of his grandparents at a young age and his mother was unable to care for him because she was consumed by depression. Or, I might learn the young woman waiting to be seen just found out her mother died from a drug overdose and now this youth has nowhere to live. What do I not know about you? Maybe if I took the time to slow down and listen, I could learn a lot.

MEET THEM WHERE THEY ARE, NOT WHERE YOU WANT THEM TO BE

Have you ever been in a conversation with another person and thought, "I know exactly what you need to do!" Perhaps your internal dialogue continued with, "You must do (fill in the blank), it is the right thing to do." The ability to meet people where they are and not where you want them to be is a gift. The gift in this scenario is allowing the people the opportunity to find their own way, even if it is not the way we (especially as professionals) would choose. Another element of meeting people where they are includes unconditional positive regard for the individual and the utmost respect. We may not like the decisions they make, but we respect them as individuals and will not judge or condemn them for the choices they have made along the way.

DO NOT FEED THE BEARS

What does "do not feed the bears" mean? Have you ever tried to feed a bear, not literally of course! Maybe you had treats in your pocket and kept feeding that figurative bear! You watched as the bear continued to devour the treats you offered, a hungry bear always wants more, the bear is insatiable! About those bears, bears come in all shapes, sizes, and ages. Bears can be in the form of your child, spouse, significant other, family members, bosses, coworkers, patients, and students. Feeding the figurative bear can begin as an innocent activity but consider proceeding with caution!

A bear feeding session may look like a straightforward conversation between two individuals. However, along the way, one of the individuals does not believe the other individual is listening or validating their thoughts or concerns. The bear starts to grumble, and the bear feed is about to ensue. A bear's favorite treats are fighting words! Fighting words can include statements such as, "You never listen!", "You don't care!", or "Have you heard even one word I have said?" Fighting words can also take the form of speaking in absolutes, using terms like always and never. Fighting words can also take the form of sarcasm.

Sarcasm comes from the Greek word, *sarkazein* which literally means to tear flesh. Bears LOVE sarcasm! Sarcasm can kill a relationship in seconds. Sarcasm can be seen as the lethal use of humor meant to demean and disrespect individuals. If you find yourself saying "just kidding" or I am "just teasing," then you should not have said anything. Sarcasm has no place in therapeutic and/or respectful communication. As previously mentioned, bears enjoy sarcasm and will always ask for more, so do not feed any bear sarcasm.

The next time you are faced with a growling and hungry bear, please take a moment to "Stop. Think. Plan." Ask yourself while you are thinking, "What Kee Concepts could I employ here to stop this bear feed?" or even better "What Kee Concepts could I employ to avoid feeding the bear in the first place?" The aforementioned Kee Concepts can be essential to avoid feeding the bear. The final concept to be covered here is also a critical component of getting out of a bear feeding!

Back Out of the Power Struggle

Last, but not least, is the Kee Concept of *back out of the power struggle*. As we learned in *do not feed the bears*, it is very easy to find yourself in communication with a hungry bear. Before the bear feeding goes too far, you can back out of the power struggle. By gathering all of the Kee Concepts in our communication bag of tools, we can come from a place of respect by listening and validating and backing out of the power struggle. Remind yourself that you may not know what is going on with this individual and you need to meet them where they are, not where you want them to be. If we practice communication from a place of love and respect, we may find ourselves communicating in a way all parties believe they have been heard and what they have to say matters.

IMPLICATIONS FOR NURSING EDUCATION AND PRACTICE

Practice using Kee Concepts in your day-to-day interactions with individuals you encounter, including your spouse, significant other, children, students, and patients. As you begin to incorporate these concepts into your daily conversations and interactions you will likely appreciate the potential for improving your communication. Establishing rapid rapport is advantageous for all communication and can be important in overcoming barriers. Two potential barriers experienced in rural healthcare include, but are not limited to, rural dwellers tendency toward self-reliance and possible mistrust of persons deemed to be outsiders. Use of Kee Concepts can provide a foundation upon which to establish a relationship and gain trust, potentially improving the willingness of the rural dweller to access healthcare earlier, before they are in crisis.

We recommend Kee Concepts be taught in nursing school starting early and frequently. Encouraging opportunities to practice the concepts throughout the education program will reinforce these tenants of communication. We have found periodic supervision via simulation a useful environment to practice, discuss, and enhance the use of these valuable communication concepts. Kee Concepts not only affect our communication with students but can also be helpful in communication with colleagues, thus encouraging a positive learning and leading environment.

We have included Kee Concepts in undergraduate and graduate nursing courses at Montana State University. Anecdotally, we have heard from current and former students with feedback on how valuable the concepts have been in both their professional and personal communication. We recently heard from a former student who is now a supervisor and leader in the ICU at a local hospital. She is about to start her graduate program working toward her Doctor of Nursing Practice degree as an acute care nurse practitioner. She contacted us out of the blue to say thank you for sharing the Kee Concepts. She believed these helpful tools allowed her to be more successful as an RN. She reported she uses her Kee Concepts daily in interactions with colleagues, administration, and most importantly patients. We encourage you to try Keep Concepts in your next interaction. You may be surprised what you learn and pleased when you can end a conversation not with apologies, but instead with a good feeling in your mind, gut, and heart.

Incorporating any or all of the Kee Concepts into the use of the scales and tools used to assess and intervene with suicidal youth may be valuable. Youth in crisis are acutely aware of the potential outcomes they may encounter based on how they answer the questions on any one of the scales we as healthcare providers may employ to assess their suicidal risk. If the youth believes the healthcare provider is coming from a genuine place of positive regard and respect, the healthcare provider may get more honest answers when asking hard questions. In turn, those honest answers and the rapid establishment of a mutually respectful relationship may allow healthcare provider to better intervene, and perhaps, save a life.

CONCLUSION

Suicide rates in rural youth outpace rates found in their urban counterparts. Despite targeted research focused on rural youth suicide risk assessment and intervention, the rates of suicide continue to increase in rural areas across the United States. The authors of this chapter encourage augmentation of evidence-based assessment tools and interventions with the Kee Concepts of Communication. We believe the Kee Concepts may prove especially useful for adults and healthcare providers working with rural youth.

Implications for nursing practice include the integration of Kee Concepts in nursing education as well as in gatekeeper trainings. Additional learning may be realized by designing simulation scenarios with a standardized patient incorporating opportunities to practice Kee Concepts at the bedside. Finally, the chapter authors would like to formally assess the perception of healthcare providers using Kee Concepts as well as the perceptions of patients receiving care from a provider practicing Kee Concepts. A research study specifically designed to assess perceptions of Kee Concepts may provide valuable feedback for continued refinement of the communication concepts as well as dissemination of potential benefits to a wider audience.

In closing, Kee Concepts are keys for communication learned through years of observation and interaction with youth and their families. The concepts are pragmatic notions easily applied to day-to-day communication and especially advantageous in a therapeutic milieu when the need to establish rapport quickly is necessary. We encourage you, the reader, to apply the concepts in your next interaction. What do you have to lose?

REFERENCES

American Heart Association & International Liaison Committee on Resuscitation. (2015). Guidelines 2015 for cardiopulmonary resuscitation and emergency cardiovascular care: An international consensus on science. *Circulation, 132*(Suppl I), s315–s367.

Bell, K. (2016). *Examining the effectiveness of gatekeeper training in suicide prevention*. Texas Women's University. https://twu-ir.tdl.org/handle/11274/9940

Centers for disease control and prevention. (2018). *Centers for disease control and prevention WISQARS leading cause of death report*. https://webappa.cdc.gov/sasweb/ncipc/leadcause.html

Centers for disease control and prevention National Center for Health Statistics. (2019). *Suicide mortality by state*. https://www.cdc.gov/nchs/pressroom/sosmap/suicide-mortality/suicide.htm

Chen, L., & Ingram, D. (2015). Quick stats: Age-adjusted rates for suicide, by urbanization of county of residence-United States, 2004 and 2013. *Mortality and Morbidity Weekly Report, 64*(14), 1.

Cramer, R., & Kapusta, N. (2017). A social-ecological framework of theory, assessment, and prevention of suicide. *Frontiers in Psychology, 8*, 1756. https://doi.org/10.3389/fpsyg.2017.01756

Cross, W., Seaburn, D., Gibbs, D., Schmeelk-Cone, K., White, A., & Caine, E. (2011). Does practice make perfect? A randomized control trial of behavioral rehearsal on suicide prevention gatekeeper skills. *The Journal of Primary Prevention, 32*(3–4), 195–201. https://doi.org/10.1007/s10935-011-0250-z

Goe, C. L. (2019). *2019 Report on health coveraged and montana's uninsured*. https://mthcf.org/wp-content/uploads/2019/06/2019-MT-Uninsured-Rate-Report_6.3.19-FINAL.pdf

Holmes, G., Clacy, A., Hermens, D., & Lagopoulus, J. (2019). The long term efficacy of suicide prevention gatekeeper training: A systematic review. *Archives of Suicide Research, 25*, 177–207. https://doi.org/10.1080/13811118.2019.1690608

Johnson, J., Harris, E., Spitzter, R., & Williams, J. (2002). The Patient Health Questionnaire for Adolescents: Validation of an instrument for the assessment of mental disorders among adolescent primary care patients. *Journal of Adolescent Health, 30*, 196–204. https://doi.org/10.1016/S1054-139X(01)00333-0

Kaiser Family Foundation. (2018). *Distribution of total population by federal poverty level*. https://www.kff.org/other/state-indicator/distribution-by-fpl/?currentTimeframe=0&sortModel=%7B%22colId%22:%22Location%22,%22sort%22:%22asc%22%7D

Kann, L., McManus, T., Harris, W., Shanklin, S., Flint, K., Wueen, B., Lowry, R., Chyen, D., Whittle, L., & Thornton, J. (2018). Youth risk behavior surveillance-US, 2017. *MMWR Surveillance Summer, 67*, 1–114. https://doi.org/10.15585/mmwr.ss6708a1. https://www.cdc.gov/healthyyouth/data/yrbs/pdf/2017/ss6708.pdf

Kroenke, K., Spitzer, R. L., & Williams, J. B. (2001). The PHQ-9. Validity of a brief depression severity measure. *Journal of Generall Internal Medicine, 16*(9), 606–613. https://doi.org/10.1046/j.1525-1497.2001.016009606.x

Long, K., & Weinert, C. (1989). Rural nursing: developing a theory base. *Scholarly Inquiry in Nursing Practice, 3*(2), 113–127.

McManara-O'Brien, K., Nicolopoulos, A., Almeida, J., Aguinaldo, L., & Rosen, R. (2019). Why adolescents attempt suicide: A qualitative study of the transition from ideation to action. *Archives of Suicide Research, 25*, 269–286. https://doi.org/10.1080/13811118.2019.1675561

Meissner, C., & Auden, H. W. (1894). *Latin phrase book*. Macmillan and Company.

Montana Department of Transportation. (2011–2015). *Fatal accident reporting system*. www.dojmt.gov

Montana DPHHS. (2019). *Montana state health assessment: 2017 A report on the health of Montanans*. https://dphhs.mt.gov/Portals/85/ahealthiermontana/2017SHAFinal.pdf

National Center for Frontier Communities. (2019). *Getting the word out on the frontier and remote designation methodology*. http://frontierus.org/what-is-frontier/

National Institutes of Health National Network of Libraries of Medicine. (2019). *Pacific northwest region: Montana*. https://nnlm.gov/pnr/about/montana

Office of Management and Budget. (2012). *Patterns of metropolittan and micropolitan population change: 2000 to 2010*. https://www.census.gov/library/publications/2012/dec/c2010sr-01.html

Posner, K., Brent, D., Lucas, C., Goulrd, M., Stanley, B., Brown, G., & Mann, J. (2011). Columbia-Suicide Severity Rating Scale (C-SSRS): Initial validty and internal consistency findings from three multisite studies with adolescents and adults. *American Journal of Psychaitry*, *168*, 1266–1277. https://doi.org/10.1176/appi.ajp.2011.10111704

Singh, A., Gopal, K., & Siahpush, M. (2002). Increasing rural-urban gradients in US suicide mortality, 1970-1997. *American Journal of Public Health*, *92*(7), 1161–1167. https://doi.org/10.2105/AJPH.92.7.1161

Sisler, S., Shapiro, N., Nakaishi, M., & Steinbuchel, P. (2020, June 22). Suicide assessment and treatment in pediatric primary care settings. *Journal of Child and Adolsecent Psychiatric Nursing*, *33*, 187–200. https://doi.org/10.1111/jcap.12282

U.S. Census Bureau. (2018a). *2010 Census urban and rural classification and urban area criteria*. https://www.census.gov/programs-surveys/geography/guidance/geo-areas/urban-rural/2010-urban-rural.html

U.S. Census Bureau. (2018b). *Quick facts: Montana*. https://www.census.gov/quickfacts/MT

U.S. Department of Agriculture. (2019). *Rural-urban commuting area codes*. https://www.ers.usda.gov/data-products/rural-urban-commuting-area-codes.aspx

Improving Health Literacy About Complementary and Alternative Therapy Among Rural Dwellers

JEAN SHREFFLER-GRANT, ELIZABETH NICHOLS,
AND CLARANN WEINERT

DISCUSSION TOPICS

- Discuss how the findings of each study included in this chapter led to the subsequent studies.
- Do you think that rural dwellers' tendency to be self-reliant and seek advice from informal sources contributes to the use of complementary and alternative medicine (CAM) as part of their health-seeking behaviors?
- How can the intervention discussed in the *Healthcare Choices: Be Safe* and *Be Wise* section of this chapter affect the healthcare choices made by older rural adults?
- How can nurses use the results of the studies discussed in this chapter to benefit the health of their rural clients/patients?

INTRODUCTION

Adequate health literacy is necessary in today's healthcare marketplace so that consumers are able to understand and evaluate the information regarding conventional or allopathic healthcare (Institute of Medicine [IOM], 2004). Health literacy is defined in *Healthy People 2010* as "the degree to which individuals have the capacity to obtain, process, and understand basic health information and services needed to make appropriate health decisions" (U.S. Department of Health and Human Services, 2000, Section 11–12).

Health literacy is even more important for evaluating complementary and alternative medicine (CAM). Healthcare consumers usually have some assistance from providers to interpret information about allopathic care and often receive instructions and advice to guide healthcare decision-making and action taking. This is less likely with CAM. These therapies are often self-prescribed or self-directed in nature and are less regulated or controlled by governmental agencies or allopathic providers. Further studies have found that often there is limited communication between consumers and allopathic providers about consumers' use or potential use of CAM (Eisenberg et al., 1993, 1998; Rodondi et al., 2019; Vallerand et al., 2003).

During the past several decades, the use of CAM in the United States has grown significantly (Barnes et al., 2008; Eisenberg et al., 1993, 1998; IOM, 2005; National Center for Complementary and Integrative Health [NCCIH], 2020). CAM has become an important component of the U.S. healthcare system as consumers, including those living in rural areas, increasingly use CAM as an adjunct to or substitute for conventional healthcare (Arcury et al., 2004; Astin, 1998; Eisenberg et al., 1998; Harron & Glasser, 2003; McFarland et al., 2002). Some people use CAM instead of allopathic care because of the lower cost of CAM, which is particularly evident during downturns in the economy (Tanner, 2009). The NCCIH (2020) defines CAM as healthcare approaches that are not typically part of conventional medical care or that may have origins outside of usual Western practice. They include natural products such as herbs, vitamins, and other dietary supplements and mind and body practices such as yoga, meditation, and acupuncture. The CAM therapies and products are not considered part of allopathic care in part because there is insufficient evidence that they are safe and effective. Types of CAM range from therapies provided by practitioners such as naturopathic physicians and acupuncturists to self-care practices, such as herbs and magnets.

Approximately 35% to 40% of adults in the United States reported having used some form of CAM in the past 12 months (Barnes et al., 2004, 2008; Clarke et al., 2015; NCCIH, 2020). In addition, roughly one in nine (11.8%–12%) children used CAM in the past 12 months (Barnes et al., 2008; Black et al., 2015). Not surprisingly, use among children whose parents used CAM was significantly higher (23.9%) than among children whose parents did not use CAM (5.1%). When cost concerns cause a delay in seeking allopathic care, CAM is more likely to be used by both adults and children than when cost is not a concern (Barnes et al., 2004). Despite the widespread use and acceptance of CAM in the general population, consumers are reluctant to inform allopathic providers that they used CAM (Eisenberg et al., 1993, 1998).

On the basis of the literature, the demographics of those in the general U.S. population who use CAM vary; but in general, CAM is used more often for chronic than acute health conditions and use is more common among women than men, younger adults than older, those with higher incomes and more education, and those living in the West than in other parts of the country (Astin, 1998; Astin et al., 2000; Cherniack et al., 2001; Eisenberg et al., 1998). Studies have found that individuals with chronic illness have a variety of reasons for using CAM, including (a) symptom relief, (b) ineffectiveness of allopathic treatments, (c) side effects of allopathic treatments, (d) dissatisfaction with allopathic care, (e) concerns about adverse effects of allopathic care, (f) desire for control, and (g) the ready availability of CAM (Johnson, 1999; Johnson et al., 2016; Montbraind & Laing, 1991; Rao et al., 1999; Vincent & Furnham, 1996).

Despite extensive literature searches, no empirical studies on health literacy specifically about CAM could be located at the time when this research team began its work. There is also very limited evidence in general about how much CAM users know about the products and treatments they use, what sources of information they use, or how they evaluate and use the information they have or acquire (IOM, 2005). Evidence is also lacking about how consumers in the United States decide when and how to use CAM and whether to comply with instructions from CAM providers or product labels. One study found that while 80% of older study participants reported using two or more CAM therapies, their self-rated knowledge about most of the therapies was very low (King & Pettigrew, 2004). The IOM cited three primary sources of information that consumers use about CAM: word of mouth, the Internet, and health food stores. The few studies evaluating the quality of information available from these sources suggested that quality may be a concern.

The purpose of this chapter is to present a summary of a series of research studies conducted by a team of investigators at the Colleges of Nursing at Montana State University (MSU) and the University of North Dakota on the use of CAM by older rural dwellers. The results of these projects raised several researchable questions regarding the health literacy levels about CAM among older rural adults, particularly rural adults with chronic illnesses. The results are relevant to the second Rural Nursing Theory theoretical statement identified by Long and Weinert (1989; also see Chapter 2) and further discussed and updated by Lee and McDonagh (2018; also see Chapter 4) and Lee and Winters (2018; also see Chapter 1). Self-reliance and use of informal networks for advice and care are the characteristics of rural residents that influence their health-seeking behaviors. These characteristics can also affect the choices that rural adults make when deciding about the use of complementary or alternative therapies.

HEALTHCARE CHOICES: A STUDY OF COMPLEMENTARY THERAPY USE AMONG OLDER RURAL DWELLERS

At the time this study was conducted, multiple well-known studies had demonstrated that use of CAM was growing among the general population in the United States, but little was known about the use of these therapies among rural residents. Most of the national studies did not report where study participants lived, and some used only urban participants. To address this gap in the literature, the *Healthcare Choices* study was conducted with older adults living in sparsely populated rural areas in Montana and North Dakota (Shreffler-Grant et al., 2005). The purpose of the study was to explore the use of, cost of, and satisfaction with the quality and effectiveness of CAM from the perspectives of the older rural adult participants. The study was conducted during 2000 to 2003 and funded by National Center for Complementary and Alternative Medicine (NCCAM) (R15AT09501). A descriptive survey design was used to generate data from a random sample of older adults in 19 rural communities in Montana and North Dakota. An interview instrument was developed to elicit data addressing the specific aims and was piloted prior to use in a 20th community. Telephone interviews were conducted with 325 older adults. Participants ranged in age from 60 to 98 years ($m = 71.7$). Most of the participants (67.7%, $n = 202$) reported having one or more chronic illnesses. Only 17.5% ($n = 57$) reported using CAM providers, whereas 35.7% ($n = 116$) used self-prescribed CAM practices. When these two categories of use were combined, a total of 45.2% of the participants used some form of CAM, or used CAM providers, self-prescribed CAM practices, or both. This finding demonstrated that these older rural residents were using as much or more CAM than participants in national studies (36%–40%) that included all adult age groups.

Relevant to the issue of health literacy about CAM, the participants in this study most often learned about the CAM therapies by word of mouth from relatives or friends, consumer marketing, or reading, rather than from healthcare professionals (Shreffler-Grant et al., 2005). Much of the CAM used by participants of this study was self-prescribed, raising questions about whether the participants had sufficient knowledge and information for safe and effective use of the CAM products. In addition, a majority (64.6%, $n = 210$) of the participants reported that they had at least one significant acute or chronic health problem and 32.3% ($n = 105$) had two or more significant health problems. The research team wondered about the potential for adverse drug–herb or drug–vitamin interactions with this population of vulnerable older adults, who likely were taking multiple prescription medications and had aging, impaired physiological responses.

Healthcare Choices: Older Rural Women

Additional analyses were conducted on a portion of the data set generated in the first *Healthcare Choices* study to answer the following research question: What factors predict the use of CAM among older rural women (Shreffler-Grant et al., 2007)? Men were excluded from this analysis because too few men in the larger data set used CAM, which is consistent with the literature about CAM use. Potential predictors were based on the literature and observations from practice and included education, age, rurality, marital status, income, spirituality, number of chronic illnesses, and health status. Logistic regression analysis was used to examine factors associated with the use of CAM by rural women participants ($n = 156$). A total of 25.6% of the women had used CAM recently and most of the therapies they used were self-prescribed. Women most likely to use CAM were those who were fairly well educated, not currently married, and in their early older years (60–69 years of age). They had one or more significant chronic illnesses and lower health-related quality of life due to emotional concerns such as depression or stress.

Although this analysis did not yield additional information about health literacy about CAM per se, the results reinforced and expanded the findings of the main study discussed earlier. The women who reported use of CAM in this analysis used primarily self-prescribed CAM, which again raises concern about their level of knowledge about CAM. Women with one or more chronic illnesses were more likely to use CAM than those without chronic illness. Specifically, for each additional chronic illness reported, the odds of CAM use increased by 46%. By identifying characteristics of older rural women who are more or less likely to use CAM, the results can be used to tailor educational interventions to improve health literacy about CAM.

Healthcare Choices: Chronic Illness

The purpose of this study was to provide a better understanding of older rural adults' use of CAM, their perceptions of efficacy of the CAM they used, and the sources of information they used about CAM (Nichols et al., 2005). The study was conducted during 2003 to 2006 and funded by the Center for Research on Chronic Health Conditions (CRCHC) in Rural Dwellers at MSU College of Nursing (National Institutes of Health [NIH]/National Institute of Nursing Research [NINR] IP20NR07790-01). Ten participants between 60 and 80 years of age who reported using CAM in the original *Healthcare Choices* study and who had two or more chronic illnesses were interviewed by telephone. Qualitative analysis was used to organize content from the interviews and identify themes. Participants used primarily self-prescribed CAM therapies such as dietary supplements and herbs, taken to compensate for perceived dietary deficiencies. Participants were generally satisfied with the results they attributed to the CAM. With regard to health literacy about CAM, the participants attempted to use reputable sources of information about the CAM products they used, but it was clear that some used the products in an inconsistent manner and did not understand what the products were intended to do for their health. Some individuals reported seeking information about CAM from sources other than their allopathic providers due to a perception that the providers were too busy to answer their questions about CAM.

Healthcare Choices: CAM Providers in Rural Locations

The CAM providers in rural locations study was motivated by the results of the first *Healthcare Choices* study, in which the older rural adults reported limited use of CAM providers, in contrast to self-prescribed CAM. The study's purpose was to determine the availability of CAM resources in 20 small rural towns in Montana and North Dakota and to explore the contribution of one type of CAM provider, naturopathic physicians, to rural healthcare (Nichols et al., 2006). The study was conducted during 2004 to 2005 and funded by the CRCHC in Rural Dwellers at MSU College of Nursing (NIH/NINR IP20NR07790-01). CAM resource data were collected from Internet and telephone directory searches and from an online survey of naturopathic physicians in Montana. Seventy-three CAM providers were identified in the 20 towns. Most naturopaths were in population centers, but some offered outreach clinics to rural communities. Based on the results, the team concluded that local availability is not the critical factor in the use of CAM providers by older rural adults. Although there were likely fewer choices of CAM providers in these small rural towns than in larger towns or cities, there were CAM providers available if the rural residents chose to use them. Rural residents are also known to travel outside their local communities to see healthcare providers who are acceptable to them (Shreffler-Grant, 2018).

HEALTHCARE CHOICES: CAM HEALTH LITERACY

MSU CAM Health Literacy Scale

Owing to questions concerning CAM health literacy revealed in the studies discussed earlier, the research team identified the need for an intervention to improve health literacy about CAM among older rural adults, particularly those with chronic health conditions. A measure of health literacy specific to CAM was needed to determine whether the intervention was effective or not. The existing health literacy measures were not suitable for this purpose since they evaluate basic reading and math skills in a conventional healthcare context (IOM, 2004) and not the more complex aspects needed to make reasoned decisions about the use of CAM. Accordingly, the research team designed the next *Healthcare Choices* project, the purpose of which was to develop a psychometrically sound instrument to measure CAM health literacy. In this project, CAM health literacy was operationally defined as the information about CAM needed to make informed self-management decisions regarding health. The optimal outcome of CAM health literacy is informed self-management of health.

Work to develop and evaluate a new instrument spanned a number of years and was supported by two intramural grants from MSU College of Nursing (2008–2009, 2015–2017) and a federal grant from NIH/NCCAM (1R15T006609-01 2011–2013). The research team utilized DeVellis' (2003) well-established guidelines for scale development to guide the instrument development process and DeVellis served as a consultant as the instrument was developed. A conceptual model of CAM Health Literacy was first developed to clarify the concepts to be included in the new instrument (Shreffler-Grant et al., 2013). A large pool of initial items for the instrument that fit with the empirical indicators in the conceptual model was developed. The draft instrument was reviewed and critiqued by experts and focus groups to assist in evaluating content validity. Following this review, the draft instrument was administered by telephone interview to a sample of 600 randomly selected older adults living in rural areas in the northwestern quadrant of the

United States. Psychometric evaluation of the instrument using the data from the telephone interviews was conducted by a lengthy interactive process of examining the effect of individual items on reliability and validity indices. The outcome of this process is the *MSU CAM Health Literacy Scale*, a 21-item instrument with Cronbach's alpha of 0.753% and 42.27% explained variance (Shreffler-Grant et al., 2014). The scale consists of a list of statements about herbal products, a type of commonly used complementary therapy. Response options range from agree strongly to disagree strongly based on the respondent's knowledge and understanding of the item content.

The validity of the MSU CAM Health Literacy Scale was further assessed by administering the new scale and two measures of general health literacy to a convenience sample of 110 older rural adults. The general health literacy measures used were the Newest Vital Sign (Weiss et al., 2005) and a single question measure (Chew et al., 2004). The scores on the new scale and general health literacy measures were compared and revealed modest but significant correlations. The research team conducted an additional evaluation of the validity and reliability of the MSU CAM Health Literacy Scale using test–retest procedures. The MSU CAM Health Literacy Scale and two general health literacy measures were administered to a group of rural community-dwelling adults (Time 1) and then again approximately 3 weeks later (Time 2). A total of 188 adults completed both administrations. The results, in brief, supported the validity and reliability of the MSU CAM Health Literacy Scale and the stability of the scale score from Time 1 to Time 2 (Weinert et al., 2019).

Although evaluation of the scale will be an ongoing process, the MSU CAM Health Literacy Scale is now a validated and reliable measure of CAM health literacy. The scale was designed for research purposes to evaluate the effectiveness of an intervention to enhance CAM health literacy. Nurse investigators, however, may find that the scale is useful in other studies in which knowledge about safe use of CAM products or knowledge that supports effective self-care and self-management practices are relevant. The scale may also have important practice applications if used as a screening tool for rural older adults at risk for limitations in health literacy about CAM.

Healthcare Choices: Be Safe

The research team's long-term goal has been to design and implement an intervention to improve health literacy about CAM among older rural adults, particularly those with chronic health conditions. With this goal in mind, the team designed and implemented a pilot project to examine the feasibility of a skill-building intervention to enhance CAM health literacy among older rural adults (Shreffler-Grant et al., 2018). The project was entitled *Healthcare Choices: Be Safe* and was conducted with funding from the NIH, National Library of Medicine (HHS-N-276-2011-00008-C 2014–2015) and an intramural grant from MSU (2014–2015).

Skill-building modules were developed for the program that focused on concepts and skills important for CAM health literacy, how to be safe when using dietary supplements and herbal products, communication with providers, and seeking and evaluating health information. The content of the modules is focused on encouraging informed use of CAM rather than encouraging or discouraging use. The modules were presented face to face and by webinar with older adults at a senior center in one small rural community in Montana. Participants completed a survey packet including the MSU CAM Health Literacy Scale and measures of general health literacy before and after the intervention. The team determined that conducting the intervention with older adults in a small rural community was feasible, although there were challenges to overcome such as gaining entry to the rural community, recruitment and retention limitations, the cost of an on-site intervention, and limitations of local resources. The feasibly study was not intended to test the effectiveness of the intervention on CAM health literacy; however, the level of CAM health literacy among the participants increased modestly. The team utilized the lessons learned in this feasibility study in the design of a more comprehensive skill-building intervention.

Healthcare Choices: Be Wise

The *Healthcare Choices: Be Wise* research study was implemented from 2016 to 2019 with support from the NIH, NCCIH (1R15AT009097-01 2016–2019). The aims of the study were to implement the skill-building intervention with older rural adults, refine and evaluate the skill-building modules and intervention protocol, and evaluate the impact of the intervention on CAM health literacy and general health literacy. The intervention is designed to enhance CAM health literacy and general health literacy and thus promote more informed health management decisions.

The intervention was implemented with older adults in eight rural communities in two northwestern states in the United States. The intervention sessions were presented in person at Senior Centers or Senior Living Centers following congregate lunch times at each site. The intervention consisted of four skill-building educational modules, each of which was 1 to 1½ hours in length offered every other week over a 7-week period. The content of the modules included: health literacy and why it is important, how to be safe when using dietary CAM supplements and over-the-counter medicines, how to find and evaluate health information, and how to be a wise partner with one's healthcare provider. The content was based on the research team's prior studies, the conceptual model, and evidence in the literature. The modules were refined based on the findings of the prior feasibility *Healthcare Choices: Be Safe* study.

Participants completed questionnaire packets at the first session (Time 1), following the fourth session (Time 2), and 5 months after the intervention (Time 3). Descriptive statistics and general linear modeling were used for analysis. It was hypothesized that CAM health literacy and general health literacy scores at Time 2 (T2) would be higher than scores at Time 1 and Time 3. The hypothesis was based on common wisdom that knowledge gained from educational sessions would likely be most robust immediately following provision of the education. Since the intervention was intended for older adults, the hypothesis is also based on literature that indicates that some cognitive changes, including changes in memory, are a normal process of aging (Harada et al., 2013).

A total of 127 older adults completed the initial session and Time 1 questionnaire, 67 (51%) completed the intervention sessions and Time 2 questionnaire, and 52 (40.9%) completed the Time 3 questionnaire 5 months later. Of the 67 participants who completed the intervention sessions, a majority were women (77.6%), aged 76.5 years on average, white non-Hispanic (98.4%), married or widowed (64%), and with more than a high school education (61%). A majority (61.3%) of those who reported income made $35,000 or less in the prior year. Self-ratings of health were somewhat equally spread across Poor/Fair, Good, and Very Good/Excellent. Despite the fairly high levels of self-reported health status, most participants (64.6%) reported having one or more significant health problem. A majority (63.1%) indicated that they had used CAM in the past 5 years.

CAM health literacy and general health literacy scores for the 52 participants who completed the Time 1, 2, and 3 questionnaires were analyzed using multivariate general linear model analyses for repeated measures. These analyses were used to test the hypothesis. CAM health literacy scores and scores on one general health literacy measure were significantly higher at Time 2 compared to Time 1 and 3, which was as hypothesized. Scores on a second general health literacy measure increased at Time 2 and again at Time 3, contrary to the hypothesis. The declining CAM health literacy scores and scores on one general health literacy measure over time strongly suggest a need for continuing strategies to support and reinforce older adults' health literacy knowledge and skills. Continued support could include periodic "Boosters" such as review sessions of the highlights of the educational session content or a mnemonic that can aid participants to retain the information.

The Time 2 and 3 questionnaires included questions to determine the participants' satisfaction with the intervention sessions and their perspectives on the usefulness of the information presented. All evaluation questions were generally or very positive, for example, 3.5 to 4.5 on a 5-point scale, except for questions regarding the use of the computer or the Internet to seek health information which had mean scores in the 2-point range. Although most participants had access to a computer with Internet connections at the Senior Center, senior living center, and/or at home, some participants indicated that they did not use computers at all. Responses on open-ended evaluation questions were all very favorable. During implementation of the *Healthcare Choices: Be Wise* intervention, the team experienced many of the same challenges that were encountered during the prior *Healthcare Choices: Be Safe* feasibility study, including gaining entry to multiple rural communities, recruitment and retention of participants, and the time and costs associated with an on-site intervention in multiple sites. Despite facing challenges, the aims of the study were successfully achieved.

The *Healthcare Choices: Be Wise* intervention is a new intervention that resulted in enhanced CAM and general health literacy among older rural adults. With additional testing, it is anticipated that this study will make a unique and significant contribution to the state of the science regarding effective methods to improve health literacy and thus promote more informed health management decisions. Prior to the work of this research team, health literacy specific to CAM was not addressed in the literature and there had not been studies on interventions to improve this aspect of health literacy. Although the intervention was designed for and implemented with older rural adults, the content of the sessions is not specific to the rural population, hence, it may be appropriate for implementation with adults of any age regardless of where they reside.

The older rural adults in this study demonstrated that they are motivated to learn how to be safe consumers and active participants in their healthcare decision-making. The *Healthcare Choices: Be Wise* skill-building intervention involved information and active discussions to enhance health literacy skills in areas such as finding, understanding, and evaluating health-related information and knowing what questions to ask before making independent health decisions. Providing additional knowledge and skills to assist older rural adults in making safe and well-informed healthcare choices is a critical role for investigators, nurses, and other healthcare providers.

CONCLUSION

Over the past two decades, this research team conducted the series of studies discussed earlier on the use of CAM among older rural adults. This work led us to identify a need to enhance the level of health literacy about CAM among this population, particularly those with chronic illnesses. To address this need, the team subsequently developed a conceptual model of CAM health literacy as well as an instrument to measure it. Following these endeavors, we then developed and implemented a skill-building intervention to enhance CAM health literacy and general health literacy among older rural dwellers.

Healthcare consumers in any location, particularly those with chronic illnesses, make numerous decisions about healthcare and use a wide variety of self-care health products and therapies, decisions often made on their own and independent of their regular healthcare providers. This is particularly true of older rural adults, who are known to be more independent, engage in more self-care, and have less access to allopathic care than those living in urban areas (Shreffler-Grant et al., 2007). Those with chronic illnesses are also more likely to use CAM therapies (Astin, 1998; Astin et al., 2000; Barnes et al., 2004; Eisenberg et al., 1998; Shreffler-Grant et al., 2007).

Making informed decisions about the use of CAM requires a sophisticated level of health literacy on the part of the consumer. Without adequate CAM health literacy, older rural consumers may not know of all the appropriate healthcare choices that may benefit them, may fall victim to scams or unscrupulous sales practices, or may ingest potentially harmful substances. Informed use of CAM can increase health and illness management options and support well-reasoned decision-making in regard to self-care for older rural adults living with chronic illnesses.

ACKNOWLEDGMENTS

The authors wish to acknowledge the following individuals: Bette Ide, PhD, RN (deceased), professor, University of North Dakota, College of Nursing, who served as a former member of the research team; David Young DVM, PhD, professor and community resources specialist, Montana State University, Bozeman, Montana, who served as a community site consultant; and Martha Lentz, PhD, RN (deceased), professor emerita and research scientist, University of Washington, School of Nursing, Seattle, Washington, who served as a data analysis consultant.

The research studies were funded in part by the following grants: NIH, National Center for Complementary and Alternative Health/National Center for Complementary and Integrative Health (1R15AT095-01 2000–2003, 1R15T006609-01 2011–2013, and 1R15AT009097-01 2016–2019); NIH, National Library of Medicine (Contract No. HHS-N-276-2011-00008-C with University of Washington 2014–2015); Center for Research on Chronic Health Conditions at MSU College of Nursing (NIH/NINR IP20NR07790-01 2003-2005); two intramural grants (2008–2009, 2015–2017) from MSU College of Nursing; and one Intramural Faculty Excellence Grant from MSU 2014–2015.

REFERENCES

Arcury, T. A., Preisser, J. S., Gesler, W. M., & Sherman, J. E. (2004). Complementary and alternative medicine use among rural residents in western North Carolina. *Complementary Health Practice Review*, 9(2), 93–102. https://doi.org/10.1177/1076167503253433

Astin, J. (1998). Why patients use alternative medicine: Results of a national study. *Journal of the American Medical Association*, 279(19), 1548–1553. https://doi.org/10.1001/jama.279.19.1548

Astin, J., Pelletier, K., Marie, A., & Haskell, W. (2000). Complementary and alternative medicine use among elderly persons: One-year analysis of a Blue Shield Medicare supplement. *Journal of Gerontology*, 55A(1), M4–M9. https://doi.org/10.1093/gerona/55.1.M4

Barnes, P. M., Bloom, B., & Nahin, R. L. (2008). *Complementary and alternative medicine use among adults and children: United States, 2007. National health statistics reports*, No. 12. National Center for Health Statistics.

Barnes, P. M., Pewell-Griner, E., McFann, K., & Nahin, R. L. (2004). *Complementary and alternative medicine use among adults: United States, 2002*. National health statistics reports, No. 343. National Center for Health Statistics.

Black, L. I., Clarke, T. C., Barnes, P. M., Stussman, B. J., & Nahin, R. L. (2015). *Use of complementary health approaches among children aged 4-17 years in the United States: National Health Interview Survey, 2007-2012*. National health statistics reports, No. 78. National Center for Health Statistics.

Cherniack, E. P., Senzel, R. S., & Pan, C. X. (2001). Correlates of use of alternative medicine by the elderly in an urban population. *Journal of Alternative and Complementary Medicine, 7*, 277–280. https://doi.org/10.1089/107555301300328160

Chew, L. D., Bradley, K. A., & Boyko, E. J. (2004). Brief questions to identify patients with inadequate health literacy. *Family Medicine, 36*(8), 588–594. https://fammedarchives.blob.core.windows.net/imagesandpdfs/pdfs/FamilyMedicineVol36Issue8Chew588.pdf

Clarke, T. C., Black, L. I., Stussman, B. J., Barnes, P. M., & Nahin, R. L. (2015). *Trends in the use of complementary health approaches among adults: United States, 2002-2012*. National health statistics reports, No. 79. National Center for Health Statistics.

DeVellis, R. (2003). *Scale development: Theory and applications* (2nd ed.). Sage.

Eisenberg, D., Davis, R., Ettner, S., Appel, S., Wilkey, S., Van Rompay, M., & Kessler R. C. (1998). Trends in alternative medicine use in the United States, 1990–1997: Results of a follow-up national survey. *Journal of the American Medical Association, 280*(18), 1569–1575. https://doi.org/10.1001/jama.280.18.1569

Eisenberg, D., Kessler, R., Foster, C., Norlock, F., Calkins, D., & Delbanco, T. (1993). Unconventional medicine in the United States. *The New England Journal of Medicine, 328*, 246–252. https://doi.org/10.1056/NEJM199301283280406

Harada, C. N., Love, M. N., & Triebel, K. (2013). Normal cognitive aging. *Clinics in Geriatric Medicine, 29*(4), 737–752. https://doi.org/10.1016/j.cger.2013.07.002

Harron, M., & Glasser, M. (2003). Use of and attitudes toward complementary and alternative medicine among family practice patients in small rural Illinois communities. *The Journal of Rural Health, 19*(3), 279–284. https://doi.org/10.1111/j.1748-0361.2003.tb00574.x

Institute of Medicine. (2004). *Health literacy: A prescription to end confusion*. National Academies Press.

Institute of Medicine. (2005). *Complementary and alternative medicine in the United States*. National Academies Press.

Johnson, J. (1999). Older rural women and the use of complementary therapies. *Journal of Community Health Nursing, 16*(4), 223–232. https://doi.org/10.1207/S15327655JCHN1604_2

Johnson, P. J., Kozhimannil, K. B., Jou, J., Ghildayal, N., & Rockwood, T. H. (2016). Complementary and alternative medicine use among women of reproductive aga in the United States. *Womens Health Issues, 26*(1), 40–47. https://doi.org/10.1016/j.whi2015.08.009

King, M. O., & Pettigrew, A. C. (2004). Complementary and alternative therapy use by older adults in three ethnically diverse populations: A pilot study. *Geriatric Nursing, 25*(1), 30–37. https://doi.org/10.1016/j.gerinurse.2003.11.013

Lee, H. J., & McDonagh, M. K. (2018). Updating the rural nursing base. In C. A. Winters (Ed.), *Rural nursing: Concepts, theory, and practice* (5th ed., pp. 45–62). Springer Publishing Company.

Lee, H. J., & Winters, C. A. (2018). Rural nursing theory: Past, present, and future. In C. A. Winters & H. J. Lee (Eds.), *Rural nursing: Concepts, theory, and practice* (5th ed., pp. 3–15). Springer Publishing Company.

Long, K. A., & Weinert, C. (1989). Rural nursing: Developing the theory base. *Scholarly Inquiry for Nursing Practice: An International Journal, 3*, 113–127. https://doi.org/10.1891/0889-7182.3.2.113

McFarland, B., Bigelow, D., Zani, B., Newsom, J., & Kaplan, M. (2002). Complementary and alternative medicine use in Canada and the United States. *American Journal of Public Health, 92*, 1616–1618. https://doi.org/10.2105/AJPH.92.10.1616

Montbraind, M., & Laing, G. (1991). Alternative health care as a control strategy. *Journal of Advanced Nursing, 16*, 325–332. https://doi.org/10.1111/j.1365-2648.1991.tb01656.x

National Center for Complementary and Integrative Health. (2020). *Complementary, alternative, or integrative health: What's in a name?* https://www.nccih.nih.gov/health/complementary-alternative-or-integrative-health-whats-in-a-name

Nichols, E., Sullivan, T., Ide, B., Shreffler-Grant, J., & Weinert, C. (2005). Health care choices: Complementary therapy, chronic illness, and older rural dwellers. *Journal of Holistic Nursing, 23*(4), 381–394. https://doi.org/10.1177/0898010105281088

Nichols, E., Weinert, C., Shreffler-Grant, J., & Ide, B. (2006). Complementary and alternative providers in rural locations. *Online Journal of Rural Nursing and Health Care*, 6(2), 40–46. http://rnojournal .binghamton.edu/index.php/RNO/article/view/154

Rao, J., Mihaliak, K., Kroenke, K., Bradley, J., Tierney, W., & Weinberger, M. (1999). Use of complementary therapies for arthritis among patients of rheumatologists. *Annals of Internal Medicine*, 131, 409–416. https://doi.org/10.7326/0003-4819-131-6-199909210-00003

Rodondi, P., Bill, A., Danon, N., Dubois, J., Pasquier, J., l'Endroit, F. M., Herzig, L., & Burnand, B. (2019). Primary care patients' use of conventional and complementary medicine for chronic low back pain. *Journal of Pain Research*, 10(12), 2101–2112. https://doi.org/10.2147/JPR.S200375

Shreffler-Grant, J. (2018). Acceptability: One component in choice of healthcare provider. In C. A. Winters & H. J. Lee (Eds.), *Rural nursing: Concepts, theory, and practice* (5th ed., pp. 233–243). Springer Publishing Company.

Shreffler-Grant, J., Hill, W., Weinert, C., Nichols, E., & Ide, B. (2007). Complementary therapy and older rural women: Who uses and who does not? *Nursing Research*, 56(1), 28–33. https://doi .org/10.1097/00006199-200701000-00004

Shreffler-Grant, J., Nichols, E., & Weinert, C. (2018). Bee SAFE, A skill-building intervention to enhance CAM health literacy: Lessons learned. *Health Promotion Practice*, 19(3), 475–481. https://doi .org/10.1177/1524839917700612

Shreffler-Grant, J., Nichols, E., Weinert, C., & Ide, B. (2013). Montana State University conceptual model of complementary and alternative medicine (CAM) health literacy. *Journal of Health Communication: International Perspectives*, 18(10), 1193–1200. https://doi.org/10.1080/10810730.3013.778385

Shreffler-Grant, J., Weinert, C., & Nichols, E. (2014). Instrument to measure health literacy about complementary and alternative medicine. *Journal of Nursing Measurement*, 22(3), 489–499. https://doi .org/10.1891/1061-3749.22.3.489

Shreffler-Grant, J., Weinert, C., Nichols, E., & Ide, B. (2005). Complementary therapy use among older rural adults. *Public Health Nursing*, 22(4), 323–331. https://doi.org/10.1111/j.0737-1209.2005.220407.x

Tanner, L. (2009, January 13). With economy sour, consumers sweet on herbal medicines. *Associated Press*. http://www.foxnews.com/printer_friendly_wires/2009Jan13/0,4675,MeltdownSupplement Sales,00.html

U.S. Department of Health and Human Services. (2000). *Healthy people 2010, section 11-2: Health communication objective*. https://www.-healthypeople.gov

Vallerand, A. H., Fouladbakhsh, J. M., & Templin, T. (2003). The use of complementary/alternative medicine for self-treatment of pain among residents of urban, suburban, and rural communities. *American Journal of Public Health*, 93, 923–925. https://doi.org/10.2105/AJPH.93.6.923

Vincent, C., & Furnham, A. (1996). Why do patients turn to complementary medicine? An empirical study. *British Journal of Clinical Psychology*, 35, 37–48. https://doi.org/10.1111/j.2044-8260.1996 .tb01160.x

Weinert, C., Shreffler-Grant, J., & Nichols, E. (2019). Psychometric evaluation of the MSU CAM Health Literacy Scale. *Complementary Therapies in Medicine*, 42, 156–157. https://doi.org/10.1016/j.ctim .2018.11.007

Weiss, B. D., Mays, M. Z., Martz, W., Castro, K. M., DeWalt, D. A., Pignone, M. P., Mockbee, J., Hale, F. (2005). Quick assessment of literacy in primary care: The newest vital sign. *Annals of Family Medicine*, 3(6), 514–522. https://doi.org/10.1370/afm.405

Nursing Education

Educating nurses for rural practice is the focus of this section. Section IV includes three new chapters and four updated chapters from the fifth edition. New chapters describe the development and implementation of an interprofessional education program for rural health care professionals (Chapter 23), competencies for rural nurse practitioners (Chapter 24), and a transcultural service-learning immersion experience for undergraduate nursing students (Chapter 27).

Updated chapters address present-day implications for rural education, practice, and policy (Chapter 21); strategies, benefits, and challenges of placing nursing students in rural hospitals for their clinical rotations (Chapter 22); the development and psychometric evaluation of the Rural Knowledge Scale (Chapter 25); and strategies to develop and sustain a rural nursing workforce (Chapter 26).

Implications for Education, Practice, and Policy

JEAN SHREFFLER-GRANT AND MARLENE REIMER[1]

DISCUSSION TOPICS

- Discuss opportunities and experiences in nursing education programs that can best prepare graduates for rural practice.
- What are several current societal or secular trends that may affect rural health, rural nursing practice, and Rural Nursing Theory?
- How can national, regional, or local health policies affect rural healthcare in a positive and less positive manner?

INTRODUCTION

As an applied discipline, nursing has traditionally measured the relevance of theory by the extent to which it can inform practice, education, and healthcare policy. Our purpose in this chapter is to make more explicit the relevance of key elements of the rural theory base. We include selected educational, practice, and healthcare policy implications of the key concepts and theoretical statements as reported by Long and Weinert (1989; also see Chapter 2), Lee and McDonagh (2018; also see Chapter 4), and Lee and Winters (2018; also see Chapter 1). We explore how these implications may need to change as Rural Nursing Theory is revised and extended. We also present exemplars from the United States, Canada, and Australia to illustrate how the key concepts and theoretical statements can inform education, practice, and healthcare policy that address rural populations and their health across international borders.

---

1. Deceased.

RURAL NURSING THEORY

Implications of the First Theoretical Statement

How a group of citizens perceive health, manage their health, and seek healthcare has broad implications for education, practice, and policy that transcend national borders. The first theoretical statement is "Rural dwellers define health primarily as the ability to work, to be productive, to do usual tasks" (Long & Weinert, 1989, p. 120). The interrelated concepts associated with this statement are work beliefs and health beliefs; health is defined in relation to work, and health needs are secondary to work needs.

EDUCATION

On the basis of the original Rural Nursing Theory work, the first theoretical statement suggests that nursing programs should include the concept of role performance as health in curricula so that nurses include actual or potential effects of a health problem on the ability to work and to do usual tasks in their assessments and plans of care. Nursing educators should also offer opportunities for students to learn how clients' definitions of health can influence their health and illness management behaviors.

PRACTICE

In the practice arena, the first theoretical statement suggests that rural health services should be oriented, structured, and timed to fit with the rhythm of work and role performance. In addition, the benefits of preventive care may be better communicated by framing them according to what will assist rural dwellers to continue to work and do their usual tasks. Data from both Canada and the United States demonstrate the need to find new ways to approach preventive care among rural dwellers, based on trends in rural health indicators such as obesity, hypertension, smoking, lack of regular healthcare visits, and growing rates of suicide and substance use disorders (Pong et al., 2009; Rural Health Information Hub, 2020).

POLICY

Policy implications of the original work include establishing funding mechanisms whereby health services can be offered near where people work that are scheduled around the cycle of rural work. Rural residents may not seek timely health services if work must be delayed or disrupted to seek care (Sellers et al., 1999).

The original theory development work on definitions of health, as well as beliefs about work and health, was conducted in the United States. Research participants were principally Caucasian rural dwellers, the majority population in the Rocky Mountain and High Plains area in which this work was conducted (88.9% of the current Montana population is Caucasian; U.S. Census Bureau, 2019). The original work was not intended to characterize these concepts for American Indians, the primary minority population in the same rural areas (6.7% of the Montana population, U.S. Census Bureau, 2019). Canadian research on health beliefs of rural dwellers, as reported by Winters et al. (2013) and Lee and Winters (2018; also see Chapter 1), was also drawn primarily from Caucasians living in the western part of the country. As noted by Lee and Winters (2018, also see Chapter 1), further research is warranted to explore American Indians and Aboriginal people living in rural areas define health and how their conception of health is the same as or different from the dominant population. In any case, it is unlikely that one definition of health or one set of health beliefs would emerge that would characterize health beliefs among different Aboriginal communities or tribes, any more than it is likely that one definition would be true for Caucasian groups of different cultures.

As discussed by Lee and Winters (2018; also see Chapter 1), rural dwellers' views of health may now be more diverse across different geographical areas, age and ethnic groups, occupations, and circumstances than when the original theory development work was conducted; so it may require a reconceptualization of definitions of health, work beliefs, and health beliefs. Of particular note are the subpopulations among rural dwellers.

Martin (1997) pointed out that farming and ranching are now experienced more as a lifestyle than as an occupation, thus calling for different approaches to affect behavioral change beyond simply appealing to individuals' motivations to continue working. More than two decades ago, Blank (1999) claimed that traditional farming and ranching had become a lifestyle choice. Since many other forms of rural living are available to Americans besides farming and ranching, and since most food and commodity crops are now produced on large industrial farms, Blank postulated that the American family farm is a lifestyle that many Americans can no longer afford. The changes Blank mentioned to support the claim have only accelerated in the intervening 20+ years. Another example of a potential need to reframe rural dwellers' definitions of health can be found within rural subpopulations where unemployment has now persisted for multiple generations. Defining health based on the ability to work may not be relevant for those who have never had regular work (Long, 1993). Some rural areas are now more racially and ethnically diverse than in the past. Culturally based beliefs about what it means to be healthy are likely to result in different definitions of health among racial and ethnic groups. Migration of urban residents to rural areas has resulted in a subpopulation of exurban rural dwellers who bring their urban values and expectations about health and healthcare with them (Troughton, 1999). The graying of rural areas is well documented in the literature, as people age in place and younger people migrate out for employment and other opportunities (Jaffe, 2015; McLaughlin & Jensen, 1998; Ricketts et al., 1999). With improved healthcare and healthier lifestyles, people are living many more years postretirement than they once did. How health is defined among this rural population may well have nothing to do with what we traditionally think of as work but instead may be more consistent with the concept of health as role performance or ability to do usual tasks. Healthy older adults may define health as the ability to actively participate in leisure, voluntary activities, and travel. Older adults in poor health may define health as nothing more than the ability to complete their activities of daily living. Further research and exploration are warranted to refine the definitions of health for these multiple rural subpopulations.

Implications of the Second Theoretical Statement

The second theoretical statement is "Rural dwellers are self-reliant and resist accepting help or services from those seen as 'outsiders' or from agencies seen as national or regional 'welfare' programs" (Long & Weinert, 1989, p. 120; also see Chapter 2). Related key concepts are self-reliance, outsider, insider, old-timer, and newcomer.

EDUCATION

The second theoretical statement underlines the importance of a participative, community development approach in which rural dwellers identify and design health initiatives to fit with their own needs and resources. This approach is consistent with the second theoretical statement as originally conceptualized, as well as with the proposed newer subtheme of symptom–action–timeline (SATL) and the new concept involving choices discussed by Lee and McDonagh (2018; also see Chapter 4). The importance of working in partnership with rural dwellers and communities is an essential content for nursing curricula so that graduates can and will apply the principles of community development and participatory action in rural practice. Skills essential for partnership development and maintenance should also be included in nursing curricula. As a middle range theory of rural health-seeking behavior evolves, students and scholars should derive and validate the theory in partnership with rural residents themselves so that it is consistent with their local needs and beliefs.

PRACTICE

Goeppinger (1993) was an early proponent of creating partnerships as a core intervention strategy in health promotion with rural populations at both individual and aggregate levels. Considering the rural tendency to make do and what Weissert et al. (1994) referred to as the "asymmetry of information between citizens and health professionals . . . about what constitutes good care" (p. 366) in traditional care models, empirical testing of the partnership model in promoting the health of rural residents is needed. A Canadian example of a tool to support participative community development for rural citizens is a workbook that was tested in Manitoba, Canada (Ryan-Nicholls, 2004). The workbook was designed to help rural citizens assess the health of their communities and identify goals and strategies to improve the sustainability of rural communities. In the United States, Findholt (2004) studied how rurality influenced community participation in health promotion initiatives. She found that having a structured process for the initiative appeared to compensate for some of the resource and experiential limitations in rural communities. Communities, for example, that had limited experience and success with previous planning efforts were not hindered in their current efforts because they had structured support and resources from a state-level office of rural health. The Rural Health Information Hub (2020) has an evidence-based toolkit available online to guide rural communities as they develop local community health programs for health promotion and disease prevention.

POLICY

The question of what healthcare resources are necessary and sufficient in rural and remote areas, given the distance to other sources of care, continues as a focus of debate and policy shifts for which evidence for decision-making is scarce. Although innovations such as telehealth, collaborative provider networks, and financial reforms have addressed limited rural health resources, major constraints persist due to the lack of sufficient population to justify a full mix of acute care, long-term care, and supported residential and home care services (Bradford et al., 2016; Keyzer, 1995, Ricketts, 2000). In a study of home care resources for rural families with cancer, Buehler and Lee (1992) found that the more rural the family, the more limited and inadequate the formal resources available to assist them. These investigators also found that the longer the dying trajectory and the greater the deterioration of the person's health, the more resources became inadequate and the greater became the burden to the caregiver. These findings illustrate one of many policy questions that have emerged: the relationship between length of illness and sustainability of resources through the trajectory of illness in rural versus urban environments. A mix of formal and informal resources and the resiliency of each to prolonged illness vary, but few studies have systematically addressed this phenomenon. Schantz (2018; also see Chapter 17) discussed the challenges of providing palliative care in the United States for rural dwellers with chronic illnesses. Inpatient and community-based palliative care services are often limited or nonexistent in many rural areas as are hospice or end of life services. Medicare regulations require that a patient must demonstrate a steady decline in health status in order to qualify for hospice services while this is not the usual trajectory for all chronic conditions. Advanced cardiac and lung disease, for example, is often characterized by periods of "fragile stability" (p. 271) that can easily be disrupted by things as simple as an overly salty diet or minor respiratory infection. For rural patients with chronic conditions, acute exacerbations often result in repeated hospitalizations that could have been prevented if skilled home-based palliative care were available.

The Australian Rural Health Strategy adopted in 1994 (Keyzer, 1995) called for "relocation of resources away from services based on existing facilities towards services based on expressed demand" (p. 28). The strategy included changes that would shift power bases from traditional rural primary and hospital care delivery to a system that relied much more on nurse practitioners and interdisciplinary collaboration. More than two decades later, however, tension still exists in Australia and elsewhere between the economic arguments for downsizing and closure of rural facilities versus advocacy for aging in place, new life-saving treatments that require pretransfer interventions at local healthcare facilities, and other new technologies such as telehealth that minimize the need for travel to urban locations for healthcare (Bolin et al., 2015; Mueller, 2001; National Rural Health Association, 2020a; Ricketts, 2000).

In the United States, the critical access hospital (CAH) has gained broad support as an alternative to the closure of local rural hospitals and has been implemented in rural areas across the nation. CAHs are in remote areas and are limited to short-stay lower-intensity services in exchange for more flexibility in staffing and other licensure requirements and more favorable Medicare reimbursement as compared with traditional rural hospitals. The underlying goal is to shift the facility's emphasis from inpatient and surgical services to emergency, outpatient, primary, and long-term care, which are services that may be more sustainable in remote rural areas because they better match the needs of area residents (Shreffler et al., 1999). One of the prototypes for this national model of care was a grassroots effort initiated by a partnership of rural citizens and legislators in a remote rural area in Montana. There are currently 48 CAHs (84% of the total nongovernmental hospitals) in Montana and 1,352 CAHs nationwide (Flex Monitoring Team, 2020). Although the CAH model has successfully maintained acute care in many rural areas, recently there has been an escalation of rural hospital closures across the nation, including some CAHs (NRHA, 2020b). Causes of rural hospital closures are varied and include reduced Medicare reimbursement, a declining rural economy, provider shortages, and location in states that did not expand Medicaid under the Affordable Care Act (ACA). Several legislative initiatives are being proposed to address the closure crisis (NRHA, 2020c).

National health policy reform in the United States and elsewhere has the potential to greatly affect the health-seeking behaviors of rural dwellers. In the United States, the Patient Protection and ACA, also referred to as Obamacare, was passed into law in 2010 and has continued to be controversial since. Despite repeated congressional efforts to repeal and replace it, most ACA provisions remain in force. Since implementation, many leaders have agreed that the ACA's provisions have benefited rural consumers and the rural healthcare system (Avery et al., 2016; Hofer et al., 2011; Newkirk & Damico, 2014). American rural dwellers are much more likely to be uninsured or underinsured than urban dwellers, which limits their access to health insurance and healthcare services. The intent of the ACA was to increase access to insurance coverage and to reduce insurance costs through purchasing networks, which was advantageous for self-employed or under-employed individuals. The ACA also prohibits pre-existing condition exclusions. There are also provisions that address the workforce shortage crisis in rural areas and eliminate some payment inequities for rural providers (Greenwood-Erickson & Abir, 2017; Roubein, 2017).

Beginning in 2020, the COVID-19 pandemic has led to unprecedented challenges in the provision of health services and has the potential to alter health-seeking behaviors of everyone regardless of where they reside. In rural areas specifically, public health departments charged with managing testing, contact tracing, and the like often serve large geographic regions that can strain limited resources (Centers for Disease Control and Prevention, 2020). Long-standing systemic health and social inequities put some rural dwellers at increased risk of getting COVID-19 or having severe illness. In the United States, small rural hospitals that were in precarious financial positions before the pandemic have been further challenged by an actual or potential influx of COVID patients while temporarily curtailing elective healthcare to reduce exposure risks (National Public Radio, 2020; Sheps Center for Health Services Research, 2020; Siegler, 2020). Rural hospitals that did not actually admit patients with coronavirus still faced additional expenses for extra equipment, supplies, and staff necessary to prepare for possible patients. Although uncertain at this time, it is possible that rural hospitals, public health departments, and other healthcare service providers will obtain relief from one of the coronavirus emergency funding bills passed into law.

Implications of the Third Theoretical Statement

Finally, the third theoretical statement is "Health care providers in rural areas must deal with a lack of anonymity and much greater role diffusion than providers in urban or suburban settings" (Long & Weinert, 1989, p. 120; also see Chapter 2). A related theme mentioned by Long and Weinert that characterizes rural nursing is "a sense of isolation from professional peers" (p. 120).

EDUCATION

Implicit in the third theoretical statement is that students planning or potentially interested in rural practice should be given opportunities to develop skills to function in a generalist role or what McLeod et al. (1998) referred to as a multispecialist role that is characteristic of rural nursing practice. Offering undergraduate students a rural elective experience is one such strategy, particularly when it not only involves placement in a rural site but also seminars on rural health and practice issues. Students with an interest in rural practice should have opportunities to develop strategies to cope with or overcome practice isolation, such as skill development in the use of mentors, consultants, and telehealth applications. Through full engagement with their communities, nurses who are newcomers in rural areas may begin to appreciate the familiarity of life in a rural community and gradually may be seen as insiders rather than outsiders, which may mitigate the negative aspects of lack of anonymity and practice isolation. Some nurses, of course, are already insiders, having come from the community. The sense of practice isolation may be less acute for them, but the practical issues of limited access to educational opportunities and ready consultation are nevertheless present to varying degrees.

PRACTICE AND POLICY

Lack of anonymity, role diffusion, and practice isolation may contribute to recruitment difficulties and high turnover of rural healthcare professionals and result in shortages of providers in rural practice settings. Here too, policy makers can look to innovative approaches and exchange of best practices. For example, the Rural Physician Action Plan in Alberta recognized that (a) medical students from rural areas were more likely to go into rural practice, but (b) rural applicants were often disadvantaged in the interview and the selection processes for medical school because of the lack of sophistication in interviewing and preparation of materials (Health Workforce for Alberta, 2017; I. Pfeiffer, personal communication, March 4, 2004). An experienced recruiter was hired to help rural applicants prepare for admission interviews. Thus, they went to a root cause with what appear to be positive results.

Stewart et al. (2011) conducted a study to identify factors that predicted intent to leave practice positions among RNs in rural and remote settings in Canada. The investigators found that some predictors were amenable to interventions that may prevent turnover among rural nurses. Workplace and community predictors of turnover relevant to the third relational statement are lower local community satisfaction, higher perceived workplace stress, lower satisfaction with autonomy in the workplace, lower satisfaction with workplace scheduling, and a desire to seek further education. Also, being a newcomer to the rural practice setting and community was a significant predictor of intent to leave.

An innovative strategy for addressing shortages of nurses and other healthcare providers in rural areas can be seen in the growth of educational outreach efforts via distance-learning technology to rural areas. Rural residents or insiders who are more likely to select rural practice upon graduation can access all or part of educational programs without leaving their rural communities for significant periods of time. Another successful approach for recruitment of health professionals in rural areas has been educational scholarships or fellowships for rural residents or grow your own programs (Hyder & Amundson, 2017; Petersen et al., 2018).

CONCLUSION

The radical changes necessary to shift education, practice, and policy to benefit rural health require a strong theory base and depth of understanding of rural health and practice that can emanate only through experience and research. Those who focus on rural health are used to thinking in terms of local contextual factors and the unique nature of a single rural area, region, or nation. Through engagement in cross-border collaborative research and scholarly work on Rural Nursing Theory, we and our respective teams have deepened our understanding of the extent to which larger issues of healthcare reform are also shifting. At the end of the day, the relevance of Rural Nursing Theory and concepts as described in this book will likely be measured by its ability to evolve and change as new knowledge shapes it and its ability to positively influence education, practice, and healthcare policy and thereby improve the health of rural citizens on both sides of the border.

REFERENCES

Avery, K., Finegold, K., & Xiao, X. (2016). *ASPE issue brief: Impact of the Affordable Care Act coverage expansion on rural and urban populations.* Department of Health and Human Services. https://aspe.hhs.gov/system/files/pdf/204986/ACARuralbrief.pdf

Blank, S. C. (1999). The end of the American farm. *The Futurist, 33*(4), 22. https://www.questia.com/magazine/1G1-54349265/the-end-of-the-american-farm

Bolin, J. N., Bellamy, G. R., Ferdinand, A. O., Vuong, A. M., Kash, B. A., Schulze, A., & Helduser, J. W. (2015). Rural Healthy People 2020: New decade, same challenges. *The Journal of Rural Health, 31*(3), 326–333. https://doi.org/10.1111/jrh.12116

Bradford, N. K., Caffery, L. J., & Smith, A. C. (2016). Telehealth services in rural and remote Australia: A systematic review of models of care and factors influencing success and sustainability. *Rural and Remote Health, 16*(4), 1–23. https://doi.org/10.22605/RRH3808

Buehler, J. A., & Lee, H. J. (1992). Exploration of home care resources for rural families with cancer. *Cancer Nursing, 15,* 299–308. https://doi.org/10.1097/00002820-199215040-00008

Centers for Disease Control and Prevention. (2020). *Coronavirus Disease (COVID-19), Rural communities.* https://www.cdc.gov/coronavirus/2019-ncov/need-extra-precautions/other-at-risk-populations/rural-communities.html

Findholt, N. (2004). *The influence of rurality on community participation in a community health development initiative.* Unpublished doctoral dissertation, Oregon Health & Science University, Portland.

Flex Monitoring Team. (2020). *Critical access hospital locations.* http://www.flexmonitoring.org/data/critical-access-hospital-locations

Goeppinger, J. (1993). Health promotion for rural populations: Partnership interventions. *Family and Community Health, 16*(1), 1–10. https://doi.org/10.1097/00003727-199304000-00004

Greenwood-Erickson, M., & Abir, M. (2017, January 22). Rural America could be hardest hit by repeal of Obamacare. *Newsweek.* http://www.newsweek.com/rural-america-hardest-hit-repeal-obamacare-544813

Health Workforce for Alberta. (2017). *About health workforce for Alberta.* http://www.rpap.ab.ca

Hofer, A. N., Abraham, J. M., & Moscovice, I. (2011). Expansion of coverage under the Patient Protection and Affordable Care Act and primary care utilization. *Milbank Quarterly, 89*(1), 69–89. https://doi.org/10.1111/j.1468-0009.2011.00620.x

Hyder, S. S., & Amundson, M. (2017). Hospital medicine and fellowship program in rural North Dakota: A multifaceted success story. *Wisconsin Medical Journal, 116*(4), 218–220.

Jaffe, S. (2015). Aging in rural America. *Health Affairs, 34*(1), 7–10. https://doi.org/10.1377/hlthaff.2014.1372

Keyzer, D. M. (1995). Health policy and rural nurses: A time for reflection. *Collegian, 2*(1), 28–35.

Lee, H. J., & McDonagh, M. K. (2018). Updating the rural nursing base. In C. A. Winters (Ed.), *Rural nursing: Concepts, theory, and practice* (4th ed., pp. 45–62). Springer Publishing Company.

Lee, H. J., & Winters, C. A. (2018). Rural nursing theory: Past, present, and future. In C. A. Winters & H. J. Lee (Eds.), *Rural nursing: Concepts, theory, and practice* (5th ed., pp. 3–15). Springer Publishing Company.

Long, K. A. (1993). The concept of health: Rural perspectives. *Nursing Clinics of North America, 28*(1), 123–130.

Long, K. A., & Weinert, C. (1989). Rural nursing: Developing the theory base. *Scholarly Inquiry for Nursing Practice: An International Journal, 3,* 113–127. https://doi.org/10.1891/0889-7182.3.2.113

Martin, S. R. (1997). Agricultural safety and health: Principles and possibilities for nursing education. *Journal of Nursing Education, 36*(2), 74–78. https://doi.org/10.3928/0148-4834-19970201-07

McLaughlin, D. K., & Jensen, L. (1998). The rural elderly: A demographic portrait. In R. T. Coward & J. A. Krout (Eds.), *Aging in rural settings: Life circumstances & distinctive features* (pp. 15–43). Springer Publishing Company.

McLeod, M., Browne, A. J., & Leipert, B. (1998). Issues for nurses in rural and remote Canada. *Australian Journal of Rural Health, 6,* 72–78. https://doi.org/10.1111/j.1440-1584.1998.tb00287.x

Mueller, K. J. (2001). Rural health policy: Past as prelude to the future. In S. Loue & B. E. Quill (Eds.), *Handbook of rural health* (pp. 1–23). Kluwer Academic/Plenum.

National Public Radio. (2020). *Rural hospital CEO preps for rise in covid-19 cases.* https://www.npr .org/2020/04/04/827435996/rural-hospital-ceo-preps-for-rise-in-covid-19-cases

National Rural Health Association. (2020a). *About rural health care.* https://www.ruralhealthweb.org/ about-nrha/about-rural-health-care

National Rural Health Association. (2020b). *NRHA save rural hospital action center.* https://www.rural healthweb.org/advocate/save-rural-hospitals

National Rural Health Association. (2020c). *End the rural hospital closure crisis.* https://www.ruralhealth web.org/NRHA/media/Emerge_NRHA/Advocacy/Government%20affairs/2020/2020-Rural-Hospital-Closure-Request.pdf

Newkirk, V., & Damico, A. (2014). *The affordable care act and insurance coverage in rural areas. Kaiser Family Foundation.* http://kff.org/uninsured/issue-brief/the-affordable-care-act-and-insurance-coverage-in-rural-areas

Petersen, P., Sharp, D. B., & Pare, J. M. (2018). Developing and sustaining the rural nursing workforce through collaborative education models. In C. A. Winters & H. J. Lee (Eds.), *Rural nursing: Concepts, theory, and practice* (5th ed., pp. 345–357). Springer Publishing Company.

Pong, R. W., Desmeules, M., & Lagace, C. (2009). Rural–urban disparities in health: How does Canada fare and how does Canada compare to Australia? *Australian Journal of Rural Health, 17*(1), 58–64. https://doi.org/10.1111/j.1440-1584.2008.01039.x

Ricketts, T. C. (2000). The changing nature of rural health care. *Annual Review of Public Health, 21,* 639–657. https://doi.org/10.1146/annurev.publhealth.21.1.639

Ricketts, T. C., Johnson-Webb, K. D., & Randolph, R. K. (1999). Populations and places in rural America. In T. C. Ricketts (Ed.), *Rural health in the United States* (pp. 7–24). Oxford University Press.

Roubein, R. (2017, April 18). Groups warn of rural health "crisis" under Obamacare repeal. *The Hill Extra.* http://thehill.com/policy/healthcare/329546-groups-warn-of-rural-health-crisis-under-obamacare-repeal

Rural Health Information Hub. (2020a). *Rural community health toolkit.* https://www.ruralhealthinfo .org/toolkits/rural-toolkit

Rural Health Information Hub. (2020b). *Rural health disparities.* https://www.ruralhealthinfo.org/ topics/rural-health-disparities

Ryan-Nicholls, K. (2004). Rural Canadian community health and quality of life: Testing of a workbook to determine priorities and move to action (Preliminary Report). *Rural and Remote Health, 4*(278), 1–10. http://www.rrh.org.au/-articles/subviewnew.asp?ArticleID=278

Schantz, J. A. (2018). Palliative care for rural chronically ill adults. In C. A. Winters & H. J. Lee (Eds.), *Rural nursing: Concepts, theory, and practice* (5th ed., pp. 267–277). Springer Publishing Company.

Sellers, S. C., Poduska, M. D., Propp, L. H., & White, S. I. (1999). The health care meanings, values, and practices of Anglo-American males in the rural Midwest. *Journal of Transcultural Nursing, 10,* 320–330. https://doi.org/10.1177/104365969901000410

Sheps Center for Health Services Research, University of North Carolina. (2020). Most rural hospitals have little cash going into COVID. *Findings Brief, NC Rural Health Research Program.* https://www .ruralhealthresearch.org/alerts/346

Shreffler, M. J., Capalbo, S. M., Flaherty, R. J., & Heggem, C. (1999). Community decision-making about critical access hospitals: Lessons learned from Montana's medical assistance facility program. *The Journal of Rural Health, 15*(2), 180–188. https://doi.org/10.1111/j.1748-0361.1999.tb00738.x

Siegler, K. (2020). *Small-town hospitals are closing just as coronavirus arrives in rural America.* https://www .npr.org/2020/04/09/829753752/small-town-hospitals-are-closing-just-as-coronavirus-arrives-in-rural-america

Stewart, N. J., D'Arcy, C., Kosteniuk, J., Andrews, M. E., Morgan, D., Forbes, D., MacLeod, M. L. P., Kulig, J. C., & Pitblado, J. R. (2011). Moving on? Predictors of intent to leave among rural and remote RNs in Canada. *The Journal of Rural Health, 27*(1), 103–113. https://doi.org/10.1111/ j.1748-0361.2010.00308.x

Troughton, M. J. (1999). Redefining "rural" for the twenty-first century. In W. Rampy, J. Kulig, I. Townshend, & V. McGowan (Eds.), *Health in rural settings: Contexts for action* (pp. 21–38). University of Lethbridge.

U.S. Census Bureau. (2019). *Quick facts Montana*. https://www.census.gov/quickfacts/fact/table/MT/PST045219

Weissert, C. S., Knott, J. H., & Stieber, B. E. (1994). Education and the health professions: Explaining policy choices among the states. *Journal of Health Politics, Policy and Law, 19*, 361–392. https://doi.org/10.1215/03616878-19-2-361

Winters, C. A., Thomlinson, E. H., O'Lynn, C., Lee, H. J., McDonagh, M. M., Edge, D., & Reimer, M. (2013). Exploring rural nursing theory across borders. In C. Winters (Ed.), *Rural nursing: Concepts, theory, and practice* (4th ed., pp. 35–47). Springer Publishing Company.

CHAPTER 22

Clinical Placements in Rural Hospitals: Expanding Nursing Students' Knowledge, Skills, and Attitudes Toward Rural Healthcare

Lori Hendrickx, Heidi A. Mennenga, Laurie Johansen, and Nicole Gibson

DISCUSSION TOPICS

- What are the opportunities that result from placing nursing students in rural hospitals for clinical experiences?
- What are the challenges related to placing nursing students in rural hospitals for clinical experiences?
- How can rural hospital clinical placement affect recruitment and retention in rural healthcare facilities?
- What are some strategies for increasing nursing student exposure to rural healthcare?

INTRODUCTION

Predictions that the current nursing shortage will continue and most likely intensify as the demand for nurses grows have resulted in a variety of recommendations for strategies to reduce the shortage and meet the demands for additional nurses. In 2017, the U.S. Department of Labor projected a 16% growth rate in the need for registered nurses for 2014 to 2024, compared to an average growth rate of 7% for all occupations (U.S. Department of Labor, 2017). Multiple authors and organizations (American Association of College of Nursing, 2017) have reported the need for additional nurses. Media exposure regarding the nursing shortage has increased national awareness and has resulted in increased numbers of applicants to nursing education programs. The AACN (2017) has reported that several statewide initiatives are being developed to address the nursing shortage; however, challenges continue.

Despite the growing numbers of nursing school applicants, the number of graduates from nursing programs has not sufficiently increased to meet the demand for registered nurses. In many cases, nursing school applicants are turned away due to a shortage of faculty and inadequate numbers of clinical sites or financial constraints. AACN (2017) reported that a faculty shortage and inadequate numbers of clinical education sites were potential barriers to meeting the demand for healthcare providers. Insufficient numbers of clinical sites are an issue faced by many nursing programs that educate students primarily in more urban hospital settings. These urban institutions often have multiple nursing programs competing for clinical time, resulting in the inability to accept more students or add additional clinical groups to the facilities already saturated with students.

In the midst of our current global pandemic, a heightened awareness of the need for emergency preparedness increases the demand for nurses to create cultures of preparedness in all healthcare settings. McSweeney-Feld and Lane (2019) emphasized the need for community-based preparedness approaches through collaborative measures using community networks. Rural hospitals can provide nursing students with experiences surrounding the interprofessional collaboration of acute care settings with community networks through community/public health agencies. Such experiences create opportunities for nursing students to implement population health interventions not only from the role as a public health nurse but also through the role of rural nurses in a variety of clinical settings. In this chapter, we describe opportunities for clinical in rural hospitals, implementation of one new program, and benefits and challenges of placing students in rural facilities for their clinical rotations.

Opportunities for Rural Hospitals

In an effort to respond to the nursing shortage, marketing strategies have resulted in substantial increases in the numbers of entering college freshmen declaring nursing as a major. In the past 15 years, South Dakota State University (SDSU) has responded to the increased demand for nursing graduates by increasing the numbers of students accepted from 48 to 64 per semester on one campus, admitting additional students twice a year rather than once a year on another campus, adding two accelerated program sites with the potential for 80 students per year, and adding an additional standard program campus with 40 students per year. These changes resulted in an increase in the number of students accepted yearly from 128 to 312. Despite the large increase in students accepted, in 2011 only one-third of qualified students applying to the SDSU College of Nursing's main campus were accepted on their first application (Hendrickx, 2011). Additional expansion of the nursing program has not occurred in part due to the lack of additional clinical placement sites.

The majority of nursing students at SDSU have traditionally received their clinical education at larger hospitals in a major city, competing with several other nursing programs for clinical placement. Clinical experiences needed to be expanded to include evenings and weekends and changes in the calendar were made so that some groups could do clinical in the summer or early in January before other programs were in session. While these adjustments did result in increased availability of clinical experiences for students, another possible solution was to explore clinical opportunities in smaller, more rural healthcare facilities.

Implementation

SDSU has five semesters in the nursing program with clinical in all the semesters. The first semester clinical experience is in a general medical–surgical setting with emphasis on basic nursing care and physical assessment skills. Several years ago, the first semester coordinator met with nursing directors in two rural hospitals to explore the possibility of placing these beginning students in their facilities for clinical. At the time, there were no other nursing programs doing clinical in these hospitals. Agreements were reached with the two rural facilities, and a pilot program for 1 year was completed.

Current nursing instructors from SDSU accompanied the students as clinical faculty for the expansion into the rural hospitals. Clinical group size was limited to eight students for one clinical instructor. After successful implementation of the pilot program, the use of rural hospitals was expanded as the nursing program increased in size.

There were a number of considerations in the selection of appropriate rural clinical sites. The proximity to campus was considered with all sites being within an hour's drive. The main campus of SDSU is located near the Minnesota border, so hospitals in both South Dakota and Minnesota were considered. Transportation was provided for the faculty member and the students through the campus motor pool fleet.

The size of the facility and average daily census needed to be adequate to accommodate eight students. This did not necessarily mean that there needed to be eight patients in the inpatient setting, just that there were learning opportunities for eight students. Students were usually assigned patients in the inpatient area first and then other learning opportunities were identified. All of the hospitals had active outpatient departments where students could help admit a patient for an outpatient procedure, follow the patient through the procedure, and then provide postprocedural care. Students also rotated through dialysis units, cardiac rehabilitation, and accompanied nurses on home health visits. Some of the hospitals had long-term care facilities attached so students were rotated through the long-term care setting as well as the hospital setting.

As the number of clinical groups increased, the need for additional clinical instructors increased as well. Clinical instructors were selected from the existing faculty first. Administrators in the rural hospitals were concerned that the instructor be familiar with their facility so initially faculty members were approached who had previously worked in one of the rural hospitals. As additional instructors were needed, further discussion revealed that two area rural hospitals had staff nurses in the educator track of SDSU's graduate program. These graduate students were then added as clinical instructors in the hospitals where they had worked as staff nurses. One additional method for recruitment of clinical instructors was having faculty members serve as preceptors for graduate students in the educator track. The graduate student spent one semester in the rural hospital setting doing clinical with a current faculty member. After graduation, these students were more comfortable doing clinical in one of the rural sites. Several of the rural hospitals being used for clinical experiences had instructors who were previously employed by the hospital or assisted with clinical in a rural hospital during graduate school, which resulted in increased trust between the college faculty and the hospital personnel and eased the transition for the clinical instructor and the nursing staff. Since two states were being used, having clinical instructors who had practiced in the hospitals resulted in instructors already holding licensure in their respective states.

Ongoing communication between the hospital and college staffs was maintained through two primary methods. The clinical instructor remained the primary resource for the hospital staff regarding changes in the curriculum, learning needs of the students and responsibilities of the nursing staff in the education of the students. The semester coordinator made periodic site visits to each site to stay in touch with the clinical instructors and the administrators at the clinical site. The semester coordinator addressed any needs of the hospital staff that arose in addition to serving as a mentor for the clinical instructors. The onsite interaction was identified as crucial by the nursing administrators at the clinical sites.

An additional consideration was the day of the week to hold clinical. Since rural hospitals often have surgeons or specialists who are on site only on certain days of the week, it was found to be beneficial to hold clinical experiences on those days as much as possible. For example, patient census was often found to be higher on the day the surgeon had procedures scheduled but typically by Friday some hospitals had discharged most of their patients.

Evaluation

Evaluation of the clinical experiences was done informally each semester and formally through interviews with the nurse managers. Clinical instructors met with the semester coordinator to provide feedback into the type of learning experiences available and appropriate adjustments were made. Face-to-face interviews were done with the nursing managers from the clinical sites. The managers were asked to identify the benefits and challenges associated with having nursing students in their rural healthcare facility.

Benefits

The use of rural facilities for clinical experiences results in many benefits not only for students but also for clinical instructors, patients, staff, and administrators. The managers reported that since rural facilities often have all patients located on a single floor regardless of diagnosis, students have easy access to patients of all ages with many different health problems. A variety of experiences and exposure to other departments also await the student in a rural facility. In a single clinical day, students could observe dialysis, participate in outpatient procedures, and assist in other departments in addition to caring for their primary patient. Additionally, since rural facilities do not typically have intravenous (IV) teams or lift teams, students were often able to perform these types of tasks and participate more in direct patient care.

Respondents indicated that the variety of diagnoses and experiences in one area also presented the clinical instructor with more diverse teaching opportunities. For example, if one student was caring for a patient with pneumonia who had crackles in his or her lungs, the instructor may have all the students listen to the patient's lung sounds, whereas another student may have a surgical patient where wound care could be completed. The clinical instructor could also choose to review the pathophysiology of the different diagnoses to which students were exposed during a single clinical day while at a clinical postconference. The variety of experiences offered by a rural facility allowed the clinical instructor to review a range of diagnoses and improve student's understanding of various illnesses. Nurse managers indicated that students also benefited from an increased understanding of the role of the nurse generalist and the level of autonomy that is prevalent in rural hospitals.

Students and clinical instructors are not the only benefactors of the use of rural facilities for nursing education. Respondents indicated that patients also benefited from having students in the rural facility. Since rural facilities are often underused for nursing education, patients often comment on how much they enjoy the one-on-one attention they gain from having a student care for them.

The nurse managers stated that nursing staff were also given the opportunity to mentor students, provide leadership, and share experiences. The presence of students in the clinical setting may also prompt nurses to increase their standard of care as they strive to model evidence-based practices. One nurse manager commented that her nurses "really have to be on their toes and think about what they are doing" when working with students. She commented further that nurses in a rural facility do not get as much exposure to nursing students and faculty and that this is an excellent learning opportunity for the staff as well as the students.

Additionally, results indicated that administrators can use the students' exposure to rural facilities as a recruitment tool. Students often do not consider employment after graduation in a smaller facility, especially if they have never been exposed to the rural environment throughout their education. However, once exposed to the challenges and variety offered by a rural setting, students may seek employment opportunities after graduation. One administrator stated that their last three nurses hired had all been students at that rural facility during a clinical experience.

Challenges

With all the benefits that correspond to the use of rural hospitals for clinical sites, there are also challenges to overcome. As noted by Newhouse (2005), smaller patient bases, along with a variety of acuity levels, are usually experienced in rural hospital clinical sites. This can result in the rise and fall of patient census. Our interviews with nurse mangers paralleled this challenge of a fluctuating census. Patient census was reported to vary from negligible to maximum census while accommodating nursing students. Utilization of a variety of nursing departments does allow facilities the capability of accommodating nursing students while experiencing a fluctuating census, in order to meet student and patient needs.

Constraints with space also presented nurse managers with accommodation barriers for nursing students. Conference rooms, as well as locker rooms, can be modestly available, with the demand for usage extending beyond the capacity of the rural hospitals, even without considering the addition of the nursing students. A desire to provide an environment conducive to learning in a postconference setting can take ingenuity. This ingenuity led to postconferences being held in break rooms and unused patient rooms if conference rooms were not available.

Nurse managers noted the challenge of maintaining communication between SDSU College of Nursing faculty and rural hospital staff. Visits by the semester coordinator helped display the commitment of the College of Nursing to collaborate with rural facilities. In addition, a predominant concern noted was the familiarity of the nurse faculty member with the rural hospital. It was evident that administrators needed to feel comfortable with the level of faculty knowledge about the rural hospital. Respondents reported that utilizing instructors from the facility increased comfort levels by assuring knowledge of the mission and vision of the facility, current policies and procedures, patient types, and staffing patterns.

IMPLICATIONS FOR EDUCATION, RESEARCH, AND PRACTICE

Implications for Education and Research

The use of rural hospitals for clinical placement in nursing education is an effective way to provide quality clinical educational experiences to beginning nursing students while relieving some of the clinical congestion from saturated urban settings. At SDSU, the use of rural hospitals has been expanded into the second semester for medical–surgical experience and has resulted in 8 to 10 fewer clinical groups in the larger urban setting each semester. Expanding clinical experiences into rural hospitals has enabled the nursing program to provide additional clinical placement sites as the nursing program increases its enrollment.

Providing clinical experiences in the rural setting enables nursing students to see the importance of the generalist role of the rural nurse and appreciate greater role diffusion. Nursing students are often surprised at the variety of learning opportunities and patient-care situations afforded them in the rural hospitals. This variety of experiences allows the nursing student to appreciate the role of the rural nurse and the flexibility required to care for such a broad range of patients. Nursing practice in a rural hospital requires a specific skill set and range of knowledge that has been described as broader and involving a higher level of responsibility in comparison to urban settings (Strasser & Neusy, 2010). Several of our students who begin their clinical experiences in a rural hospital request to return to a rural setting in their final semester for their preceptorship experience, citing the variety of experiences as the predominant reason for the request.

Increased awareness of the possibilities in rural health can also be promoted through other means. For example, in order to encourage educators to expand clinical education into rural areas, an "Academic Bush Camp" was designed and participants learned about rural health opportunities through experiential learning and workshops. Results indicated that the camp increased awareness of opportunities and has led to increased willingness to place students in a rural clinical experience (Page et al., 2016).

Another strategy to promote rural health would be the implementation of a rural primary care clinical experience. Primary care is often an underutilized setting for undergraduate clinical experiences. The primary care setting can offer a unique experience and provide students with the opportunity to view the opportunities and challenges of rural healthcare. Additionally, students may be more likely to view registered nurses who are practicing to the full scope of their license in various roles, such as providing independent nurse visits, serving as care managers, or conducting medication management (Flinter et al., 2017). Since the majority of practicing registered nurses have not received education or training in primary care competencies, providing a primary care clinical experience may enrich the educational preparation of nursing students (Bauer & Bodenheimer, 2017).

Implications for Practice

Involving nursing students in rural hospital clinical experiences provides an opportunity for rural hospitals to promote their facilities. Rural hospitals have historically struggled to recruit and retain caregivers, with rural nurse vacancy rates significantly higher than urban areas (Cramer et al., 2006; Skillman et al., 2015). While many recruitment strategies have been tried, much of the research in this area suggests that exposure to rural hospitals for clinical placements is a major factor in recruitment of healthcare personnel to rural settings and that students often respond positively to their rural healthcare experiences. Research indicates that there are three primary factors associated with students choosing to practice in rural settings: having a rural background, positive clinical experiences in a rural setting, and targeted training for rural practice (Bigbee & Nixon, 2013; Skillman et al., 2015; Strasser & Neusy, 2010; Walters et al., 2016).

Providing rural clinical experiences for undergraduate nursing students has been promoted as a recruitment strategy for rural hospitals. Neill and Taylor (2002) reported that qualitative evaluation of rural clinical placement indicated a positive student response with increased interest in rural nursing following graduation. Other studies have resulted in recommendations for providing rural training and including rural content in the curriculum to improve recruitment and retention (Daniels et al., 2007; Devine, 2006; Orda et al., 2017).

Thrall (2007) identified best practices for recruiting nurses into rural practice that include establishing links with area colleges to provide clinical education and possibly providing funding assistance for employees to attend nursing school in exchange for working at the hospital for a period of time following graduation. Rural hospitals can also develop nurse residency or internship programs for nursing students. These internship opportunities provide additional experiences in rural hospitals that are competing with urban centers that may have similar programs. In South Dakota, several rural administrators have approached the first semester coordinator at South Dakota Rural Health Association meetings to indicate their interest in providing clinical experiences for SDSU nursing students. While some of these rural facilities are located a significant distance from the main campus, it may be possible to consider an overnight or extended experience where students could be housed locally and minimize travel time.

Orda et al. (2017) established a rural internship accreditation program for medical interns. Training in remote geographical locations resulted in an improvement in rural staffing, which led to a decrease in the reliance on locum staffing. The rural training program was recognized as essential for successful recruitment and retention of providers interested in practice in remote areas.

The rural hospitals used for clinical experiences at SDSU have all reported a positive experience with nursing students completing clinical in their facilities. Clinical instructors have had similar positive experiences. While anecdotal data and clinical evaluations from students indicate a positive response to rural clinical placement, additional research is warranted to describe their perceptions of rural clinical experiences and the preparation these experiences provide for subsequent clinical rotations and eventual nursing practice.

Implications for Clinical Placement for Advanced Practice Registered Nurses

Graduate nursing education programs support students to pursue lifelong education and advance their nursing degree with many options available. It is well documented in the literature that nurses and healthcare providers who have a rural connection or experience are more likely to practice in a rural setting and rural areas continue to be impacted by primary care provider shortages. A specific advanced nursing education option for nurses seeking to advance their education and impact rural populations through practice in primary care is the nurse practitioner degree. The SDSU College of Nursing currently offers a family nurse practitioner (FNP) program with masters, postgraduate certificate, and doctoral degree options. In alignment with the SDSU College of Nursing mission focus on rural and underserved populations, the demographics of the state of South Dakota and surrounding Upper Midwest states, and need for more rural primary care providers, the FNP program requires rotations in rural primary care.

The clinical coordinators for the FNP students work collaboratively with local and regional healthcare organizations to support and secure clinical providers who are academically and experientially qualified to precept FNP students. FNP student placement accounts for student preferences, organizational preferences, and program and individual student learning outcomes. Students placed in a rural location with a preceptor are often exposed to increasing opportunities to practice in expanded roles of managing acute and chronic disease, performing clinical procedures, covering emergency room shifts, providing onsite care to patients in long-term care settings, and answering after-hours calls.

Partnering students with interests in or connections to rural primary care with rural primary care providers has resulted in students seeking employment in a rural setting within the sponsoring healthcare organization for the SDSU FNP program.

CONCLUSION

Rural hospitals have traditionally not been selected as clinical placement sites for nursing education and are an untapped resource for nursing programs needing additional clinical resources. These facilities can provide a wide variety of opportunities for patient care and expose the nursing student to the wealth of experiences that rural healthcare provides. Results from the experiences at SDSU have been positive and should encourage the exploration of rural healthcare facilities for nursing clinical experiences.

REFERENCES

American Association of College of Nursing. (2017). *Fact sheet: Nursing shortage.* http://www.aacnnursing.org/Portals/42/News/Factsheets/Nursing-Shortage-Factsheet-2017.pdf?ver=2017-10-18-144118-163

Bauer, L., & Bodenheimer, T. (2017). Expanded roles of registered nurses in primary care delivery of the future. *Nursing Outlook, 65,* 624–632. https://doi.org/10.1016/j.outlook.2017.03.011

Bigbee, J., & Mixon, D. (2013). Recruitment and retention of rural nursing students: A retrospective study. *Remote and Rural Health, 13,* 2486. http://www.rrh.org.au/journal/article/2486

Cramer, M., Nienaber, J., Helget, P., & Agrawal, S. (2006). Comparative analysis of urban and rural nursing workforce shortages in Nebraska hospitals. *Policy, Politics, & Nursing Practice, 7*(4), 248–260. https://doi.org/10.1177/1527154406296481

Daniels, Z. M., VanLiet, B. J., Skipper, B. J., Sanders, M. L., & Rhyne, R. L. (2007). Factors in recruiting and retaining health professionals for rural practice. *Journal of Rural Health, 23*(1), 62–71. https://doi.org/10.1111/j.1748-0361.2006.00069.x

Devine, S. (2006). Perceptions of occupational therapists practicing in rural Australia: A graduate perspective. *Australian Occupational Health Journal, 53*(3), 205–210. https://doi.org/10.1111/j.1440-1630.2006.00561.x

Flinter, M., Hsu, C., Cromp, D., Ladden, M., & Wagner, E. (2017). Emerging new roles and contributions to team-based care in high-performing practices. *Journal of Ambulatory Care Manager, 40*(4), 287–296. https://doi.org/10.1097/JAC.0000000000000193

Hendrickx, L. (2011, May). *Facing a shortage of clinical sites? Rural hospitals can meet your needs.* Paper presented at the Midwest Healthcare Educators' Academy, Grand Forks, North Dakota.

McSweeney-Feld, M. H., & Lane, S. J. (2019). Disaster preparedness in turbulent times: Lessons in building a culture of readiness. *Aging Today, 40*(4), 9.

Neill, J., & Taylor, K. (2002). Undergraduate nursing students' clinical experiences in rural and remote areas: Recruitment and retention. *Australian Journal of Rural Health, 10*(5), 239–243. https://doi.org/10.1046/j.1440-1584.2002.00482.x

Newhouse, R. P. (2005). Exploring nursing issues in rural hospitals. *The Journal of Nursing Administration, 35*(7/8), 350–358. https://doi.org/10.1097/00005110-200507000-00007

Orda, U., Orda, S., Gupta, T., & Knight, S. (2017). Building a sustainable workforce in a rural and remote health service: A comprehensive and innovative rural generalist training approach. *Australian Journal of Rural Health, 25,* 116–119. doi:10.1111/ajr.12306

Page, A., Hamilton, S., Hall, M., Fitzgerald, K., Warner, W., Nattabi, B., & Thompson, S. (2016). Gaining a proper sense of what happens out there: An Academic Bush Camp to promote rural placements for students. *Australian Journal of Rural Health, 24*(1), 41–47. https://doi.org/10.1111/ajr.12199

Skillman, S., Hager, L., & Frogner, B. (2015). *Incentives for nurse practitioners and registered nurses to work in rural and safety net settings.* http://depts.washington.edu/fammed/chws/wp-content/uploads/sites/5/2016/03/CHWS_RTB159_Skillman.pdf

Strasser, R., & Neusy, A. (2010). Context counts: Training health workers in and for rural and remote areas. *Bulletin of the World Health Organization, 88*(10), 777–782. https://doi.org/10.2471./BLT.09.072462

Thrall, H. (2007). Best practices for recruiting rural nurses. *Hospitals & Health Networks, 81*(12), 47–50.

U.S. Department of Labor. (2017). *Job outlook for registered nurses.* http://www.bls.gov/ooh/healthcare/registered-nurses.htm

Walters, L., Seal, A., McGirr, J., Stewart, R., DeWitt, D., & Playford, D. (2016). Effect of medical student preference on rural clinical school experience and rural career intentions. *Rural and Remote Health, 16*, 3698. http://www.rrh.org.au/journal/article/3698

CHAPTER 23

Where You Live Matters: Bringing Interprofessional Education to the Rural Healthcare Workforce

D. "DALE" M. MAYER AND DARIN BELL

DISCUSSION TOPICS

- Define interprofessional education (IPE) and interprofessional collaborative practice (IPCP) and identify two benefits for both IPE and IPCP.
- Describe how IPE and IPCP would benefit rural settings; specifically, patients and families and rural healthcare professionals and rural communities.
- Identify two strategies for the development of IPE and IPCP activities for a rural setting and write objectives for these activities.
- List two specific actions you can take to promote IPE and IPCP locally.

INTRODUCTION

Interprofessional collaborative practice (IPCP) and interprofessional education (IPE) are rapidly gaining recognition as critical for the provision of high-quality, cost-effective care. However, while the impact of IPCP is widely recognized, the development of IPE methods in rural settings is not often considered in the training of healthcare professionals (HCPs). This chapter describes the authors' experiences bringing IPE to rural HCPs and learners, specifically medical residents, physicians, nursing students, and nurses at critical access hospitals (CAH) and rural clinics. As educators and clinicians, we discuss our experiences bringing IPE to the rural healthcare workforce and review the opportunities and challenges we have encountered. We also share ideas for how to bring IPE to rural sites and discuss implications for education, research, and practice, because where you live matters.

Interprofessional Practice and Education

The need for team-based collaborative care was advocated for in the Declaration of Alma-Ata (International Conference on Primary Health Care, 1978), but in the subsequent four decades, there have been a limited number of studies that have explored the relationship between IPCP and health outcomes. However, Lutfiyya et al. (2019) reported the majority of recent studies found a positive relationship between the two. According to Baik (2017), team-based care has three core attributes: interprofessional collaboration, patient-centered approach, and integrated care process. In rural settings, with limited resources, it is logical to expect the benefits of IPCP would be magnified, although there is a paucity of literature supporting this idea.

IPE has been a buzzword for many years. An often-cited definition is that IPE "occurs when students from two or more professions learn about, from and with each other to enable effective collaboration and improve health outcomes" (World Health Organization, 2010, p. 7). The National Center for Interprofessional Practice and Education (NEXUS) has a mission to "support evaluation, research, data, and evidence that ignites the field of interprofessional practice and education and leads to better care, added value and healthier communities" (NEXUS, 2020, para 5). The National Center is now differentiating *new IPE*, which emphasizes the importance of interprofessional *practice* and education (IPE); thus, accentuating the need to focus on both practice and education to enable HCPs to work collaboratively on teams to ensure high-quality healthcare at the lowest cost in all settings (NEXUS, 2020).

Rural Healthcare

There are 1,350 CAH located in the United States (Rural Health Information Hub, 2019). Unlike hospitals located in urban settings, CAHs, which are located in rural areas, have limited fiscal and human resources and operate under the following conditions: CAHs are required to have 25 or fewer inpatient beds, be located 35 miles or more from the nearest hospital, maintain an average length of stay of 96 hours or less, and provide emergency services around the clock (Rural Health Information Hub, 2019). CAHs provide acute and ambulatory care, labor and delivery services, and some CAHs may offer home care services and general surgery (Mayer & Winters, 2016). Unlike hospitals located in urban settings, CAHs have limited fiscal and human resources. It is recognized that rural HCPs encounter challenges, including professional isolation (also see Chapter 26, Developing and Sustaining the Rural Nursing Workforce Through Collaborative Educational Models), lack of anonymity (also see Chapter 5, Lack of Anonymity: Changes for the 21st Century), role diffusion (also see Chapter 8, The Distinctive Nature and Scope of Rural Nursing Practice: Philosophical Bases), and limited access to continuing education (CE) (also see Chapter 9, Understanding the Lived Experiences of the Rural Bedside Nurse: A Global View).

Approximately 19% of the population of the United States lives in rural areas (U.S. Census Bureau, 2017). However only 12% of the physician workforce practice in rural areas, and the number of primary care providers per capita (including physicians, nurse practitioners, and physician assistants) decreases, the more rural the setting (Larson et al., 2020; Rosenblatt et al., 2010). These facts illustrate a substantial mismatch in resource needs versus allocation. Similarly, newly licensed nurses are also not "flocking to rural setting[s] to practice" (Forneris, 2019, para 5). Forneris reported that in 2017 only 15.2% of newly graduated rural nurses (RNs) were employed in hospitals of 100 beds or less, and only 6.8% started their careers in hospitals with 50 or less beds. RNs must be "expert generalists" (Mayer & Winters, 2016, p. 75), which means they have expertise in a wide range of skills that apply to all age groups and a variety of healthcare issues. Nursing students who have lived in rural settings and been assigned to rural hospitals for clinical rotations may be more interested in practicing in a rural setting (Forneris, 2019).

Every minute counts in an emergency cases, and such cases can be particularly stressful for rural HCPs given limited exposure to life-threatening situations. The recall of knowledge and skills reviewed and practiced on a biennial basis, that is, CPR, can fade over time due to infrequent application of learned emergency skills and protocols in rural settings (Stellflug & Lowe, 2018). Doctors cannot *do it all* in rural settings and must depend on nurses and other health professions to provide high-quality care for patients. Rural HCP's roles often overlap in their scope of practice with their colleagues' roles, especially in emergency situations. For example, a nonpharmacist may need to dispense medications, while a nurse stabilizes a patient before the physician arrives. Such situations speak to knowing the skills and strengths of your team and the importance of collaborative teamwork, which supports the third theoretical statement associated with Rural Nursing Theory (Lee & Winters, 2018).

There is also a growing mismatch between the large number of rural elders in need of healthcare and the small numbers of HCPs seeking employment in rural settings. This mismatch necessitates teamwork and collaborative care in rural settings in order to provide the highest quality care possible in the context of limited resources. Healthcare disparities are magnified when it comes to older people. According to the 2012–2016 American Community Survey (ACS) data, there were 46.2 million older people in the United States and 10.6 million of them in areas designated as rural (U.S. Census Bureau, 2019). In Montana, both the total and the rural populations are aging with 25.4% of the total state population over age 60; 49.6% of people over age 65 live in rural areas, while 50.4% live in more urban parts of the state. The fastest growing age group is those 85 and older, with projections that this age group will be more than triple by 2050 (Houser et al., 2018). We have a perfect storm given the aging of rural Americans in conjunction with HCP shortages common in rural communities. Evidence about the rural workforce speaks to a need to bring IPE and IPCP to rural settings during medical and nursing education, especially if we expect graduates to work as collaborative teams in practice settings after licensure.

In the medical and nursing education literature, there are several predictors of likelihood to practice in a rural area after completion of training (Forneris, 2019; MacQueen et al., 2018). Some predictors are inherent to the background of the individual and their personal circumstances, and some are influenced by educational factors. The primary background characteristic that increases likelihood for rural practice is if the trainee is originally from a rural location. Educational factors in medical education include training in a rural location, especially with a rural focus or track, and training in primary care, most notably the specialty of family medicine. Because of these factors and our background and experience, we focus our discussion of IPE training in the context of education for nursing students and family medicine residents in programs with a rural focus. To better understand this context, it is valuable to have a general knowledge of medical and nursing education and the ways in which this education is both similar and different.

Education and Certification for Physicians and Rural Nurses

Medical education differs from nursing education in both timing and structure. Most medical training programs in the United States require a bachelor's degree, followed by 4 years of medical school. After medical school, there are 3 to 7 years of residency training in an area of medical specialty, after which there are optional fellowships available for further sub-specialization (Association of American Medical Colleges, 2020). Most medical schools are consistent in their curricular structure, based in part on accreditation requirements, and the timing of the three steps of the U.S. Medical Licensing Exam (USMLE) for medical doctor (MD) or the three levels of the Comprehensive Osteopathic Medical Licensing Examination of the United States (COMLEX-USA) for Doctor of Osteopathic Medicine (DO). The first 2 years are largely classroom based, with a heavy emphasis on basic sciences, anatomy, physiology, and the pathologic basis of disease states. The next 2 years are clinically focused, with specific clinical rotations through the major medical specialties. There are some variations, but the majority follow closely to this format (AAMC, 2020). The USMLE is a three-step examination, with each step taking place over one or more days. Passing all three parts of either the USMLE or COMLEX-USA is required to be licensed to practice medicine independently in the United States (National Board of Medical Examiners, 2020; National Board of Osteopathic Medical Examiners, 2020).

Some postgraduate training in an accredited residency program is required by all 50 states to receive a license to practice medicine. However, the length of training and a requirement for completion of residency vary state-to-state. No states currently allow a newly graduated physician to become licensed directly out of medical school and begin practice as a general practitioner (GP), without any further training (Federation of State Medical Boards, 2018). Some GPs remain in practice in many states, having been grandfathered in prior to residency training requirements, or after partially completing residency training, but they are few (Young et al., 2019). In rural settings, the GP model has largely been replaced by family medicine as a board-certified area of medical specialization. Family medicine was developed as a medical specialty with its own board of specialization in 1969 (American Board of Family Medicine, 2020a). To become board certified in family medicine requires completion of a 3-year residency training program accredited by the Accreditation Council for Graduate Medical Education (ACGME). Completion of a residency program makes a candidate eligible to sit for the Family Medicine Board Examination to become certified by the American Board of Family Medicine (American Board of Family Medicine, 2020b).

The nursing profession has not reached consensus about the minimum requirements for entry into practice as an RN. However, the American Association of Colleges of Nursing (AACN, 2000) and other professional organizations have affirmed that a bachelor of science in nursing (BSN) degree is the minimum educational requirement for practice as an RN although hospital-based diploma and associate degree registered nursing programs are still in existence. Regardless of their educational preparation, all nursing students educated to be RNs take the same licensing exam, the NCLEX-RN®, upon completion of their pre-licensure educational program. National efforts to increase the number of BSN-prepared RNs have been supported by numerous organizations including the Magnet® recognition program (American Nurses Credentialing Center, n.d.), which outlines a path to nursing excellence. In a landmark report, the Health and Medicine Division (2010) recommended that 80% or greater of the RN workforce have a BSN or higher degree in nursing by the year 2020. Not surprisingly, these national efforts have led to an increase in enrollment in BSN programs (AACN, 2000). Given efforts to increase the RN workforce, nursing education took steps to develop accelerated BSN programs that recruit students with a bachelor's degree in another field to enroll in a shortened (12–15 months) nursing program. Graduates of accelerated nursing programs are eligible to take the NCLEX-RN licensing exam.

RNs have many options to consider for graduate education; they may enroll in master's and doctoral educational programs in nursing or related fields. Similar to medical board certification, RNs may sit for national certification after receiving a master's or practice doctoral degree (DNP) as an APRN in one of four APRN roles: certified nurse practitioner (CNP), certified nurse midwife (CNM), certified registered nurse anesthetist

(CRNA), and clinical nurse specialist (CNS) (AACN, n.d.). RNs with clinical expertise in a particular area may choose to become certified by a professional organization after demonstrating competency in that specialty. Certifications are available for multiple specialties including oncology, critical care, leadership, and geriatrics, to list a few. Nurses can continue their education to receive a research doctoral degree (Doctor of Philosophy / PhD). Table 23.1 compares the education and certification process for medical and nursing education for those seeking to become an RN.

Education for Rural Practice

A common model for rural training among family medicine residency programs is to have a rural focus at an urban-based program. This often includes a requirement of one or more months spent at rural sites, but most training occurs at a larger institution. A second model is the rural training track (RTT), which is often set up along a 1:2 model, with the first year of residency at a larger institution, and the last 2 years at a smaller rural hospital. There are approximately 40 RTTs or RTT-like programs in family medicine (Rural Training Track Collaborative, 2020). RTTs have a 73% success rates of placing doctors in rural communities (Patterson et al., 2013), but generally train only one to two residents at a time, due to limited teaching capacity and resources.

A hybrid approach to training rural doctors has been adopted at the Family Medicine Residency of Western Montana (FMRWM), where one of the authors (DB) currently works. The primary training site is in Missoula, Montana, with an alternate training site for years two and three in Kalispell, Montana. The alternate site qualifies by population

TABLE 23.1 Medical and Nursing Education and Certification

Medical Education	Nursing Education
Bachelor's Degree (4 years)	**Diploma** (3 years) (*phasing out) **Associate Degree** (3 years) **Bachelor's Degree** (4 years) NCLEX-RN for nursing license
Medical School (4 years) *MD/DO* USMLE Steps 1–3 or COMLEX-USA levels 1–3	**Graduate Education** Multiple options **Master's degree** (multiple options – see APRN titles below)
Residency Training (3–7 years) Board Certification Examination	**Doctoral Degree** DNP Research doctorate (PhD)
Board Certification Independent Licensure	**Board Certification for APRNs:** CNM, CNP, CNRA CNS **Specialty Certification options** for clinical expertise in wide range of topics (geriatrics, palliative care, nursing education, oncology clinical nurse leader, etc.)

CNM, certified nurse midwife; CNP, certified nurse practitioner; CNS, clinical nurse specialist; COMLEX-USA, Comprehensive Osteopathic Medical Licensing Examination of the United States; CRNA, certified registered nurse anesthetist; DNP, Doctorate of Nursing Practice; DO, Doctor of Osteopathy; MD, Doctor of Medicine; NCLEX-RN, National Council Licensure Exam–Registered Nurse; USMLE, United States Medical Licensing Examination.

as an RTT, although by availability of medical resources, it is significantly less rural. FMRWM has also developed a rural education network of 16 remote and frontier sites, and all family medicine residents from both Missoula and Kalispell are required to spend time immersed in a rural setting. Additionally, many residents fulfill several of their core-required experiences in areas such as pediatrics, surgery, sports medicine, and emergency medicine at rural locations. Rural partner sites participate in regular program sponsored professional development activities to help ensure consistently high-quality training experiences.

Some nursing programs have also developed tracks focused on rural nursing. For example, Montana State University (MSU) College of Nursing, in conjunction with the state Area Health Education Center (AHEC) and the Office of Rural Health, received grant funding to establish a rural primary care track (RPCT) (MSU, n.d.). Although the College of Nursing's graduate programs have always had a rural focus, the grant funding augments the nursing education occurring in the classroom and in clinical settings with support for student travel to rural sites for clinical and rural immersion experiences. At MSU, the RPCT is linked to the AHEC Scholars' (2019) program, which is a national program designed to prepare a diverse healthcare workforce that is equipped to work in rural and underserved areas. Health profession students who are in the AHEC Scholars program are required to complete additional learning activities focused on six topic areas: IPE, behavioral health, social determinants of health, cultural competence, practice transformation, and current and emerging health issues; and graduate with a certificate that identifies them as an AHEC Scholar.

Undergraduate nursing students at MSU frequently are assigned to clinical rotations in rural settings. These rural experiences include assisting rural school nurses with hearing and vision screenings of children, making home visits with a CAH's home/health and hospice nurse, collaborating with a county extension agent to develop walking maps for rural communities, bringing health education to staff working in long-term care settings, and working with nurse preceptors to learn about leadership and management in a CAH.

Challenges for the Rural Workforce

Rural settings are frequently considered health professional shortage areas (HPSA; Health Resources & Services Administration, 2020) and shortages generally relate to a scarcity of primary care, dental and mental health providers. In the absence of certain health professionals, there is increased necessity for interprofessional collaboration. The entire healthcare team is stretched and must rely on each other to cover different aspects of the role or service that is not available. However, HCPs trained in urban settings may be wary about practicing in a rural environment due to apprehension about workload, limited opportunities for time off, scarce access to in-person CE, professional isolation, lack of anonymity, and worries about maintaining professional boundaries (Rural Health Information Hub, 2020). Therefore, rural communities need a proactive approach to the recruitment and retention of a collaborative rural workforce and often partner with other organizations to increase efficiency, and promote best practices related to recruitment and retention. One such organization is the National Rural Recruitment and Retention Network (2016), which is a national network that connects HCPs with employment opportunities in rural and HPSAs.

Rural areas have encountered unique challenges during the COVID-19 pandemic (Centers for Disease Control and Prevention CDC, 2020) and rural HCPs need to network and collaborate with others in the community to strengthen the local healthcare infrastructure. Shortages of HCPs may be compounded by a limited number of hospital beds, specifically intensive care beds, and medical equipment. This again increases the need for interprofessional collaboration and teamwork to provide the highest possible quality care. Emergency medical services may be staffed by volunteers who must leave their home or workplace to respond to emergencies. In rural areas public health departments frequently are responsible for large geographic areas and may be staffed in large part by individuals who were not primarily trained in public health. In rural areas, it does not take many COVID-19 cases to overwhelm local resources, further straining even high-functioning interprofessional teams.

Most HCPs, including nurses, physicians, pharmacists, social workers, and others, are required to engage in annual CE as a condition of license renewal (Holuby et al., 2015). Rural HCPs may find it difficult to travel to in-person educational offerings due to geographic distances associated with travel, costs, time, and lack of staff available to fill in during their absence. Online education appears to be a good alternative to travel but in rural settings slower internet speeds often limit online educational content to text-based format. All educational contents with audio, graphics, and/or video, require high-speed internet, which may not be available in rural areas (Speed Matters, n.d.).

This pandemic, with the associated stay at home orders, forced schools and universities to convert to online classes in early 2020. These actions resulted in the exponential growth of online education. In addition, professional organizations and healthcare associations have converted annual meetings to virtual formats. As a result, access to online CE is improved, and if virtual meetings continue to be the norm, the need for rural HCPs to travel for CE and professional development opportunities may decline. However, much of the CE offerings currently available are discipline specific, with fewer opportunities for ongoing education in IPCP.

One of the authors (DMM) received funding to conduct a project to bring CE on palliative care to HCPs working in rural Montana. An educational intervention was conducted using the End-of-Life Nursing Education Consortium (ELNEC; AACN, 2020) core curriculum, which was appropriate for nurses and physicians. Attendance was open to all interested HCPs. Each CAH engaged in the project posted flyers promoting this education, and course dates were shared with the family medicine residents. In addition, pharmacists at each CAH were invited to co-present content related to pain management. However, participation of other disciplines, specifically physicians and pharmacists, was often not possible due to schedules not aligning, staffing shortages, and the lack of protected time, which may have supported attendance. The ELNEC curriculum was presented as either a one-day or one-and-a-half-day class and participants received between 7.75 and 11.25 nursing contact hours, respectively. All sessions included breakout sessions with case discussions and the sharing of participant's experiences providing care to clients with serious illnesses. A total of 42 HCPs attended this course; most were RNs, and one pharmacist co-presented pain management content. Course evaluations from the participants included comments (Table 23.2) about the need for improved communication with other members of the healthcare team.

Challenges of Implementing IPE in Rural Clinical Settings

There are many documented challenges to developing and implementing IPE programs (Wong et al., 2019). IPE can be especially difficult to develop in rural settings. Limited resources and logistical challenges exist when it comes to developing specific, interdisciplinary training activities in rural clinical sites. However, there are tools available to determine how clinical sites work together as teams, and how ready they are for IPE,

TABLE 23.2 Comments Related to IPE/IPCP From HCPs After a PC Education Course When Asked for Constructive Feedback on Improving the Course

RN Comments
Interdisciplinary approach to find good pain relief [for patient]
Include pharmacist to determine morphine equivalency
Include nonnursing staff is some sort of remembrance [after a patient dies]
Better collaboration with team members (hospitalists/MD's especially)
[The presence of] ...*physicians, social workers and other HCPs on the IDT* [at this training] *would be great*
How to build a working relationship between doctors and nurses when caring for palliative/dying patients
Training for the providers/physicians – I wish they would focus on palliative care a little earlier

SW Comment
Explore alternative pain medication [options] *with pharmacist*

Notes: Italic font indicates direct words of participants. Provider: physician, nurse practitioner, physician assistant.
IDT, interdisciplinary team; SW, social worker

such as the ACE-15 and InSITE tools, which may be useful when assessing the capacity for IPE at a given location (Sick et al., 2019; Tilden et al., 2016). Such tools may help to assess the implicit learning regarding interprofessional care that may be available at a given site.

Scheduling is one of the greatest challenges that arises with IPE in rural settings. Most nursing, medical, and other healthcare training programs are organized and scheduled independently, even within the same educational institution. Health professions programs do not communicate with each other when developing their curricular schedules and clinical experiences. As a result, there may be little overlap between where trainees are placed and when they are there. Often each individual discipline must scramble to find clinical placement sites to meet their objectives and educational needs. With the scheduling challenges programs face individually, coordinating efforts among programs is given a low priority. The scheduling challenge is magnified in smaller rural training sites, which may only host one or a few learners of any given discipline per year. Due to small size there can be a limited educational capacity, and if there are only one or two interested clinicians, then stability/availability of educators adds to that challenge. Therefore, small rural sites may vary in their ability to take learners consistently. Even if a small rural hospital or clinic hosts trainees of different disciplines, the lack of schedule coordination provides little opportunity to interact either informally or in formalized IPE programs.

Even in larger institutions, integrating learners can be a challenge in clinical settings. Nursing students and residents from the authors' programs regularly overlap at larger hospitals and clinics, along with students from multiple other disciplines. Even with the presence of IPE champions on their clinical faculty, developing ongoing clinical IPE processes in these institutions has been a multi-year effort. It has involved significant resource use and active engagement/reengagement to develop relationships and obtain buy-in from practicing clinicians and administration.

Compounding the above challenges is a relative lack of value assigned to interprofessional training on the part of practicing professionals, who may not have received significant training in IPCP and may not recognize how it currently impacts their work.

Surveys we have done with our clinical faculty indicate there is often passive agreement that IPE is important but is not something they prioritize. This holds true among rural clinical educators as well. Surveys with our rural clinical partners about curricular areas for focus, consistently rank IPE low on the list.

This relatively low perceived value of developing IPE deters individual educators from spending time and effort on IPE when engaged in clinical training. If clinical instructors in a rural setting believe they have limited time and capacity for clinical education, they may be reluctant to spend that resource on other disciplines, preferring instead to focus exclusively on their own discipline. This makes inherent sense: if you have limited capacity for education, there is a natural inclination to focus your efforts where you believe you can make the greatest impact. A focus on your own discipline allows you to pass on the greatest amount of knowledge and experience.

Overcoming IPE Challenges

We have adopted several strategies to overcome challenges to IPE throughout the nursing and medical resident training process. We discuss some of those techniques here and provide ideas for incorporating greater awareness of and engagement in IPE, regardless of clinical setting. The first part of our process is increasing IPE awareness and activities at the home institution. As discussed previously, it is easier to develop IPE opportunities where the focus is education, with IPE champions on site, and access to robust educational resources. Through inter-program and inter-institutional outreach and collaboration, the University of Montana (UM) College of Health, which houses FMRWM, and the MSU College of Nursing, Missoula campus, have created an IPE committee for the express purpose of increasing opportunities for interprofessional collaboration. This committee has been in existence for many years and includes representatives from multiple health education programs involved with undergraduate and graduate education. Efforts at these two large state universities have recently resulted in the development of the Montana University System (MUS) Institute for Interprofessional Education & Collaborative Practice (Montana University System Institute for Interprofessional Education, 2020), co-led and co-sponsored by both MSU and UM. The MUS IPE Institute is designed to connect health professions programs across Montana with clinical sites, many of which are in rural communities, to promote IPE and collaborative practice statewide (MUS IPE Institute, 2020). This commitment from two state universities speaks to the institutional dedication of time and resources that has been critical for the implementation of our ongoing IPE efforts.

We have had success with several IPE opportunities on campus. Twice a year we conduct IPE simulation days utilizing the College of Nursing simulation lab with three or four disciplines at a time, including nursing, medicine, pharmacy, athletic training, physical therapy, and speech and language pathology students. Successful cases have focused on critical care and management of emergency situations, obstetrical complications, communication with speech-impaired patients, experience with geriatric and stroke simulation equipment, and progression of on-field emergencies continuing through to definitive hospital care. We also hold twice annual, large, half-day IPE seminars for up to 250 learners at a time, with small interprofessional groups of students learning about different disciplines and participating together in tabletop and case-based learning experiences. We have developed several semester-long courses on interprofessional collaborative care, which allow students from multiple disciplines to be in classes together. FMRWM annually hosts a multidisciplinary didactic session introducing IPCP to the first-year residents and health professions students. Each of these recurring opportunities and other individual events have slowly begun to shift the culture of learning at our institutions. For example, students regularly seek opportunities to engage with other health profession students in optional experiences beyond the requirements for IPE as set forth by an increasing number of accrediting bodies and individual programs (Health Professions Accreditors Collaborative, 2019).

At FMRWM, we have also taken specific steps to increase IPE during rural clinical placements. We encourage thinking about IPE more broadly to include practicing clinicians in different disciplines, rather than only focusing on interprofessional learners; which is consistent with the National Centers new IPE perspective (NEXUS, 2020). In rural settings, interprofessional collaboration is taking place daily but is not often identified as IPE by residents and students. In rural communities, interprofessional care is often taken for granted, and working across disciplines is not readily identified as something unique or remarkable. When asked about IPE training on clinical rotation evaluations, resident physicians often report little to no formal opportunities. However, when asked if they worked directly with other HCPs, they describe regular collaboration with other disciplines.

One way the FMRWM has attempted to make informal interprofessional opportunities more valuable to learners is through the development of specific curricular goals for rural clinical rotations. Having the learner identify when they are engaged in interprofessional care and encouraging them to seek opportunities to work with other disciplines increases their awareness and engagement with IPCP. By setting curricular expectations in advance and subsequently engaging in retrospective analysis, the lessons learned from interprofessional activities can be solidified. This is maximized by building time into the schedule where learners are assigned to spend part of a day working directly with professionals from other disciplines.

At MSU College of Nursing, we collaborate with IPE champions locally and regionally to develop opportunities for students to learn from and with each other on a regular basis. Current efforts are underway to develop IPE objectives for courses in our curriculum so that collaborative interactions between health profession students become part of the culture both in the classroom and in the clinical settings. Nursing faculty voluntarily serve on local IPE committees, plan, and organize interprofessional events each semester, and teach elective IPE courses. Feedbacks of students from varied health profession programs after IPE events have been overwhelmingly positive, and their constructive criticism has been used to improve future offerings.

In our experiences, the challenge of educational resource scarcity can be overcome through training of rural preceptors as documented by Osborne et al. (2018). Many nursing students do clinical rotations in rural communities in conjunction with courses on public health and nursing leadership and management. These students get to experience the benefits of IPCP as their nursing preceptors connect them with providers and other HCPs at CAHs. With interdisciplinary training on clinical education and the value of interdisciplinary teams for improving both health outcomes and work environments, the FMRWM program has seen an increase in the acceptance and integration of overt interprofessional collaboration and education at our rural partner institutions. Providing CE credits for these training opportunities has increased engagement and participation on the part of rural preceptors. FMRWM has established an annual rural educators' conference each fall, focusing on clinical education, and increasingly on IPE and practice. Participation in this conference has grown each year, with consistent positive evaluations. Due to these efforts, we have seen a decrease in resistance to formal IPE opportunities at our rural partner sites. However, consistency with IPE-focused activities remains an ongoing challenge in rural settings.

Implications for Education, Research, and Practice

Rural clinical sites offer a potentially rich environment for interprofessional learning. They are smaller, and practitioners of different disciplines are more likely to know each other personally and work with each other on a regular basis. These personal connections likely contribute to strong collaborative relationships that benefit rural IPE activities. However, Croker and Hudson (2015) reported little to no description related to collaborative relationships in their review of 24 publications that focused on IPE in rural settings. Their conclusions encourage those publishing about IPE in rural settings to provide "explicit descriptions of the nature of educators collaborative relationships" (p. 886). These researchers make a case for including details of their collaborative relationships given that these relationships likely contribute to the overall IPE experience.

As educators we need to bring students in various health professions programs together with specific learning objectives related to actively engaging together in understanding their own role as well as developing an understanding of the roles and responsibilities of other HCPs on the team. At the end of a clinical experience, asking learners what disciplines they worked with and how they collaborated to improve patient care encourages learners to reflect on not only their role but also the holistic aspects of team-based, person-centered care. Both prospective and retrospective analyses of interprofessional collaborative care on the part of the learner can help them to identify the importance, benefits of, and interdependence of the healthcare team in the management of patients and their care. Specific training for rural educators, especially when offering CE credit, helps shift the perception of IPE and its importance in training and may open opportunities for trainees to learn from interprofessional team members while at rural sites. Rural settings provide a valuable opportunity, since due to a relative lack of resources, there is often an increased dependence on interdisciplinary team members to maximize the care for patients. However, it takes time and effort to cultivate those opportunities for the betterment of both the clinical sites and the learners rotating through rural communities.

To maximize interprofessional learning for rural practice, we recommend a combination of formal IPE, integrated into the training at the home institution, and a focused effort toward developing both formal and informal interprofessional care and learning opportunities at rural clinical sites. Resources and capabilities for formal IPE at the home institution are generally much higher than in smaller, more distant, rural clinical sites, and programs may be co-located with other health professions programs. Our experience is that with a focused group of faculty from different disciplines who are interested in developing IPE opportunities, it becomes easier to develop the administrative support, resources, and time to develop beneficial experiences, all keys to successful integration of interprofessional activities into learning (Bridges et al., 2011). Some IPE activities with documented benefit, such as interprofessional simulation training (Taylor et al., 2017), are more easily established in locations with simulation equipment and faculty familiar with the equipment, which are often located at educational institutions.

However, training with a focus on interprofessional collaborative care in rural settings has not been well studied. The studies that have been published on rural IPE most often involve seminars/discussion groups, case presentations, and community projects (Walker et al., 2018). These studies have not generally evaluated the effects of interaction with practicing HCPs in rural clinical settings. As is often the case with IPE efforts, IPE experiences in rural settings have positive outcomes in terms of ability to collaborate, managing the complexity of healthcare in rural settings and understanding and valuing the roles of different disciplines with increased respect for those providers (Walker et al., 2019). There are mixed results as to whether IPE in rural settings increases or decreases the likelihood of rural practice at the end of training (Mpofu et al., 2014). Not surprisingly, additional research is needed on the impact and outcomes associated with bringing IPE and IPCP to rural settings.

CONCLUSION

If the goals of IPE are to be met, we need to increase the ability of HCPs to engage with and learn from each other in multiple settings. Therefore, we should incorporate team-based care and promote IPE and IPCP throughout our educational programs and in all practice settings. We can promote the concept of team-based care by bringing interprofessional HCPs together to learn about the roles and responsibilities of other disciplines on the team, while developing a culture of mutual respect, with support from both educational and clinical organizations.

Bringing interprofessional practice and education to the rural workforce is beneficial for both interdisciplinary HCPs and rural residents in need of healthcare close to home. As people age, they tend to utilize more healthcare services and rural Americans want to receive healthcare close to home. The lack of human and fiscal resources in rural settings requires the healthcare team to collaborate in order to provide high-quality healthcare. Formal IPE and IPCP training can better prepare HCPs to provide efficient and cost-effective team-based healthcare.

REFERENCES

Accreditation Council for Graduate Medical Education. (2020, July 1). *ACGME program requirements for graduate medical education in family medicine.* https://www.acgme.org/Portals/0/PFAssets/ProgramRequirements/120_FamilyMedicine_2020.pdf?ver=2020-06-29-161615-367

American Association of Colleges of Nursing. (n.d.). *APRN education.* https://www.aacnnursing.org/Teaching-Resources/APRN

American Association of Colleges of Nursing. (2000). *The baccalaureate degree in nursing as minimal preparation for professional practice* [Position Statement]. AACN. https://www.aacnnursing.org/News-Information/Position-Statements-White-Papers/Bacc-Degree-Prep

American Association of Colleges of Nursing (2020). *About ELNEC.* https://www.aacnnursing.org/ELNEC/About

American Board of Family Medicine. (2020a). *History of ABFM.* https://www.theabfm.org/about/ABFM-history

American Board of Family Medicine. (2020b). *Am I board eligible?* https://www.theabfm.org/become-certified/am-i-board-eligible

American Nurses Credentialing Center. (n.d.). *ANCC magnet recognition program.* https://www.nursingworld.org/organizational-programs/magnet/

Area Health Education Center. (2019). *AHEC scholars and core topics.* https://www.nationalahec.org/index.php/scholars-home

Association of American Medical Colleges. (2020). *Curriculum reports.* https://www.aamc.org/data-reports/curriculum-reports/interactive-data/academic-level-length-distribution-us-and-canadian-medical-schools

Baik, D. (2017). Team-based care: A concept analysis. *Nursing Forum, 52*(4), 313–322. https://doi.org/10.1111/nuf.12194

Bridges, D. R., Davidson, R. A., Odegard, P. S., Maki, I. V., & Tomkowiak, J. (2011). Interprofessional collaboration: Three best practice models of interprofessional education. *Medical Education Online, 16,* 6035. Advance online publication. https://www.tandfonline.com/doi/pdf/10.3402/meo.v16i0.6035

Centers for Disease Control and Prevention. (2020). *Rural communities.* https://www.cdc.gov/coronavirus/2019-ncov/need-extra-precautions/other-at-risk-populations/rural-communities.html

Croker, A., & Hudson, J. N. (2015). Interprofessional education: Does recent literature from rural settings offer insights into what really matters? *Medical Education, 49*(9), 880–887. https://doi.org/10.1111/medu.12749

Federation of State Medical Boards. (2018). *State specific requirements for initial medical licensure.* https://www.fsmb.org/step-3/state-licensure/

Forneris, L. (2019, November 21). *Time for new perspective: Rural nursing workforce.* National Rural Health Association. https://www.ruralhealthweb.org/blogs/ruralhealthvoices/november-2019/time-for-new-perspective-rural-nursing-workforce

Health and Medicine Division. (2010). *The future of nursing: Leading change, advancing health.* National Academies Press.

Health Professions Accreditors Collaborative. (2019, February 1). *Guidance on developing quality interprofessional education for the health professions.* https://healthprofessionsaccreditors.org/wp-content/uploads/2019/02/HPACGuidance02-01-19.pdf

Health Resources & Services Administration. (2020). *Health professional shortage areas (HPSAs).* https://bhw.hrsa.gov/shortage-designation/hpsas

Holuby, F. S., Pellegrin, K. L., Barbato, A., & Ciarleglio, A. (2015). Recruitment of rural healthcare professionals for live continuing education. *Medical Education Online, 20*(1), 1–3. https://doi.org/10.3402/meo.v20.28958

Houser, A., Fox-Grage, W., & Ujvari, K. (2018). *Across the states: Profiles of long term services and support.* https://www.aarp.org/content/dam/aarp/ppi/2018/08/across-the-states-profiles-of-long-term-services-and-supports-full-report.pdf

International Conference on Primary Health Care. (1978). Declaration of Alma-Ata. World Health Organization [WHO]. *WHO Chronicle, 32*(11), 428–430. https://www.who.int/publications/almaata_declaration_en.pdf?ua=1

Larson, E. H., Andrilla, C. H. A., & Garberson, L. A. (2020). *Supply and distribution of the primary care workforce in rural America: 2019.* [Policy Brief]. WWAMI Rural Health Research Center, University of Washington.

Lee, H. J., & Winters, C. A. (2018). Rural nursing theory: Past, present, and future. In C. A. Winters & H. J. Lee (Eds.), *Rural Nursing; Concepts, Theories, and Practice* (5th ed., pp. 3–15). Springer Publishing Company.

Lutfiyya, M. N., Chang, L. F., McGrath, C., Dana, C., & Lipsky, M. S. (2019). The state of the science of interprofessional collaborative practice: A scoping review of the patient health-related outcomes based literature published between 2010 and 2018. *PLOS ONE, 14*(6), e0218578. https://doi.org/10.1371/journal.pone.0218578

MacQueen, I. T., Maggard-Gibbons, M., Capra, G., Raaen, L., Ulloa, J. G., Shekelle, P. G., Miake-Lye, I., Beroes, J. M., & Hempel, S. (2018). Recruiting rural healthcare providers today: A systematic review of training program success and determinants of geographic choices. *Journal of General Internal Medicine, 33*(2), 191–199. https://doi.org/10.1007/s11606-017-4210-z

Mayer, D., & Winters, C. (2016). Palliative care in critical access hospitals. *Critical Care Nurse, 36*(1), 72–78. https://doi.org/10.4037/ccn2016732

Montana State University. (n.d.). *Rural primary care nursing track.* http://healthinfo.montana.edu/rural-primary-care/index.html

Montana University System Institute for Interprofessional Education & Collaborative Practice. (2020). *Welcome to the Montana IPE institute.* https://montanaipe.org

Mpofu, R., Daniels, P. S., Adonis, T. A., & Karuguti, W. M. (2014). Impact of an interprofessional education program on developing skilled graduates well-equipped to practice in rural and underserved areas. *Rural and Remote Health, 14*(3), 2671. https://www.rrh.org.au/journal/article/2671

National Board of Medical Examiners. (2020). *Taking the USMLE.* https://www.nbme.org/taking-assessment/united-states-medical-licensing-examr-usmler

National Board of Osteopathic Medical Examiners. (2020). *COMLEX-USA the pathway to osteopathic medical practice & licensure in the United States.* https://www.nbome.org/exams-assessments/comlex-usa/

National Center for Interprofessional Practice and Education. (2020). *About the national center*. https://nexusipe.org/informing/about-national-center

National Rural Recruitment and Retention Network. (2016). *Healthcare jobs across the nation*. https://www.3rnet.org/

Osborne, M. L., Tilden V. P., & Eckstrom, E. (2018). Training health professions preceptors in rural practices: A challenge for interprofessional practice and education. *Journal of Interprofessional Care*. Advance online publication. https://doi.org/10.1080/13561820.2018.1458707

Patterson, D. G., Longenecker, R., Schmitz, D., Phillips, R. L., Skillman, S. M., & Doescher, M. P. (2013). *Rural residency training for family medicine physicians: Graduate early-career outcomes, 2008-2012*. [Policy Brief]. WWAMI Rural Health Research Center, University of Washington School of Medicine Department of Family Medicine. https://depts.washington.edu/fammed/rhrc/publications/policy-brief-rural-residency-training-for-family-medicine-physicians-graduate-early-career-outcomes-2008-2012/

Rosenblatt, R. A., Chen, F. M., Lishner, D. M., & Doescher, M. P. (2010). *The future of family medicine and implications for rural primary care physician supply*. Final Report #125, WWAMI Rural Health Research Center, University of Washington School of Medicine Department of Family Medicine Final Report #125. https://depts.washington.edu/uwrhrc/uploads/RHRC_FR125_Rosenblatt.pdf

Rural Health Information Hub. (2019). *Critical access hospitals*. https://www.ruralhealthinfo.org/topics/critical-access-hospitals

Rural Health Information Hub. (2020). *Recruitment and retention for rural health facilities*. https://www.ruralhealthinfo.org/topics/rural-health-recruitment-retention

Rural Training Track Collaborative. (2020). *Explore rural health professions education*. https://rttcollaborative.net/rural-programs/

Sick, B., Radosevich, D. M., Pittenger, A. L., & Brandt, B. (2019). Development and validation of a tool to assess the readiness of a clinical teaching site for interprofessional education (InSITE). *Journal of Interprofessional Care*. Advance online publication. https://doi.org/10.1080/13561820.2019.1569600

Speed Matters. (n.d.). *Distance learning*. https://speedmatters.org/distance-learning

Stellflug, S. M., & Lowe, N. K. (2018). The effect of high fidelity simulators on knowledge retention and skill self-efficacy in pediatric advanced life support courses in a rural state. *Journal of Pediatric Nursing, 39*, 21–26. https://doi.org/10.1016/j.pedn.2017.12.006

Taylor, S., Fatima, Y., Lakshman, N., & Roberts, H. (2017). Simulated interprofessional learning activities for rural health care services: Perceptions of health care students. *Journal of Multidisciplinary Healthcare, 10*, 235–241. https://doi.org/10.2147/JMDH.S140989

Tilden, V. P., Eckstrom, E., & Dieckmann, N. F. (2016). Development of the assessment for collaborative environments (ACE-15): A tool to measure perceptions of interprofessional "teamness." *Journal of Interprofessional Care, 30*(3), 288–294. https://doi.org/10.3109/13561820.2015.1137891

U.S. Census Bureau. (2017). What is *rural America*? https://www.census.gov/library/stories/2017/08/rural-america.html#:~:text=Urban%20areas%20make%20up%20only,Census%20Bureau%20%2D%20Opens%20as%20PDF

U.S. Census Bureau. (2019). *Older population in rural America*. https://www.census.gov/library/stories/2019/10/older-population-in-rural-america.html

Walker, L., Cross, M., & Barnett, T. (2018). Mapping the interprofessional education landscape for students on rural clinical placements: An integrative literature review. *Rural and Remote Health, 18*(2), 4336. https://doi.org/10.22605/RRH4336

Walker, L. E., Cross, M., & Barnett, T. (2019). Students' experiences and perceptions of interprofessional education during rural placement: A mixed methods study. *Nurse Education Today, 75*, 28–34. https://doi.org/10.1016/j.nedt.2018.12.012

Wong, P. S., Chen, Y. S., & Saw, P. S. (2019). Influencing factors and processes of interprofessional professional education (IPE) implementation. *Medical Teacher*. Advance online publication. https://doi.org/10.1080/0142159X.2019.1672864

World Health Organization. (2010). *Framework for action on collaborative practice*. https://apps.who.int/ iris/bitstream/handle/10665/70185/WHO_HRH_HPN_10.3_eng.pdf;jsessionid=9357A262470D 1F3511647B942EEB0574?sequence=1

Young, A., Chaudhry, H. J., Pei, X., Arnhart, K., Dugan, M., & Steingard, S. A. (2019). FSMB Census of Licensed Physicians in the United States, 2018. *Journal of Medical Regulation*, *105*(2), 7–23. https:// doi.org/10.30770/2572-1852-105.2.7

CHAPTER 24

Explicating Family Nurse Practitioner Competencies for Rural Practice

STACY M. STELLFLUG AND KAILYN MOCK

DISCUSSION TOPICS

- Discuss how rural healthcare needs influence the education and skills of family nurse practitioners (FNP)?
- How can professional competencies improve care in rural settings?
- Describe how the identified competencies in the scale may be used to assess FNP Education and Practice?

INTRODUCTION

There are approximately 50 million people or 20% of the U.S. population living in rural areas (U.S. Census Bureau, 2018). The definition of rural is dependent on the source. Definitions for rural can be as complex as the number of people per square mile and as simple as anything not considered urban. Common characteristics of definitions of rural include a higher number of older adults, children, unemployment, and poverty (Zhu et al., 2015). Individuals living in rural areas are more likely to participate in agricultural work, which has been considered one of the most dangerous professions by Occupational Health Safety Agency (OSHA, 2018).

Healthcare delivery systems in rural areas face many challenges in meeting the needs of the communities they serve. Many rural areas rely on critical access hospitals (CAHs) to meet the healthcare needs of the population. The CAHs program is a federal U.S. program established in 1997 as part of the Balanced Budget Act (Rural Health Information Hub, 2018). The program offers support to small hospitals in rural areas to serve residents that would otherwise have to travel long distances for emergency care. CAHs must adhere to several guidelines including but not limited to having no more than 25 hospital beds, an average length of stay of less than 96 hours, and the CAHs must be physically located more than 35 miles from another hospital (Rural Health Information Hub, 2018). An exception can be granted for the distance rule for areas with poor roads and/or difficult terrain. A decreased number of beds and short length of stay requirements can pose difficulties for the CAHs especially during influenza season or if a global pandemic occurs. Rural CAHs are often unable to provide specialized healthcare services and frequently struggle to provide even basic care services.

Preparation of healthcare providers for entry into practice in a rural setting is essential to meet the needs of CAHs and the rural communities they serve. In this chapter challenges inherent to entering practice in a rural setting will be presented. The chapter also includes a discussion of the ability of family nurse practitioners (FNPs) to fulfill the role of rural healthcare provider. Finally, the development of the Rural Family Nurse Practitioner Competency Inventory (RFNPCI) as a tool to hone FNP curriculum, assess FNP practice, and target continued education and professional growth will be described.

BACKGROUND

Attracting and retaining providers in rural settings has been historically difficult. FNPs are positioned to fill a need that has long been a struggle to meet. FNPs comprise the second largest group of healthcare providers in the United States (Agency for Healthcare Research and Quality, 2012). They are more likely than their physician counterparts to work in rural communities and more likely to serve as providers for patients enrolled in Medicaid or paying out of pocket for care, especially in rural areas (U.S. Health Resources and Service Administration, 2014). FNPs are well positioned to assume the role of healthcare provider in any rural/frontier county in the United States. However, the healthcare facilities in these rural counties often are looking for more than a primary care provider. In resource-limited counties with fiscally minded CAHs, hiring a provider who can cover the clinic, ED, and inpatient care may not only be desirable but necessary. Educating FNPs to meet specific needs of rural care is fundamental for colleges of nursing as well as the CAH, the community, and the success of the FNP.

Rural healthcare can be demanding but also very rewarding for the FNPs who choose to practice in the rural setting. Defining practice competencies for FNPs in a rural setting has been elusive. Competencies refer to the mobilization of complex knowledge of how to act in a particular situation (Pepin et al., 2018). Competencies can be seen through integration of specific knowledge, skills, and attitudes acquired through learning (Tardif, 2006). Previous research in FNP practice competency has largely focused on specialty care and care in urban settings. Often FNPs in specialty care and/or urban settings work with a distinct specialty area or population, thus defining essential competencies for the practice is finite. By contrast, FNPs in rural settings must be prepared to provide care to individuals from a wide range of backgrounds, ages, and presenting problems. A rural FNP is often asked to wear multiple hats. The rural FNP may find themselves providing care for individuals in the ED, patients admitted to the hospital, and in the clinic setting, typically in the same day. Rural FNPs must be clinically competent in a number of specialty areas.

STUDY TO IDENTIFY RURAL FAMILY NURSE PRACTITIONERS COMPETENCIES

A wide skillset and knowledge base are necessary to function as an FNP in a rural setting. Currently, there are no established knowledge or skill competencies available to guide FNP education, assess FNP abilities prior to hire, or assess FNPs as they progress toward competency. The primary purpose of this study was to identify rural FNP competencies by a Delphi panel of practicing Rural FNP experts. The research objective was accomplished by using a Delphi panel of rural FNPs who are currently working in CAHs in the state of Montana.

Conceptual Framework

A lack of established knowledge and skill competencies can pose a barrier to education, professional advancement, and professional self-fulfillment. This is especially true in the rural healthcare setting. Competencies are necessary to not only function but survive in rural settings and may provide the key to attracting and maintaining FNPs in positions that have otherwise been difficulty to fill. Competence in providing care in a rural setting requires FNPs to gain the required knowledge and skills and attain a level of confidence or self-efficacy. Long and Weinert's Rural Nursing Theory along with Bandura's Self-Efficacy Theory were used to inform and guide the process of explicating FNP competencies for rural practice.

Long et al. (1997) described the role of the rural nurse generalist as well as the advanced education of such generalists at Montana State University (MSU). Recognizing the special needs of a rural population through the seminal work of Long and Weinert's Rural Nursing Theory, MSU faculty developed an advanced practice education program based in Rural Nursing Theory (Long & Weinert, 1989). Rural FNPs must be educated in a way they can be comfortable with a significant amount of uncertainty and possess the ability to be flexible to respond to whatever walks through the door next. Role diffusion is a concept that has been explored within the context of Rural Nursing Theory in an unpublished master's thesis completed by MSU faculty member Jane Scharff (1987). Scharff (1987) noted the rural hospital nurse must be a jack of all trades within the realm of numerous healthcare disciplines. The role diffusion concept is applicable to the rural FNP as well and serves as a theoretical and practical component of the education of FNPs in rural settings. Explication of the competencies necessary for rural practice has not been previously addressed, nor has assessment of the rural FNPs confidence in their skill and knowledge set. Defining and assessing rural FNP competencies is essential to the success of an FNP in a rural community.

Self-efficacy is an individual's belief in how capable they are to execute and achieve a task (Bandura, 1997, 2006). Self-Efficacy Theory has its origins in Social Cognitive Theory as proposed by Albert Bandura. The theory consists of three factors that influence self-efficacy: behaviors, environment, and personal/cognitive factors (Bandura, 1997). Self-efficacy develops from experiences in which participants are able to reach goals through persevering, overcoming obstacles, and observing others succeed through sustained efforts (Bandura, 1997). A strong sense of self-efficacy may allow an individual to mobilize their motivation and cognitive resources to provide action. When low levels of self-efficacy are present, the likelihood is high an individual will not attempt to act.

The ultimate goal for the development of an RFNPCI would be to guide education and curricular development for FNPs wanting to serve in rural settings. The competency inventory could also be used to assess FNP student's confidence with skills deemed necessary to practice in a rural setting as they progress through their program of study. The use of Bandura's Self-Efficacy Theory allows for self-assessment and targeted interventions when necessary.

Methods

Competencies have been defined as complex responses based on combining and mobilizing internal resources such as knowledge, skills, and attitudes with external resources then applying the competencies to specific types of situations. To identify competencies in rural FNP practice, a Delphi method was employed. Rand Corporation developed the Delphi method in the 1950s as a way to forecast the effect of technology on warfare (RAND Corporation, 2019). The Delphi method involves a group of experts who reply to questionnaires and receive feedback as a statistical representation of the group response (RAND Corporation, 2019). The process is repeated in an attempt to reduce the range of response and arrive at what can be considered expert consensus (RAND Corporation, 2019).

A total of six FNPs practicing in a rural setting and/or a CAH comprised the initial expert panel. The expert FNPs were asked via a Research Electronic Data Capture (REDCap) survey to consider their practice in a rural setting and then answer several questions. Study data were collected and managed using REDCap data capture tools hosted at the Institute of Translational Health Sciences at University of Washington. REDCap is a secure, web-based application designed to support data capture of research studies and is supported by the National Center for Advancing Translational Sciences of the National Institutes of Health under Award Number UL1 TR002319 (Harris et al., 2009). The content is solely the responsibility of the authors and does not necessarily represent the official views of the National Institutes of Health. The survey questions to be considered were:

1. What are the top five knowledge topics for rural practice you wish you had learned in FNP school but did not?
2. What are the top five skills necessary for rural practice you wish you had learned in FNP school but did not?
3. What are the top five resources you use in your practice you would recommend to EVERY FNP graduate entering practice?
4. What do you know now about rural practice that you wish you knew when you started your practice as a rural FNP?

From the expert panel response, a list of 90 skills, knowledge content, and practice resources necessary for rural practice were identified. The list then went back to the expert panel for review. From the list, 10 items were removed as they were deemed to be redundant. The list of 80 items was sent back to the expert panel of six FNPs for review. Further suggestions for clarification and redundancy resulted in an additional three items being removed. Group consensus resulted for the remaining 77 items. Additionally, the expert panel suggested categorization of the items into one of three categories based on where the items would be performed or the information that would be necessary to practice in the particular setting. The three categories were identified as advanced life support (ALS) items, urgent/emergent items, and clinic-related items.

The list of 77 items was used to create an inventory titled the RFNPCI, which was then electrically sent via REDCap to a list of 48 FNPs practicing in rural sites in Montana. The results from the practicing FNPs in rural sites in Montana are presented as follows.

Measures

DEMOGRAPHIC CHARACTERISTICS

Demographic data collected included participant age, ethnicity, gender, highest level of nursing education obtained, and current employment status as an FNP. Demographic information collected about practices sites included approximate population of the town, practice site type, and practice site size. The demographic information was collected as a part of the overall survey.

Rural Family Nurse Practitioner Competency Inventory

The inventory consisted of 77 items representative of skills, knowledge, and resources identified by an expert panel of practicing rural FNPs. Participants in this round of inventory assessment were asked to *rate how important you believe the following skills and knowledge are for a new graduate FNP to possess when entering practice in a rural setting* on a 5-point Likert scale. Items rated as 0 on the Likert scale correlated to a rating of *not important at all* to a score of 5 indicating very *important*. There were no degree labels for numbers falling between 0 and 5. Possible score ranges were 0 to 5 with a higher mean score suggesting the participants felt the item was important for new graduate FNPs entering into practice in rural settings. Ranking of the items allowed for determination of items importance as well as preferences over other items. The scale scores were interpreted in the following manner:

5.00–4.50 = High Importance
4.49–3.50 = Substantial Importance
3.49–2.50 = Moderate Importance
2.49–1.50 = Low Importance
1.49–1.00 = No Importance

Data Analysis

International Business Machine (IBM) Statistical Package for the Social Science (SPSS) Version 26 was used for data analysis. Descriptive statistics were calculated for the demographic variables. The calculation of the mean and *SD* was calculated for each of the 77 items. The competencies were then ranked from highest to lowest according to mean within each of the three practice areas identified (ALS, urgent/emergent, and clinic). If there was a tie, the competency with the lowest *SD* was ranked first. If the mean and *SD* were the same, the item appearing most often in the expert panels initial list of competencies was ranked first.

Results

DEMOGRAPHICS

Twenty participants completed the RFNCPI survey. The sample was comprised of FNPs currently practicing in a rural setting in Montana. On average, the participants were 47.9 years of age and had been in practice for approximately 11.3 years. Participants were predominately white (90.5%), female (76.2%), educated at the Master of Nursing (MN) or Master of Science in Nursing (MSN) level (66.7%), and employed full time (81%) (see Table 24.1). The majority of FNPs reported practicing in a town with a population of <5,000 people (47.6%). Most FNPs reported worked in community health clinics (23.8%) followed by private practice of three or more providers (14.3%) or a clinic affiliated with a CAH (14.3%). On average, the FNPs saw 66.5 patients per week. See Tables 24.1 and 24.2.

Rural Family Nurse Practitioner Competency Inventory

The RFNPCI inventory items fell into one of three distinct practice realms, ALS, emergent/urgent, and clinic related care. The items were analyzed based on their assignment to their respective care area. Results from the survey's sent to rural FNPs are presented below.

RFNPCI-ADVANCED LIFE SUPPORT

A total of 11 of 16 items ranked in the *high to substantial importance* (5.0–3.5) categories. The items in Table 24.3 represent high-acuity low-frequency situations, while many of

TABLE 24.1 Participant Demographics (*n* = 20)

Characteristic	M	SD
Age	47.9	10.4
Years in practice	11.3	6.7
	n	%
Race		
White	19	90.5
American Indian or Alaska Native	1	4.8
Gender		
Male	4	19
Female	16	76.2
Education		
MN or MSN	14	66.7
DNP	4	19
Doctor of Philosophy	2	9.5
Employment as an FNP		
Full time	17	81
Part time	3	14.3

DNP, Doctor of Nursing Practice; FNP, family nurse practitioner; MN, Master of Nursing; MSN, Master of Science in Nursing.

TABLE 24.2 Practice Site Demographics (*n* = 20)

Characteristic	M	SD
Number of patients seen weekly	66.5	34.9
	n	%
Population of town		
< 5,000	10	47.6
5,001–10,000	4	28.5
>10,000	6	28.6
Primary practice site type		
Private: 1–2 providers	4	19
Private: 3+ providers	3	14.3
Community health clinic	5	23.8
CAH-affiliated clinic	3	14.3
CAH ED	2	9.5
Urban clinic	1	4.8
Other	1	4.8

CAH, critical access hospital.

TABLE 24.3 RFNPCI-ALS Items, Ranked Items Range, Mean, *SD*, and Variance (*n* = 20)

	Range	*M*	*SD*	Variance
For each of the following items, rate how important you believe the following skills and knowledge are for a new graduate FNP to possess when entering practice in a rural setting. The new graduate FNP should be able to/possess:				
Recognize and treat respiratory distress in a pediatric patient	1	4.90	0.31	0.1
Recognize and treat a patient in cardiopulmonary arrest	4	4.55	0.95	0.89
Recognize and treat pediatric cardiac arrest	3	4.55	0.95	0.89
Recognize and treat pediatric shock	3	4.45	0.76	0.58
Current pediatric advanced life support certification	3	4.40	0.88	0.78
Current advanced cardiac life support certification	3	4.40	0.83	0.78
Assess and manage cervical spine-related trauma	3	4.20	1.01	1.01
Stabilize a newborn for transport to a higher level of care	3	3.75	1.12	1.25
Place an intraosseous needle for fluids and medications	3	3.75	1.02	1.04
Taken advanced trauma life support in the past 12 months	3	3.74	1.00	0.98
Insert an advanced airway in a patient with respiratory arrest	4	3.50	1.32	1.74
Manage a ventilated patient prior to transfer	4	3.35	1.23	1.50
Provide imminent childbirth and postdelivery maternal care	4	3.20	1.15	1.33
Do rapid sequence intubation	4	3.20	1.32	1.75
Current neonatal resuscitation program certification	4	3.20	1.28	1.64
Current stroke provider certification	4	3.15	0.58	0.88

ALS, advanced life support; FNP, family nurse practitioner; RFNPCI, Rural Family Nurse Practitioner Competency Inventory.

the expert panel members believed all of the items were important, they recognized the inability to cover every conceivable patient presentation in FNP education and the need to prioritize items that are *must know* versus those considered *nice to know* prior to entering practice in a rural setting. Two of the five items that scored below 3.5 addressed obstetrical care. Many of the rural FNP experts mentioned few CAHs provide obstetrical care, thus care of a birthing woman and/or post care of a neonate would be deemed uncommon occurrences in their practice settings.

RFNPCI-EMERGENT/URGENT

A total of 15 items were assigned to the emergent/urgent care category. Of the items identified, seven were deemed to be of *high to substantial importance*, see Table 24.4. The remaining eight items were reviewed by the expert panel. Expert FNPs agreed while the items may be important, they could be learned later on the job. The ability to do the items falling below a mean of 3.5 would also depend on access to resources. Some facilities have limited equipment and may not have ultrasound, advanced imaging, or even equipment necessary for procedures like paracentesis or thoracentesis as well as sexual assault examination kits.

RFNPCI-CLINIC

The largest subset of RFNPCI items was found in the clinic category. A total of 51 items were identified by the rural FNP expert panel. Of the 51 items, 36 were identified as *high to substantial importance*. Of the 15 items falling below a mean of 3.5, rural FNPs again noted the items can be learned on the job as well as with time and experience. Again, the theme of lack of access to some technologies and equipment also play a role in rating many of the items lower. The results from the RFNPCI-Clinic survey are presented in Table 24.5.

TABLE 24.4 RFNPCI-Emergent/Urgent Care Items, Ranked Items Range, Mean, *SD*, and Variance (*n* = 20)

	Range	*M*	*SD*	Variance
For each of the following items, rate how important you believe the following skills and knowledge are for a new graduate FNP to possess when entering practice in a rural setting. The new graduate FNP should be able to/possess:				
Consult with other providers in arrangement of transfer of care	0	5.00	0.00	0.00
Communicate with prehospital units	2	4.70	0.66	0.43
Assess a patient with suicidal ideation	2	4.70	0.57	0.33
Assess and treat acute epistaxis	2	4.40	0.75	0.57
Splint or cast a fractured bone	2	4.40	0.75	0.67
Assess and manage a peritonsillar abscess	3	4.26	0.99	0.98
Measure compartment pressure in an extremity	4	3.55	0.15	1.31
Place a gastrointestinal tube for feeding or decompression	4	3.45	1.50	2.26
Reduce a fracture of a long bone	4	3.35	1.27	1.61
Perform a sexual assault examination	3	3.25	1.07	1.15
Interpret a bedside ultrasound (FAST) exam	4	3.05	1.23	1.52
Perform a bedside ultrasound (FAST) exam	4	3.05	1.23	1.52
Perform and/or direct procedural sedation	4	3.05	1.43	2.05
Perform a thoracentesis	4	2.68	1.20	1.45
Perform a paracentesis	4	2.65	1.18	1.40

FNP, family nurse practitioner; RFNPCI, Rural Family Nurse Practitioner Competency Inventory.

TABLE 24.5 RFNPCI-Clinic Items, Ranked Items Range, Mean, *SD*, and Variance (*n* = 20)

	Range	*M*	*SD*	Variance
For each of the following items, rate how important you believe the following skills and knowledge are for a new graduate FNP to possess when entering practice in a rural setting. The new graduate FNP should be able to/possess:				
Order pertinent diagnostic tests	0	5.00	0.00	0.00
Assess and treat a patient with acute pain	0	5.00	0.00	0.00
Complete a comprehensive exam	0	5.00	0.00	0.00
Complete a comprehensive history	0	5.00	0.00	0.00
Assess patient response to a therapeutic intervention	1	4.95	0.22	0.05
Order pertinent non-pharmacologic therapies	1	4.95	0.22	0.05
Order pertinent pharmacologic therapies	1	4.95	0.22	0.05
Assess and treat a patient with anxiety	1	4.90	0.31	0.10
Consult specialist to receive feedback/guidance on a plan of care	2	4.90	0.45	0.20
Initiate interventions for patients with potential exposure to violence, neglect and/or abuse	2	4.89	0.46	0.21
Perform incision, drainage, irrigation, and packing of a wound/abscess	1	4.89	0.31	0.10
Interpret diagnostic tests	2	4.85	0.49	0.24
Interpret an electrocardiogram of the heart	1	4.85	0.37	0.13
Perform an orthopedic exam of a patient with hip pain	1	4.85	0.37	0.13
Assess for potential violence, neglect or abuse	2	4.85	0.49	0.24
Assess and treat a patient with depression	1	4.85	0.37	0.13
Assess and treat a patient with chronic pain	2	4.80	0.52	0.27
Perform simple skin closure	1	4.80	0.41	0.17
Perform an orthopedic exam of a patient with knee pain	2	4.80	0.52	0.27
Perform an orthopedic exam of a patient with shoulder pain	3	4.75	0.72	0.51
Interpret a chest x-ray	2	4.70	0.57	0.33
Perform a skin lesion removal	1	4.70	0.47	0.22
Perform a skin lesion biopsy	1	4.65	0.49	0.24
Assess and treat skin lesions (plantar warts, decubitus care, etc.)	2	4.65	0.49	0.24
Assess and treat a patient with a bipolar illness	2	4.60	0.60	0.36
Removal of a foreign body	2	4.50	0.76	0.58
Perform a toenail removal	2	4.50	0.76	0.58
Perform a digital block	2	4.50	0.83	0.68
Assess the eye with fluorescein dye	2	4.50	0.76	0.60

(continued)

TABLE 24.5 RFNPCI-Clinic Items, Ranked Items Range, Mean, *SD*, and Variance (*n* = 20) (*continued*)

	Range	*M*	*SD*	Variance
Interpret plain x-ray films of long bones	2	4.44	0.70	0.50
Interpret plain x-ray films of the wrist	2	4.40	0.68	0.46
Interpret plain x-ray films of the ankle	2	4.40	0.68	0.46
Remove a cast	5	4.30	1.26	1.59
Revise a wound for closure	3	4.25	0.85	0.72
Assess and mange a patient desiring contraceptive	5	4.20	1.70	2.91
Incise and drain a Bartholin cyst	3	4.15	0.99	0.98
Perform a joint injection	3	4.15	0.99	0.98
Debride a minor burn	4	4.10	1.071	1.15
Perform ultraviolet examination of skin and or secretions	4	4.00	1.12	1.26
Perform joint aspirations	3	3.95	1.05	1.10
Perform office spirometry	5	3.95	1.43	2.05
Place hormone implants	4	3.85	1.23	1.50
Perform pulmonary function testing	4	3.70	1.34	1.80
Insert an intrauterine device	4	3.55	1.28	1.63
Dilate and examine the eye	4	3.40	1.27	1.62
Perform incision of a thrombosed hemorrhoid	4	3.25	1.20	1.46
Perform a slit lamp examination of the eye	4	3.20	1.47	2.17
Perform tonometry to assess intraocular pressure	4	2.95	1.31	1.73
Interpret a Cat Scan of the chest	4	2.80	1.32	1.75
Interpret a Cat Scan of the abdomen	4	2.75	1.37	1.88
Interpret a Cat Scan of the pelvis	5	1.85	1.60	2.56

FNP, family nurse practitioner; RFNPCI, Rural Family Nurse Practitioner Competency Inventory Data presented in Tables 24.3, 24.4, and 24.5 were shared and discussed with the rural FNP expert panel. Panel members recommended focusing on items with means of 3.5 and above. As repeatedly noted, there are skills, knowledge, and resources that are *must know* in a rural setting and those that are *nice to know* or can be learned on the job. The original RFNPCI of 77 items was pared down to 54 items. The 54 items were determined to be of *substantial to high importance*. The 54 items fall across three practice areas and include seven ALS Items, 11 emergent/urgent items, and 36 clinic items. Next steps and the implications for nursing education and practice are discussed in the following.

NEXT STEPS AND IMPLICATIONS FOR RURAL FAMILY NURSE PRACTITIONER PRACTICE

We suggest the next step in the process of explicating the identified competencies may include presentation of the inventory to chief operating officers and chief medical officers involved in the process of interviewing and hiring FNPs to fill the needs in their rural communities. Specifically, we want to know how important the identified competencies are to healthcare leaders responsible for hiring FNPs in rural settings. Feedback from rural administrative leaders may result in some modifications and/or additions of items to the inventory. The rural FNP experts would be consulted for their input on additional items or modification of existing items. Once these data have been obtained, we would propose the presentation of the RFNPCI to graduate nursing faculty and nursing education leaders for consideration of both current curricula and future modifications in curricula to meet the identified competencies.

Psychometric testing of the RFNPCI with current graduate students at various points in their program working toward their FNP would also be a critical component to assess the RFNPCI. Once the competencies are integrated into the FNP curricula, regular assessment of FNP students with the RFNPCI as they progress through their program of study could provide valuable insight and guidance in the process of preparing the next generation of rural FNPs.

CONCLUSION

The identification and compilation of rural FNP competencies is an area of interest that has not previously been explored in the extant literature. Through the eyes and minds of expert rural FNPs, we have identified an inventory that may be useful in education design and assessment. The identified RFNPCI can provide a starting point for both the design of advanced practice nursing education and the evaluation of students as they progress through the curricula specifically designed to meet the needs of a rural generalist FNP prepared to step into the role of provider in a rural setting.

We appreciate the inventory is not static and will likely evolve significantly over time to meet the changing needs of rural dwellers and the communities in which they reside. A case in point, as we completed the data collection for this inventory, the United States along with the global community experienced a pandemic of unprecedented levels. The RFNPCI does not specifically address pandemic response, disaster preparedness, or the use of telehealth technologies. Further discussion with rural FNP experts to identify the skills and knowledge necessary to address a novel illness as well as the effects it can have on an already taxed healthcare system with limited resources is vital.

Based on findings from this exploration as well as the ever-changing environment of healthcare, evaluation of the inventory every 2 to 3 years will be essential. Changes in technology, economies, politics, and pandemics effect even the most rural locales across the globe. Providing healthcare in rural settings requires a wide breadth of knowledge and skills that can be modified and adapted to meet the needs of rural dwellers across multiple care milieus. The rural FNP educated in foundations of Rural Nursing Theory and Practice will not only be able to respond to the needs of the rural community but be able to respond in a way that is both evidence-based and adaptable at a moment's notice.

REFERENCES

Agency for Healthcare Research and Quality. (2012). *Primary care workforce facts and stats.* https://www .ahrq.gov/research/findings/factsheets/primary/pcworkforce/index.html

Bandura, A. (1997). *Self-efficacy: The exercise of control.* Freeman.

Bandura, A. (2006). Guide for constructing self-efficacy scales. In F. Pajares & T. Urdan (Eds.), *Self-efficacy beliefs of adolescents* (pp. 307–337). Information Age Publishing.

Harris, P., Taylor, R., Thielke, R., Payne, J., Gonzalez, N., & Conde, J. (2009). Research electronic data capture (REDCap)-A metadata-driven methodology and workflow process for providing translational research informatics support. *Journal of Biomedical Information, 42*(2), 377–381.

Long, K., Scharff, J., & Winters, C. (1997). Advanced education for the role of rural nurse generalist. *Journal of Nursing Education, 36*(2), 91–94.

Long, K., & Weinert, C. (1989). Rural nursing: Developing a theory base. *Scholarly Inquiry in Nursing Practice, 3*(2), 113–127.

OSHA. (2018). *Agricultural operations.* https://www.osha.gov/dsg/topics/agriculturaloperations/

Pepin, J., Goudreau, J., Lavoie, P., Belisle, M., Blanchet Garneau, A., Boyer, L., Larue, L., & Lechhasseur, K. (2018). A nursing education research framework for transformative learning and interdependence of academia and practice. *Nursing Education Today, 52,* 50–52.

RAND Corporation. (2019). *Delphi method.* https://www.rand.org/topics/delphi-method.html

Rural Health Information Hub. (2018). *Critical access hospitals (CAHs).* https://www.ruralhealthinfo.org/topics/critical-access-hospitals

Scharff, J. (1987). *The nature and scope of rural nursing: Distinctive characteristics.* Unpublished Master's Thesis, Montana State University-Bozeman.

U.S. Census Bureau. (2018). *2010 Census urban and rural classification and urban area criteria.* https://www.census.gov/programs-surveys/geography/guidance/geo-areas/urban-rural/2010-urban-rural.html

U.S. Health Resources and Service Administration. (2014). *Highlights from the 2012 national sample survey of nurse practitioners.* https://bhw.hrsa.gov/sites/default/files/bhw/nchwa/npsurveyhighlights.pdf

Zhu, X., Mueller, K., Vaughn, T., & Ullrich, F. (2015). *A rural taxonomy of population and health resource charactersitcs* (Rural Policy Breraf, Issue). https://rupri.public-health.uiowa.edu/publications/policybriefs/2015/Rural%20Taxonomy%20Brief.pdf

CHAPTER 25

Development and Psychometric Evaluation of the Rural Knowledge Scale

Heidi A. Mennenga, Laurie Johansen, Becka Foerster, and Lori Hendrickx

DISCUSSION TOPICS

- What are the strengths and limitations of the Rural Knowledge Scale?
- How does the development of the Rural Knowledge Scale contribute to the science of nursing?
- What are some potential applications for the Rural Knowledge Scale?

INTRODUCTION

Addressing gaps in student knowledge regarding rural nursing concepts can be difficult without a valid and reliable measurement tool. By identifying and addressing gaps in knowledge, nursing faculty members may be able to impact student interest and confidence in rural nursing practice, potentially increasing their desire to practice in rural healthcare settings upon graduation. This chapter describes the process for developing an instrument to assess nursing student knowledge of rural nursing practice and conducting psychometric evaluation of the newly developed Rural Knowledge Scale. The final 27-item version of the Rural Knowledge Scale demonstrated acceptable psychometric properties and can be utilized to identify gaps in student knowledge related to rural nursing practice and rural healthcare issues. By identifying and addressing gaps, students' interest and confidence in rural nursing practice may be impacted and result in more nurses who are interested in practicing in rural settings.

BACKGROUND

There are 60 million people living in rural America (United States Census Bureau, 2019). However, only 16% of RNs working in the United States are currently employed in rural settings (Health Resources and Service Administration [HRSA], 2013). With approximately

2.9 million RNs in the United States, it is imperative to have enough nurses caring for people living in rural areas (United States Department of Labor, 2019). In 2010, the National Advisory Council on Nurse Education and Practice (NACNEP) projected a 36% shortage of RNs by 2020. However, in 2017, the HRSA Heath Workforce projected a surplus supply of RNs by 2030. Despite this, the projected numbers of RNs by 2030 differed across various regions of the United States, noting geographic differences and disparities while underscoring the complexity of ensuring adequate distribution of RNs throughout the United States. With optimism for future projections for adequate numbers of RNs, Snavely (2016) cautions the United States to prepare for a nursing shortage in the coming years due to the aging baby boomer population with a rise in chronic care needs and an increased demand for quality care provided by RNs and the healthcare workforce. The employment projections from the Bureau of Labor Statistics (2012) also support this shortage. The RN workforce is projected to increase, yet through new RN positions and replacement of vast numbers of RNs retiring, a significant need for an additional 203,700 new RNs yearly is predicted.

Several sources caution against being overly optimistic when it comes to the future nursing workforce. Fahs (2012) suggested careful regard for the future availability of RNs in rural healthcare facilities with historic patterns showing greater shortage of RNs in rural locations when compared to their urban counterparts. Likewise, HRSA (2013) also reported even with the growth rate in the nursing workforce, urban areas continue to have higher per capita rates of nurses with no specific data available on the number of RNs traveling away from their rural communities to more urban areas for employment. To meet the continued healthcare needs and unique challenges of the rural population, rural healthcare facilities need to have the ability to recruit and retain an adequate number of RNs now and in the future.

Although the nursing workforce projections are promising for the country as a whole, findings in the literature revealed challenges faced specifically by rural healthcare facilities as they struggle to recruit and retain RNs and other healthcare professionals (Mester, 2018). Rural populations consistently deal with a misdistribution of healthcare professionals, with fewer healthcare professionals per capita than urban areas (Rural Health Information Hub, 2018). Data from the National Sample Survey of RNs revealed an increase in the percentage of RNs living in rural areas who commute for employment, increasing from 14% in 1980 to 37% in 2004, adding to the misdistribution of RNs in rural areas (Skillman et al., 2007). Additionally, a study by Johansen et al. (2018) found RNs cited many reasons for living in rural communities yet choosing to commute to larger communities for employment rather than working in their home community.

In 2016, the NACNEP linked the challenges with recruiting and retaining nurses to the increased challenges of socioeconomic and health disparities with the rural population. Because of these challenges, rural nurses especially require a comprehensive knowledge base, a feeling of commitment to their community and the population they serve, and the ability to innovate with limited resources (NACNEP, 2016; Probst et al., 2019).

In addition to an available workforce, it is also vital for rural healthcare professionals to understand the dynamics of the rural population. People living in rural areas have health disparities that add to the complexity of their healthcare needs. There is an increased prevalence of disease and rates of premature death in rural populations (Centers for Disease Control and Prevention [CDC], 2017a). For example, rural women dwellers self-reported higher rates of obesity and rural adolescent dwellers were found more likely to smoke tobacco (Rural Health Research & Policy Centers, 2014). Higher overall rates of death exist in rural areas (CDC, 2017b). The reality is the nursing workforce in the rural areas of the United States cares for a population with a significantly different, and often more complicated, health status compared to their urban counterparts.

Discernment of the employment decisions surrounding RNs working in rural health-care settings is essential to establish effective future recruitment and retention strategies to meet the workforce needs of rural healthcare settings. Thoughtful consideration is necessary when taking into account nurses' choices to not practice nursing in rural settings because of a lack of familiarity with the unique aspects of rural nursing. The Rural Nursing Theory by Long and Weinert (1989) originally shed light on the vast role diffusion needed for a nurse to successfully practice in a rural healthcare setting. Recent research by Medves et al. (2015) continued to support the broad scope of practice of the rural nurse and added that the rural nurses truly practice in a specialty area of their own. Nurses' decisions to seek employment in rural healthcare settings may be impacted by their lack of confidence or decreased comfort levels practicing as nurse generalists. This lack of confidence or decreased comfort level sometimes stems from no previous exposure to the nurse generalist role as well as an unfamiliarity with the unique aspects and expectations that exist in rural nursing practice. Hunsberger et al. (2009) completed a qualitative study of nurses in rural Canada. They found nurses practicing in rural settings were stressed by the nurse generalist role and stress was exacerbated by the narrow base of resources available to them. These study findings indicated the need to prioritize education for nurses practicing, or considering practice, in rural healthcare settings by building intentional rural nursing practice considerations into nursing curricula.

Academic institutions play a key role in preparing nurses for their potential roles in rural communities. Nursing students, whether they intend to seek employment in rural or urban areas, need knowledge of healthcare resources for rural areas and an understanding of sociocultural and lifestyle characteristics of patients living there. Literature shows the value of providing curricular content on rural healthcare to help prepare students to care for rural dwellers in and out of the rural setting (Rutledge et al., 2014). Programs educating nurses, especially those programs serving rural areas, have a role in providing education that prepares nurse generalists through both course content and clinical experiences alike. Acquiring knowledge, skills, and attitudes to meet the needs of the rural population are essential for nurses to feel comfortable seeking employment in rural healthcare facilities. Studies revealed a need for curricular content specific to rural health and firsthand experiences within rural healthcare settings in order to apply appropriate skills unique to rural nursing practice (Molinari et al., 2011; Stasser & Neusy, 2010).

As noted by the American Association of Colleges of Nursing (2008), baccalaureate-prepared nurses should graduate having had adequate exposure to the practice of nursing across the life span and in a variety of healthcare venues. Moreover, clinical opportunities provided nursing students effect the nursing workforce, Rural immersion experiences provide opportunities for nursing students to gain an understanding of the role of the rural nurse generalist (Hendrickx et al., 2018) and can positively impact the future recruitment of nurses to rural healthcare facilities (Coyle & Narsavage, 2012). Rural hospital managers were surveyed following nursing student exposure to rural clinical sites. They reported that exposing students to the mixture of patient situations and collaborative opportunities available in rural healthcare settings was instrumental for baccalaureate-prepared nurses to understand the role of the rural nurse generalist. Study findings by Daniels et al. (2007) showed that nurses having some background or prior experiences in rural settings led to a desire to return to those communities. As previously noted, workforce issues continue to be a difficult reality in rural healthcare facilities and ensuring adequate numbers of qualified RNs prepared to practice in rural areas is a priority. Molinari and Monserud (2008) found many nurses chose to live in a rural community because of their family ties to the community. While summarizing previous systematic reviews about interventions to retain nurses in rural areas, Mbemba et al. (2013) found successful strategies included the creation of organized interactions between nursing students and healthcare professionals in rural settings. They also found success in recruiting students who had previously lived in the rural community and had some form of connection to practicing in a rural setting. The rural community and the rural healthcare system create a context important to the future recruitment and retention of nurses and other healthcare professionals.

NURSING STUDENT KNOWLEDGE OF RURAL NURSING CONCEPTS

The knowledge level of baccalaureate nursing students regarding rural nursing concepts is not known; therefore, addressing gaps in knowledge is difficult. By identifying and addressing gaps in knowledge, nursing faculty members may be able to impact student interest and confidence in rural nursing practice, potentially increasing their desire to practice in rural healthcare settings upon graduation. In a review of the literature, no existing instruments measuring knowledge about rural nursing practice were identified.

Purpose of Research

The purpose of this research was to develop an instrument to assess nursing student knowledge of rural nursing practice and conduct psychometric evaluation of the newly developed Rural Knowledge Scale.

Methodology

The Rural Knowledge Scale was developed in three phases: concept clarification, item development, and psychometric testing.

CONCEPT CLARIFICATION
Since no instruments measuring knowledge about rural nursing practice were found, the authors determined the need to develop an instrument. The Rural Nursing Theory (Long & Weinert, 1989) and common themes found in the literature review were used to develop an initial 24-item Rural Knowledge Scale.

ITEM DEVELOPMENT
Based on a literature review and concepts in the Rural Nursing Theory, the initial 24-item tool was developed and divided into six sections:

- Rural environment (two items)
- Rural health risk/issue (four items)
- Rural healthcare access (two items)
- Rural healthcare technology (two items)
- Rural nursing practice (four items)
- Rural characteristics (10 items)

A panel of five experts on rural nursing, several nationally known, was invited to review the instrument for content validity. The initial 24-item instrument had an acceptable scale content validity index of 0.89. The individual items all had a content validity index of 0.6 or above and were retained in the scale. Based on the comments from the panel of five rural nursing experts, three additional items were added, resulting in a 27-item Rural Knowledge Scale.

PSYCHOMETRIC TESTING

Approval was obtained from the institutional review board to conduct psychometric testing on the Rural Knowledge Scale. Undergraduate baccalaureate students at one Midwestern university were asked to complete the 27-item instrument. Participants were enrolled across the five semesters of the nursing program.

Instrument

The 27 items on the Rural Knowledge Scale are organized into six sections, based on the Rural Nursing Theory: rural environment, rural health risk/issue, rural healthcare access, rural healthcare technology, rural nursing practice, and rural characteristics. The 27-item instrument uses a 5-point Likert scale with possible responses ranging from "not at all knowledgeable" to "very knowledgeable." The use of a 5-point Likert scale includes a neutral point, so participants can express their true reactions (Polit & Beck, 2011).

Results

Statistical analysis was completed using IBM Statistical Product and Service Solutions (SPSS) Statistics Software version 23 (IBM Corporation, Armonk, New York). Descriptive demographic statistics and total scores on the Rural Knowledge Scale were calculated. Factor analysis using principal axis factoring was conducted on the Rural Knowledge Scale.

According to Tabachnick and Fidell's (2012) recommendation that more than 200 participants should be used for instrument development, an adequate sample size was obtained. The convenience sample ($N = 347$) was predominantly female (87.4%), White (83.8%), and under the age of 25 (66.8%). Possible scores on the Rural Knowledge Scale range from 27 to 135. A score of 81 would indicate neutrality, with a score greater than 81 indicating increased knowledge about rural issues. For this research study, scores on the overall instrument ranged from 27 to 135, with a mean of 90.2 ($SD = 20.89$), and indicated students self-reported they were generally knowledgeable about rural issues.

The Kaiser–Meyer–Olkin Measure of Sampling Adequacy was 0.942 for the scale, indicating factor analysis could be performed (Tabachnick & Fidell, 2012). Extraction of factors was determined by the examination of the scree plot and consideration of eigenvalues greater than 1. The scree plot for the total scale indicated one factor would be appropriate, signifying all items were interrelated. All items had loadings of more than 0.40 and were retained (Table 25.1) (Polit & Beck, 2011).

Reliability for the total scale was determined by calculating a Cronbach's alpha with a result of 0.96. According to Polit and Beck (2011), a Cronbach's alpha greater than 0.70 is desirable for a new instrument. Based on this guideline, the Rural Knowledge Scale demonstrates excellent internal consistency.

Limitations

This research has limited generalizability since it occurred with a homogeneous student sample from one school of nursing. Because this nursing school is in a predominantly rural state, more nursing students may come from rural backgrounds. Students who

TABLE 25.1 Factor Loadings for Rural Knowledge Scale

Item	Factor Loading
Longer distances	0.662
Travel conditions	0.628
Availability of transportation	0.686
Occupational safety	0.780
Weather exposure	0.709
Health literacy	0.772
Underinsurance or lack of insurance	0.727
Availability of healthcare services	0.732
Availability of primary care providers	0.726
Availability of specialists	0.721
Impact of public policy on rural healthcare	0.684
Telehealth availability	0.558
Availability of equipment	0.592
Confidentiality and anonymity	0.601
Availability of professional development	0.681
Expert generalist role	0.686
Recruitment/retention of nurses	0.677
Delays in seeking treatment	0.742
Social support networks	0.719
Strong work ethic	0.717
Determination	0.727
Frugality	0.707
Lack of privacy	0.703
Church affiliation/religious	0.694
Resourcefulness	0.775
Self-reliance	0.748
Insider/outsider differentiation	0.765

participated in this study were more likely to have been exposed to rural healthcare issues either through clinical experience in rural facilities or in simulation activities with a rural focus. The Rural Knowledge Scale should also be validated with other populations, such as practicing RNs.

IMPLICATIONS FOR RURAL HEALTH AND NURSING EDUCATION

Rural healthcare facilities and nursing education programs share responsibility for preparing nursing students to practice in a rural setting. The shortage of nurses in rural areas is well documented in the literature. Recent studies have identified positive strategies that may be used to encourage nurses to remain in rural areas to practice (Calleja et al., 2019). Healthcare facilities can target recruitment efforts toward high school students who demonstrate an interest in healthcare careers by offering incentives such as tuition reimbursement and guaranteed placement upon graduation. The literature supports the use of grow-your-own programs focused on long term efforts to introduce healthcare as a career option and assist in skill development. Collaborative community efforts can help recruit and retain rural residents in healthcare careers in their home communities (Rural Health Information Hub, 2019). Rural facilities can also use the Rural Knowledge Scale as an assessment tool for new hires to measure understanding of rural issues prior to practice in a rural area. Having this background information will allow the facility to shape an orientation program that supports newly hired nurses by building on strengths in knowledge about rural healthcare and reinforcing areas of weakness. Having a good understanding of the issues facing rural healthcare should improve the transition from the nursing education environment to actual nursing practice in a rural community.

Although nursing students from rural areas may have a broader knowledge of rural healthcare issues, nursing education programs should include content on rural healthcare in the curriculum for all students. Nursing students from urban areas are often unaware of the richness of a rural clinical rotation and find the varied opportunities and generalist nature of rural healthcare provide a well-rounded educational experience (Hendrickx et al., 2018). Using the Rural Knowledge Scale to assess nursing students' knowledge prior to delivery of educational content on rural healthcare can provide valuable information to nursing faculty or clinical instructors about the level of understanding of rural issues prior to course development and implementation.

CONCLUSION

Practicing in rural healthcare settings requires an understanding of the generalist role. Rural practice can be a complex experience in which the nurse must provide care to patients across the life span, who are experiencing a multitude of conditions. Additionally, the rural experience may vary based on individual facility setting. These factors may result in a difficult transition for a newly hired nurse with no rural healthcare background. Providing an educational experience that prepares a nurse for rural practice can be a vital component of a successful move into rural practice. Successful educational experiences can be enhanced with the Rural Knowledge Scale. The final 27-item version of the Rural Knowledge Scale demonstrated acceptable psychometric properties and can be utilized to identify gaps in student knowledge related to rural nursing practice and rural healthcare issues. By identifying and addressing gaps, students' interest and confidence in rural nursing practice may be impacted and result in more nurses who are interested in practicing in rural settings.

REFERENCES

American Association of Colleges of Nursing. (2008). *The essentials of baccalaureate education for professional nursing practice*. http://www.aacnnursing.org/portals/42/publications/baccessentials08.pdf

Bureau of Labor Statistics. (2012). *The 30 occupations with the largest projected employment growth, 2010–20*. https://www.bls.gov/news.release/ecopro.t10.htm

Calleja, P., Adonteng-Kissi, B., & Romero, B. (2019). Transition support for new graduate nurses to rural and remote practice: A scoping review. *Nurse Education Today*, 76, 8–20. https://doi.org/10.1016/j.nedt.2019.01.022

Centers for Disease Control and Prevention. (2017a). *Health-related behaviors by urban-rural county classification – United States, 2013*. https://www.cdc.gov/mmwr/volumes/66/ss/ss6605a1.htm

Centers for Disease Control and Prevention. (2017b). *Leading causes of death in nonmetropolitan and metropolitan areas: United States, 1999-2014*. https://www.cdc.gov/mmwr/volumes/66/ss/ss6601a1.htm

Coyle, S. B., & Narsavage, G. L. (2012). Effects of an interprofessional rural rotation on nursing student interest, perceptions, and intent. *Online Journal of Rural Nursing and Health Care*, 12(1), 40–48. http://rnojournal.binghamton.edu/index.php/RNO/article/view/42

Daniels, Z., VanLeit, B., Skipper, B., Sanders, M., & Rhyne, R. (2007). Factors in recruiting and retaining health professionals for rural practice. *The Journal of Rural Health*, 23(1), 62–71. doi:10.1111/j.1748-0361.2006.00069.x

Fahs, P. (2012). RN labor supply bubble: What does it mean for rural health care? *Online Journal of Rural Nursing and Health Care*, 12(1), 1–2. https://doi.org/10.14574/ojrnhc.v12i1.153

Health Resources and Service Administration. (2013). *The U.S. nursing workforce: Trends in supply and education*. https://bhw.hrsa.gov/sites/default/files/bhw/nchwa/projections/nursingworkforcetrendsoct2013.pdf

Health Resources and Service Administration. (2017). *Supply and demand projections of the nursing workforce: 2014-2030*. https://bhw.hrsa.gov/sites/default/files/bhw/nchwa/projections/NCHWA_HRSA_Nursing_Report.pdf

Hendrickx, L., Mennenga, H., & Johansen, L. (2018). The use of rural hospitals for clinical placements in nursing education. In C. A. Winters & H. J. Lee (Eds.), *Rural nursing: Concepts, theory, and practice* (5th ed., pp. 325–334). Springer Publishing Company.

Hunsberger, M., Baumann, A., Blythe, J., & Crea, M. (2009). Sustaining the rural workforce: Nursing perspectives on worklife challenges. *The Journal of Rural Health*, 25(1), 17–24. doi:10.1111/j.1748-0361.2009.00194.x

Johansen, L. J., Evanson, T. A., Ralph, J. L., Hunter, C., & Hart, G. (2018). Experiences of rural nurses who commute to large communities. *Online Journal of Rural Nursing and Health Care*, 18(2), 224–265. http://dx.doi.org/10.14574/ojrnhc.v18i2.540

Long, K. A., & Weinert, C. (1989). Rural nursing: Developing the theory base. *Research and Theory for Nursing Practice*, 3(2), 113–127.

Mbemba, G., Gagnon, M., Paré, G., & Côté, J. (2013). Interventions for supporting nurse retention in rural and remote areas: An umbrella review. *Human Resources for Health*, 11(44), 1–9. 10.1186/1478-4491-11-44

Medves, J., Edge, D., Bisonette, L., & Stansfield, K. (2015). Supporting rural nurses: Skills and knowledge to practice in Ontario, Canada. *Online Journal of Rural Nursing and Health Care*, 15(1), 7–41. http://rnojournal.binghamton.edu/index.php/RNO/article/viewFile/337/272

Mester, J. (2018). Rural nurse recruitment. *Nursing Management*, 49(12), 51–53. doi:10.1097/01.NUMA.0000544468.98484.b7

Molinari, D. L., Jaiswal, A., & Hollinger-Forrest, T. (2011). Rural nurses: Lifestyle preferences and education perspectives. *Online Journal of Rural Nursing and Health Care*, 11(2), 16–26. https://doi.org/10.14574/ojrnhc.v11i2.27

Molinari, D. L., & Monserud, M. (2008). Rural nurse job satisfaction. *Rural and Remote Health*, 8(4), 1–12. https://www.rrh.org.au/journal/article/1055

National Advisory Council on Nurse Education and Practice. (2010). *The impact of the nursing faculty shortage on nurse education and practice*. https://www.hrsa.gov/sites/default/files/hrsa/advisory-committees/nursing/reports/2010-ninthreport.pdf

National Advisory Council on Nurse Education and Practice. (2016). *Preparing nurses for nurse roles in population health management*. Health Resources and Services Administration. https://www.hrsa.gov/sites/default/files/hrsa/advisory-committees/nursing/reports/2016-fourteenthreport.pdf

Polit, D., & Beck, C. (2011). *Nursing research: Generating and assessing evidence for nursing practice* (9th ed.). Lippincott Williams & Wilkins.

Probst, J. C., McKinney, H., & Odahowski, C. (2019). *Rural registered nurses: Educational preparation, workplace, and salary*. Rural & Minority Health Research Center. https://www.sc.edu/study/colleges_schools/public_health/research/research_centers/sc_rural_health_research_center/documents/ruralregisterednurses.pdf

Rural Health Information Hub. (2018). *Rural healthcare workforce*. https://www.ruralhealthinfo.org/topics/health-care-workforce

Rural Health Information Hub. (2019). *Education and training of the rural healthcare workforce*. https://www.ruralhealthinfo.org/topics/workforce-education-and-training

Rural Health Research & Policy Centers. (2014). *Rural health reform policy research center: The 2014 update of the rural-urban chartbook*. https://ruralhealth.und.edu/projects/health-reform-policy-research-center/pdf/2014-rural-urban-chartbook-update.pdf

Rutledge, C. M., Haney, T., Bordelon, M., Renaud, M., & Fowler, C. (2014). Telehealth: Preparing advanced practice nurses to address healthcare needs in rural and underserved populations. *International Journal of Nursing Education Scholarship, 11*(1), 1–9. doi:10.1515/ijnes-2013-0061

Skillman, S., Palazzo, L., Hart, L., & Butterfield, P. (2007). *Changes in the rural registered nurse workforce from 1980 to 2004*. University of Washington. http://depts.washington.edu/uwrhrc/uploads/RHRC%20FR115%20Skillman.pdf

Snavely, T. (2016). A brief economic analysis of the looming nursing shortage in the United States. *Nursing Economics, 34*(2), 98–100. https://pubmed.ncbi.nlm.nih.gov/27265953/

Stasser, R., & Neusy, A. (2010). Context counts: Training health workers in and for rural and remote areas. *Bulletin of the World Health Organization, 88*(10), 777–782. doi:10.2471/BLT.09.072462

Tabachnick, B., & Fidell, L. (2012). *Using multivariate statistics* (6th ed.). Allyn & Bacon.

United States Census Bureau. (2019). *One in five Americans live in rural areas*. https://www.census.gov/library/stories/2017/08/rural-america.html

United States Department of Labor. (2019). *Occupational employment and wages, May 2019: Registered nurses*. United States Bureau of Labor Statistics. https://www.bls.gov/oes/current/oes291141.htm

CHAPTER 26

Developing and Sustaining the Rural Nursing Workforce Through Collaborative Educational Models

POLLY PETERSEN, DAYLE SHARP, AND JUDITH PARE

DISCUSSION TOPICS

- The main character presented in Case Study 4 is Susan. Susan is torn between the challenges and opportunities of rural nursing practice. Describe at least three strategies that Susan's nurse manager could implement to support her desire for broader clinical experiences while continuing employment in a rural healthcare setting.
- Case Study 3 summarizes the story of Mary, a nurse who had an opportunity to attend a specialty education program in an urban healthcare setting. Discuss the role of nursing administrators in rural and urban settings to advocate and fund these types of residency programs. Do they have a professional obligation to support these programs? What are the benefits and potential challenges? Utilize evidence from the literature to support your views.
- Case Study 5 highlights one federal program that provides funding for nurses who are motivated to enroll in an advanced nursing education program. Select a federal or state program that offers resources for nurses in your area to earn an advanced degree while continuing to practice in a rural healthcare setting. Describe the benefits and limitations of the program in detail.
- How does a virus such as COVID-19 and its sequela affect rural nursing education and practice?

INTRODUCTION

Rural nursing varies greatly based upon geography and cultural values; however, the attitudes and attributes of rural nurses (RNs) remain constant. Many RNs have grown up in the area with family ties that result in their decision to stay and work in rural settings. However, there is a shortage of RNs in these healthcare settings. In the United States, the number of RNs per capita has remained lower in rural areas compared to urban areas from 1980 to present (Skillman et al., 2009; US Healthcare, 2015). This distributional imbalance of RNs extends past the United States to areas throughout the world, with 45% the world's population living in rural settings (The World Bank, 2018) and only 38% of the total nursing workforce working in rural areas (Dolea et al., 2010). Rural areas have more licensed practical nurses/licensed vocational nurses (LPNs/LVNs) per capita, whereas urban areas have more RNs (U.S. Department of Health and Human Services Health Resources and Services Administration, 2014). This imbalance is not expected to improve. Nationally, RN shortages are estimated to continue until 2030 with a shortage of one-half million RN jobs (Zhang et al., 2018). In a survey of U.S. nurses conducted by the Center for the Advancement of Healthcare Professionals (2017), one in four nurses responded they planned on retiring within 1 year which was a 9% increase from a survey conducted in 2015 (Health Resources and Services Administration [HRSA], 2017). This percentage of nurses who plan on retiring in 1 year has increased significantly according to a new survey conducted by American Mobile Nurses (AMN) Healthcare (2017). The survey found 73% of baby boomer nurses planned to retire within 3 years or less. There are estimated to be substantial variations across the United States for RNs in 2030 due to the large differences between their projected supply and demand. When looking at each state's 2030 RN supply minus its 2030 demand, results reveal both shortages and surpluses in the RN workforce across the United States (National Council of State Boards of Nursing, 2017). This means the U.S. healthcare system will likely face a drain of nursing knowledge and experience at a time when the aging population is growing. The impact of the nursing shortage is expected to vary across regions of the United States; the greatest impact is expected in the South (Zhang et al., 2018).

Reasons for shortages in rural settings include lack of educational opportunities and resources; lack of diversity, social support, and cultural congruence; feelings of isolation; and policies that are inconsistent to support rural healthcare. Collaborative initiatives in education and institutional support can enhance the professional characteristics of rural nurses. This chapter utilizes case studies to illustrate strategies to build capacity while offering ideas for collaborative education models that address recruitment, retention, and workforce development of rural nursing. These case studies also demonstrate a variety of scenarios to support rural nurse experiences.

CASE STUDIES

Case #1

Paula was raised in Abilene, Kansas. She dreamed of being a nurse since she was in elementary school, but her dream was not supported by family members. Her parents advised her to continue to work on the family ranch until she found a proper husband. Upon the death of her father in 2000, Paula made the difficult decision to enter the associate degree nursing program at the community college. Paula was 34 years old at the time of her graduation. She accepted a position working 11:00 p.m. to 11:00 a.m. in the ED at the local critical access hospital (CAH). Although the hours were long, this schedule allowed Paula to be an extra pair of hands on her family's cattle ranch that was left to Paula and her husband.

(continued)

(continued)

Paula would tell her coworkers at the hospital that she considered her nursing career as time-off from her job on the ranch that was becoming increasingly physically demanding. Paula developed a reputation as being hard to deal with and novice nurses would avoid asking her questions or for help for fear of bullying or retribution. Eventually, these concerns reached Paula's supervisor Jane, who happened to have graduated from nursing school with Paula. In order to better assess the dynamics on the unit, Jane decided to make regular rounds through the ED. Jane quickly realized that Paula's coworkers were correct; Paula was verbally aggressive when coworkers came to her with questions or asked for help. However, Jane observed a patient interaction involving Paula that was reminiscent of the friend and classmate that she knew from their days in nursing school. Paula was admitting a 37-year-old female with a known history of intravenous (IV) drug abuse. The patient was being admitted with complications related to hepatitis. Jane was impressed with the skill, compassion, and kindness that Paula exhibited while providing patient care. Jane reflected on how she could frame her follow-up with Paula to be a teachable moment and encourage Paula to show the same compassion and care to her coworkers that she was able to give to her patient with complex physical, emotional, and mental health needs.

CASE #2

Lucia lives in a rural area of Texas where her family migrated from Mexico so that her parents could work in the cotton fields. Her father had planned to move the family back to Mexico; however, he wanted to offer his children opportunities that were not available in their native country. Lucia has always had an interest in taking care of others. This came naturally to her, as she has been caring for family members since she was a child. She is the oldest and the first in her family to advance her education past the sixth grade. Because of her interest in caring for others, her school guidance counselor suggested that she participate in the Health Occupation Students of America (HOSA) program at her high school. In the HOSA program, she has been able to learn about nursing both in class and at a local clinic. She is excited about being in the HOSA program because when she graduates from high school, she will be a certified nursing assistant.

She is excited about working as a nursing assistant but wants to continue her education to become a nurse. She wants to talk to her parents about attending nursing school but does not know how they will pay the tuition or how she will travel to the university. Before she is able to talk with her parents, she receives an acceptance letter from the community college 45 miles from her home. She had applied to the nursing program with the encouragement of her school counselor. Lucia also applied for multiple scholarships and was pleased to receive a scholarship due to her enrollment in HOSA. With this scholarship, Lucia will be able to start her dream of attending college and someday attaining her bachelor's degree in nursing.

(continued)

(continued)

Case #3

Mary grew up in a small town in central Nebraska. She had an opportunity in the middle school to participate in a program that allowed her to volunteer at the local CAH one evening each week. As she spent time feeding Mr. Jones, a patient recovering from a stroke in the long-term care unit, she had a chance to watch the nurses and doctors at the main care station. They were smart and compassionate, and she knew she wanted to do exactly what they did.

Mary finished an associate degree program at a community college, passed her national licensure exam, and returned to her hometown to marry her high-school sweetheart. After a 2-week orientation period, Mary was assigned to working night shifts in the CAH that included a 20-bed long-term care unit and a 2-bed ED. She spent most of her time assisting the aides in turning patients, assisting others to the bathroom, and passing medications. Although Mary enjoyed the camaraderie of the team of aides that she worked with, she also felt overwhelmed to think that if there were an emergency, she alone would be responsible for the life of that patient until support came in to assist. This feeling of doom weighed on her, knowing she did not have the experience or education to handle such a situation. Mary chose to attend a 6-week critical care course offered in a large hospital 200 miles away. Mary loved the course; she worked with patients utilizing the knowledge she gained in the classroom setting and felt supported by the staff. She saw patients who were critically ill get better and return to a full life after discharge. She knew she could never go back to the rural CAH setting again; she could never transition the care she gave the patients in the critical care course without the team she had come to rely on for that care. Mary left the CAH after returning from the critical care course to work in a big city ICU.

Case #4

Susan wanted to be a nurse for as long as she could remember. Growing up on a large cattle ranch in eastern Idaho, she had learned at an early age to care for orphaned lambs, and how to pull a calf. Susan excelled in science courses in school and was accepted for early admission to the associate degree of nursing program at her local community college, which had the only nursing program within a 150-mile radius. Susan's mother wished that her daughter could have enrolled in the nursing program at the state university but the cost of the program and the distance from the ranch was too great. Susan is very close to her family and she is very proud of her contributions to the family ranch that has been the primary source of income for generations.

Susan just completed her second year as an RN in the CAH in her community and she is beginning to wonder about job opportunities that have been posted in the medical center 155 miles away. Her ultimate goal of attaining certification as an ED nurse has yet to be realized. She had registered for a certification conference twice but due to weather and cuts to the education budget, she was unable to attend either conference event. She is frustrated by the lack of a professional career ladder and support for nurses who want to participate in continuing education and pursue advanced degrees but simply do not have the time or

(continued)

(continued)

funding resources. Susan is grateful for all her parents have done to support her education and her nursing practice, but she is torn between a desire to expand her clinical experiences and her obligations to her family and their ranch.

Susan is particularly interested in broadening her experiences with advanced technology to support the needs of trauma patients. She worries about her limited experience working with patients who have multisystem needs and she is frustrated by the lack of resources the CAH has to offer. Susan commented to her mother one evening after an unplanned 16-hour shift; "Nursing is a part of who I am but, I am beginning to wonder if who I am is all that I can be?"

CASE #5

Glenn has been an RN for over 20 years and has been working as a nurse on a medical surgical unit in a small CAH in northern rural New Hampshire. He has become disheartened with the limited healthcare access in his community. He has been caring for individuals who have advanced stages of chronic disease due to lack of follow-up care. Thus, Glenn has begun to investigate options for advancing his education to become a nurse practitioner so that he can become a primary care provider for his rural neighbors. The nearest graduate program is over 100 miles away.

Glenn was approached by the chief nursing officer (CNO) of his hospital about a recent grant, Advanced Nursing Education Workforce (ANEW), offered to nurse practitioner students at the state university. She recommended he attend an online information session describing the grant and the family nurse practitioner program. He was excited to learn. The grant was offering money for him to attend college, the university had already set up agreements with preceptors in his area, and that he will take most courses online with some available synchronously at his hospital.

CASE #6

Teresa is a 66-year old ICU nurse who has more than a four-decade history of being an active member of the Baptist church in rural Georgia. Her plan had been to continue to work at the local hospital for the next 4 years and then retire with her husband and travel the country. However, in the winter of 2020, Teresa was exposed to COVID-19 while caring for patients in the ICU and 6 days after her exposure, she tested positive for the virus. Initially, Teresa's only symptom was a low-grade fever but on day 7 she developed acute shortness of breath and she was admitted to the ICU where she had worked for 42 years. Teresa was intubated for more than 26 days during her hospitalization and her recovery was complicated by a minor stroke and two pulmonary emboli. Despite the sequelae that she experienced during the acute phase of her illness, her condition stabilized, and she was discharged to home after 7 weeks of hospitalization. Although she was grateful for her recovery, this once vital, active professional's daily regimen now included physical therapy, occupational therapy, and multiple medications including anticoagulants therapy. Her primary care physician encouraged Teresa

(continued)

(continued)

to consider retiring immediately due to the risks that bedside nursing posed to her health. Teresa was devastated by the recommendation and as she had during many difficult times in her life, she turned to her pastor for guidance. Pastor Williams told Teresa that there was a grant available to establish a parish nurse program in the community and he had been looking for a nurse who might be interested in enrolling in the certification program that was being offered for licensed nurses. The program was a 12-week certification program that was offered on 12-consecutive Saturdays. The cost of the program was $1,200.00 but the grant funding covered the cost of the program and graduates would receive a certificate from a national nursing accreditation organization. Although parish nurses are not paid for the care they provide, they provide a valuable service for persons with no health insurance or whose benefits have ended. Teresa's family encouraged her to register for the program and recognize the difference she could make for the people in her underserved community. It has been 3 months since Teresa became a certified parish nurse. She is happily exhausted at the end of every day and she recognizes that this job is an ideal match for her physical limitations. Teresa will continue to need close follow-up due to the complications she experienced during her acute illness. While receiving follow-up care, parish nurse program provided Teresa with the ability to continue to utilize her nursing skills and provide care for those in her community who would be alone and isolated without these unique services.

CASE #7

Margie is the most senior member of the rural nursing staff in the CAH in northern California. Margie is old enough to retire but financially unable to do so. Four years ago, Margie's husband died suddenly after suffering a major stroke on the ranch where he had worked for more than 40 years. Margie's daughter lives in the same community but her single-parent income often is not enough to pay monthly bills. Margie's salary is now her only income. She often works additional shifts to support the needs of her daughter and grandchildren.

She just celebrated her 43rd anniversary in nursing practice and is proud she has spent her entire career in a CAH, but she worries about who will be there to take over her position. She had not met any new nurses in this new generation of nurses who have the same attitudes and values that she felt had supported her career.

RURAL NURSING WORKFORCE

Rural and frontier settings have unique characteristics. There are long distances from town to town. Members of the population have lived there for many generations and know their neighbor's lineage as well as they know their own. In fact, it may often be a shared lineage. When one of them becomes ill, they generally seek care at the local CAH. However, CAHs are in a precarious situation with potential decreases in funding related to healthcare reforms in reimbursement (Balasubramanian & Jones, 2016), fiscal instability, as well as RN and other healthcare provider shortages to care for patients.

Reasons for this shortage include the aging RN population and the inability to recruit new graduates. Chief executive officers (CEOs) from one midwestern state reported a critical RN shortage in 91 (91%) of the hospitals located in that state (Cramer et al., 2011). This mirrors the RN shortage in rural areas; 74% of rural CEOs reported a 73% shortage of RNs (MacDowell et al., 2010). In rural areas, there are 10% fewer RNs per 100,000 residents than in urban areas (HRSA, 2013; Statista Research, 2014). A comparison of RNs in rural and urban areas conducted by the National Center for Health Workforce Analysis (2014) found in urban areas there were 93.5 RNs to every 10,000 persons, in rural areas the number of RNs was 85.3 per 10,000 persons. When geographic regions experience RN shortages, hospitals often decrease RN staffing patterns and utilize LPNs or temporary RN employees who are not familiar with the area, resulting in a simultaneous drop in patient satisfaction (Cramer et al., 2011).

The average age for practicing RNs in the United States in 2013 was 50 years with 53% of the workforce over the age of 50 years (American Nurses Association, 2014). In 2010, the average age of practicing nurses was close to 55 years; 30% of rural RNs were over the age of 55 years (Pribulick et al. 2010). Many of these nurses have been clinically engaged in their profession for more than three decades, demonstrating resilience and adaptation to enormous changes in healthcare delivery. The total years of experience that these retiring RNs will take with them is estimated to be 1.7 million years (Buerhaus et al., 2017). This loss of expert, older nurses can potentially compromise quality of care and the assurance of a safe patient and staff environment.

CNOs from rural hospitals have expressed alarm at the growing trend for nurses to travel from their rural homes to work in metropolitan hospitals, also contributing to the RN shortage in CAHs. These urban facilities offer higher salaries and tuition benefits, the option to be trained in various specialty areas, and promotions that are congruent with the levels of education (Havens et al., 2012). In 2018, average salaries differed between urban and rural nurses with urban nurses making, on average, nearly $4,500 per year more than rural nurses (Probst et al., 2019). CNOs in rural settings must create practice environments that support the recruitment and retention of highly qualified RNs resulting in a qualified healthcare workforce that contributes to high patient satisfaction scores.

IMPLICATIONS

These case studies bring to the forefront issues that should be addressed related to educational support from CAHs and other rural healthcare facilities. Programs that provide RNs with knowledge to deliver current, evidence-based care, tuition support for increasing degree levels such as a Bachelor of Science in Nursing (BSN), as well as advanced education and degrees to move into a primary care provider role are needed. Opportunities for team-based healthcare development, including interprofessional education (IPE) in rural settings, and financial and professional support for diverse populations who are willing to remain in rural facilities to care for family and friends of their own community are also important options for consideration.

For there to be enough nurses to care for the rural population, recruitment and retention issues must be addressed. Kulig et al. (2015) identified three common initiatives for proposed solutions: educational opportunities, financial incentives, and enhanced infrastructure. Additional solutions to address barriers to recruitment and retention of healthcare staff in remote areas include financial incentives; the need for supportive relationships in nursing including mentoring, clinical supervision, and precepting;

information and communication technology support; and defined career pathways (Mbemba et al., 2013).

Educational Opportunities

The literature indicated that one potential solution to address the inability to recruit new RNs to the rural setting is to provide a rural clinical experience within nursing education programs. This model could be supported through a collaboration between state universities and community colleges in rural areas and beyond. These types of programs allow nursing students to have the opportunity to work with students from other healthcare educational programs including medicine, pharmacy, and physical and occupational therapy in rural situations. Some universities have understood the importance of students being exposed to other disciplines when completing their education. Universities have developed courses with students from various healthcare careers working together to understand the role of each discipline. Other programs have initiated the use of Project ECHO®. Project ECHO uses adult learning techniques and interactive video technology, to connect groups of community specialists in regular real-time collaborative sessions (Project ECHO, 2020). The sessions are designed around case-based learning and mentorship to help providers gain expertise required to provide needed services. Currently, the University of New Hampshire nursing department has students attend Extension for Community Healthcare Outcomes (ECHO) sessions focused on Medication-Assisted Treatment that is attended by individuals from the New England area from various disciplines (primary care providers, substance misuse counselors, pharmacy, social work, and counselors). Applications of such interprofessional care access networks have shown great promise in strengthening the ability of healthcare students to practice in a collaborative fashion as well as address the needs of populations with limited access to care (Wros et al., 2015). Another resource for IPE is utilization of healthcare professionals within the rural settings as instructors and mentors. The positive influence of students learning from providers but also providers learning from students enhances collaborative interactions (Pelham et al., 2016).

Area Health Education Center

Area Health Education Centers (AHEC) are committed to expanding healthcare providers in rural and underserved areas. Through the introduction of a wide variety of healthcare possibilities, they guide students toward careers in the healthcare field, assisting them with goal setting, educational planning, and critical thinking skills. AHEC works with schools, colleges, and community partners to offer culturally appropriate clinical experiences to underrepresented minority students in kindergarten through 12th grade. Working with over 1,000 community health centers, students are exposed to shadowing experiences, mentoring, recruitment, resources, and continuing education (National Area Health Education Center Organization, 2015).

AHEC continues to support nurses once they are in practice. AHEC works with local hospitals and support nurses, offering continuing education classes online and in classroom settings. Online courses allow the rural RN to obtain necessary training without having to travel long distances (National Area Health Education Center Organization, 2015). Many courses are offered including Advanced Cardiac Life Support (ACLS), Basic Life Support (BLS), and Pediatric Advanced Life Support (PALS). Face-to-face training can be done at the CAH, other community locations, or a training stimulation van traveling to the nurses.

Health Occupation Students of America

The HOSA program is a student organization recognized by the U.S. Department of Education (HOSA, 2012a). The goal of HOSA is to enhance the delivery of compassionate, quality healthcare by providing health science education to students. With the support of health occupation educators as advisors, students develop the knowledge, skills, and leadership to meet the needs of their healthcare community. In the 2015 to 2016 school year, there were over 4,000 HOSA chapters and 200,000 students had participated in HOSA (HOSA, 2012b). Along with new skills and experiences, HOSA members are also eligible for additional scholarship opportunities.

ANEW Program

The ANEW program, federally funded through the HRSA was awarded to universities throughout the United States to advance the nursing workforce in rural and underserved areas. ANEW supports innovative academic practice partnerships to prepare primary care APRN students to practice in rural and underserved settings through academic and clinical training (https://www.hrsa.gov/grants/find-funding/hrsa-17-067). Universities have identified the following areas of focus:

- Developing preceptorships in rural and underserved areas
- Workshops with continuing medical education (CME) related to clinical teaching
- Interprofessional activities
- Preceptor orientations through online modules
- Mental health and substance use
- Scholarships to students

These are just a few examples of agency educational and financial support and recruitment initiatives of students into healthcare. Many of these opportunities are not limited to those interested in careers in nursing, but rather all healthcare professions. It also introduces the concept of IPE and team building early in professional development.

Financial Incentives

While certainly much emphasis could be placed on the wage differences for rural RNs compared to those practicing in urban settings, our focus for financial incentives is on the commitment of CAHs to the RNs to maintain certifications and other educational obligations. Travel presents additional financial burdens for rural healthcare providers to maintain mandated certifications for continued accreditation as well as opportunities for continued education and degree completion. This financial burden of advancing education can be decreased through the use of online courses or offering courses via videoconferencing. Likewise, it is of value for CAH administrators to consider financial support of tuition reimbursement or consistent Internet service as individual reliability of Internet services may be a barrier for many rural residents.

The National Rural Health Association (NRHA) advocates for access to quality healthcare for rural residents and CAHs. NRHA has developed initiatives to stop Medicare cuts to rural hospitals and offer innovative delivery models for rural healthcare (NRHA, 2017). NRHA supports continued funding for professional training such as Teaching Health Center and Rural Track training programs. In addition, NRHA advocates for continued funding to the National Health Service Corps (NHSC), Community Health Center Fund, and annual healthcare policy and fellowship programs.

Collaborative educational and financial support of those interested in rural healthcare professions also includes federal government agencies. Two federal agencies that remain committed to the development of enhancing rural workforce include HRSA and the NHSC. HRSA offers scholarships to students accepted and enrolled in all levels of nursing education (HRSA Health Workforce, 2017). Students have potential to receive funding for tuition, fees, and other educational costs. In exchange, the student must work in a facility with a critical nurse shortage upon graduation.

The NHSC, a division of the HRSA (HRSA, 2017), was established in 1972 and offers healthcare to individuals in rural and underserved areas. Currently, 13.7 million people receive care from more than 13,000 clinicians serving at NHSC-approved sites in urban, rural, and tribal communities. Since the NHSC began, more than 50,000 primary care medical, dental, and mental and behavioral health professionals have provided care for rural and underserved populations (HRSA, 2020). NHSC accepts applications from individuals committed to becoming a primary care provider and who attend an accredited U.S. school to become an APRN.

Enhanced Infrastructure Through Education

Recruitment to practice in rural healthcare settings is extremely difficult. One reason for this is a lack of infrastructure support (Kulig et al., 2015). New nurses may find a lack of support from older, more experienced nurses. This lack of support may be a result of perceptions of generational differences. Older nurses perceive that younger nurses have different values and beliefs; they are interested in working environments that require specialized skills. However, a new graduate nurse may find the lack of other professional team members to be daunting; the potential anonymity is inconsistent with many educators' guidance to select a place of employment that will support a new nurse's professional growth. If the new nurse has not lived in a rural setting, the lack of social and professional cohorts is limited, resulting in feelings of isolation. Options to address these issues include development of a nurse residency programs that may enhance socialization and decrease the feelings of isolation.

Nurse Residency and Fellowship Programs

New graduate RNs require organizational support when transitioning to their professional role. To assist the new graduate nurse transition into their professional role, nurse residency programs (NRPs) designed to introduce the new graduate to critical thinking skills, confidence building, time management, and socialization can be beneficial (Graetz, 2017). Rural healthcare facilities often lack resources to develop such programs. By using NRPs, decreases can be appreciated in both nurse turnover as well as the cost to hire and train new nursing staff. The recent cost of nurse turnover for a bedside RN is $44,400 ranging from $33,300 to $56,000, which results in the average hospital losing $3.6 to $6.1 million. Unfortunately, rural hospitals have been limited in offering NRPs due to limited financial resources and positions. In Iowa, the Iowa Online Nurse Residency Program (IONRP) was established offering a cost-effective residency program that blends the values and expectations of millennials with the uniqueness of rural nursing (Forneris, 2019). This 12-month online program provides clinical immersion, mentorship, and enhanced professional competencies, enabling opportunities for advancement, meaningful contributions, and exploring change projects. The IONRP has been an effective way to offer new graduates firsthand rural nursing experience while showing new graduate nurses that rural hospitals are invested in their future.

Hospitals that have initiated NPRs have reported decreases in turnover rates and an increase in the competence of new graduate nurses (Graetz, 2017). Current orientation programs often do not include the information needed for the new graduate to transition to their new role. Due to lack of this supportive transition, the agency can accrue the cost of training additional nurses or the use of outside agency nurses, overtime, and increased recruitment processes. Costs associated with nurse turnover range from $10,000 to $88,000 (Pittman et al., 2013, p. 597).

In addition to turnover, there are concerns of competency. Berman et al. (2014) reported a gap between the actual practice of nursing and what nurses are taught in their formal education. Gaps included lack of critical thinking, communication skills, time management, assessment skills, and the ability to work as a team member. Although nursing curriculums attempt to address these gaps, limitations of time and clinical situations only prepare students in a generalist role.

The use of older nurses as mentors and preceptors for a residency program has the potential to bridge the generational gap. It provides opportunities for older nurses to share their vast knowledge of rural healthcare and begin to understand new graduates' values. Older nurse mentors can minimize the isolation felt by nurses new to the rural community and support growth in competency.

Nurse fellowship programs offer support to newly graduated APRNs. Physician residencies are mandatory, however, APRN fellowships/residencies are voluntary. Nurse practitioners enrolled in postgraduate fellowship programs, postgraduate training, and mentored experiences can have a higher level of job satisfaction (Sciacca & Reveille, 2016) with 70% completing residencies reporting they were satisfied or very satisfied (Firth & Marsan, 2017).

Graduate nursing fellowships can prepare the new graduate to be more confident and competent while contributing to the workforce. During fellowships, students can engage in weekly education, participate in quality improvement projects, and engage in specialty rotations while being mentored. Fellowship participants engage in a variety of assessment methods such as exit interviews, portfolio creation, mentor meetings, and simulation (Sciacca & Reveille, 2016)

Currently, most nurse fellowship programs are internally funded. Legislation had been proposed to allocate funding to establish residency training programs for family nurse practitioners in federally qualified health centers as part of the Affordable Care Act, however, Congress never made the appropriation. As the conversation continues and fellowships become more common among APRNs, legislation is expected to accommodate federal funding for nurses hoping to gain on-the-job training (Firth & Marsan, 2017).

Socialization and Isolation

Rural nurses experience profession isolation: geographic, social, or ideological (Williams, 2012). Geographic isolation results from being a significant distance from places of interest, conferences, or educational opportunities. Social isolation is the lack of contact with family and friends. Ideological isolation is feeling like an outcast and represented in the rural literature as the insider/outsider concept (Winters et al., 2013). Some rural settings have developed support material for individuals working in rural and remote areas. These resources focus on social isolation, pointing out one can feel isolated when moving into a new community and not knowing anyone. Resources offer suggestions that community members can serve as mentors and other ways to care for self when relocating.

Retention is affected when a nurse feels isolated and unsupported with limited opportunities to advance in their current role. If they do not feel appreciated, RNs may choose to leave for a different opportunity. It is important for rural healthcare providers to consider specific methods to reduce professional isolation. Utilization of information and communication technology can potentially reduce this type of isolation. Nursing research opportunities can also be established, support groups developed, and electronic communications can decrease the feeling of being isolated (Williams, 2012).

CONCLUSION

Although there is a gap in the literature related to global issues that influence the recruitment and retention of rural and frontier nurses, educational programs, health-care facilities, and professional organizations have a responsibility to address this gap. Professional organizations include nursing groups, hospital and state health educational cooperatives, and government agencies. Nursing leaders in rural health-care settings would benefit from utilizing opportunities to support nurses in education, whether for advanced degrees or continuing education to maintain skills and knowledge, or certification reviews. Educators and leaders in rural healthcare settings should consider support of those who are familiar with rural living and all of its implications, including lack of anonymity, isolation, socialization, and work beliefs and providing care to their community. Areas that would be appropriate to consider include enhanced infrastructure that supports nurse's transition to the rural nursing culture, along with safety and welfare in the workplace setting and education, both for continuing evidence-based knowledge development and advanced degree opportunities.

Rural nurses often feel disenfranchised from their urban colleagues. They are often placed in practice situations where there is no collective support to guide them in defining their role and the boundary of that role. The educational background of rural nurses entering practice must have a foundation in rural theory, leadership, and evidence-based practice information (Long & Weinert, 2018; also see Chapter 2). Rural nurses must demonstrate a competence in assessment and prioritization of care needs within their scope of practice. Although they may not have immediate access to evidence-based information and research, they must know how and where to access that information. CAHs, nursing education programs, and state and federal agencies can all provide those linkages and resources for rural nurses.

REFERENCES

American Mobile Nurse Healthcare. (2017). *2017 Survey of registered nurses: Viewpoints on leadership, nursing shortages, and their profession.* https://www.amnhealthcare.com/2017-rnsurvey/

American Nurses Association. (2014). *The nursing workforce 2014: Growth, salaries, education, demographics & trends.* http://www.nursingworld.org/MainMenuCategories/ThePracticeofProfessionalNursing/workforce/Fast-Facts-2014-Nursing-Workforce.pdf

Balasubramanian, S.S., & Jones, E. C. (2016). Hospital closures and the current healthcare climate: The future of rural hospitals in the USA. *Rural and Remote Health, 16,* 3935. www.rrh.org.au/journal/article/3935

Berman, A., Beazley, B., Karshmer, J., Prion, S., Van, P., Wallace, J., & West, N. (2014). Competence gaps among unemployed new nursing graduates entering a community- based transition-to-practice program. *Nurse Educator, 39*(2), 56–61. https://doi.org/10.1097/NNE.0000000000000018

Buerhaus, P., Auerbach, D., & Staiger, D. (May 3, 2017). *How should we prepare for the wave of retiring baby boomer nurses?* Health Affairs Blog. https://www.healthaffairs.org/do/10.1377/hblog20170503.059894/full/

The Center for the Advancement of Healthcare Professionals (2017). *2017 Survey of registered nurses: Viewpoints on leadership, nursing shortages, and their profession.* https://www.amnhealthcare.com/uploadedFiles/MainSite/Content/Campaigns/AMN%20Healthcare%202017%20RN%20Survey%20-%20Full%20Report.pdf

Cramer, M. E., & Jones, K. J., & Hertzog, M. (2011). Nurse staffing in critical access hospitals: Structural factors linked to quality care. *Journal of Nursing Care Quality, 26*(4). 335–343. https://doi.org/10.1097/NCQ.

Dolea, C., Stormont, L., & Braichet, J. (2010). Evaluated strategies to increase attraction and retention of health workers in remote and rural areas. *Bull World Health Organization, 88,* 379–387. https://doi.org/10.2471/BLT.09.070607

Firth, S., & Marsan, L. (2017). For NPs, residency programs gain favor. *The Journal of Advanced Practice Nursing.* https://www.asrn.org/journal-advanced-practice-nursing/1684-for-nps-residency-programs-gain-favor.html

Forneris, L. (2019, November 21). Time for new perspective: Rural nursing workforce. *Rural Health Voices.* Rural Health Association. https://www.ruralhealthweb.org/blogs/ruralhealthvoices/november-2019/time-for-new-perspective-rural-nursing-workforce.

Graetz, J. J. (2017). *A nurse residency model for rural and community hospitals: Making a difference in graduate nurse turnover rates.* http://hdl.handle.net/10755/595655

Havens, D. S., Warshawsky, N., & Vasey, J. (2012). The nursing practice environment in rural hospitals: Practice Environment Scale of the Nursing Work Index assessment. *Journal of Nursing Administration, 42*(11), 519–525. https://doi.org/10.1097/nna.0b013e3182714506

Health Occupation Students of America-Future Health Professionals. (2012a). *HOSA-Future health professionals reaches 200,000 members!* http://www.hosa.org/node/453

Health Occupation Students of America. (2012b). *Mission, purpose, goals, creed, core values.* http://www.hosa.org/mission

Health Resources and Services, Administration Bureau of Health Professions, National Center for Health Workforce Analysis. (April 2013). *The U.S. nursing workforce: Trends in supply and education,* https://www.ruralhealthinfo.org/assets/1206-4974/nursing-workforce-nchwa-report-april-2013.pdf

Health Resources and Services Administration. (2017). *Supply and demand projections of the nursing workforce 2014-2030.* https://bhw.hrsa.gov/sites/default/files/bhw/nchwa/projections/NCHWA_HRSA_Nursing_Report.pdf

Health Resources and Services Administration. (2020). *National health service corps.* https://bhw.hrsa.gov/loans-scholarships/nhsc

Health Workforce. (2017). *Nurse corps scholarship program.* https://bhw.hrsa.gov/loansscholarships/nursecorps/scholarship

Kulig, J. C., Kilpatrick, K., Moffitt, P., & Zimmer, L. (2015). Recruitment and retention in rural nursing: It's still an issue! *Nursing Leadership, 28*(2), 40–50. https://doi.org/10.12927/cjnl.2015.24353

Long, K. A., & Weinert, C. (2018). Rural nursing: Developing the theory base. In C. A. Winters & H. J. Lee (Eds.), *Rural nursing: Concepts, theory and practice* (5th ed., pp. 17–30). Springer Publishing Company.

MacDowell, M., Glasser, M., Fitts, M., Nielsen, K., & Hunsaker, M. (2010). A national view of rural health workforce issues in the USA. *Rural Remote Health, 10*(3), 1531. https://www.rrh.org.au/journal/article/1531

Mbemba, G., Gagnon, M. P., Paré, G., and Côté, J. (2013). Interventions for supporting nurse retention in rural and remote areas: An umbrella review. *Humans Resources for Health, 11,* 44. https://doi.org/10.1186/1478-4491-11-44

National Area Health Education Center Organization. (2015). *Mission & history.* https://nationalahec.org/index.php/about-us/mission-history

National Council of State Boards of Nursing. (2017). *National nursing workforce study*. https://www.ncsbn.org/workforce.htm

National Rural Health Association. (2017). *NRHA fighting for rural*. https://www.nsinursingsolutions.com/Documents/Library/NSI_National_Health_Care_Retention_Report.pdf

Pelham, K., Skinner, M. A., McHugh, P., & Pullon, S. (2016). Interprofessional education in a rural community: The perspectives of the clinical workplace providers. *Journal of Primary Health Care*, *8*(3), 210–219. https://doi.org/10.1071/HC16010

Pittman, P., Herrera, C., Bass, E., & Thompson, P. (2013). Residency programs for nurse graduates: How widespread are they and what are the primary obstacles to further adoption? *Journal of Nursing Administration*, *43*(1), 597–602. https://doi.org/10.1097/01.NNA.0000434507.59126.78

Probst, J. C., McKinney, S. H., & Odahowski, C. (2019). *Rural registered nurses: Educational preparation, workplace, and salary*. Rural & Minority Health Research Center. https://www.sc.edu/study/colleges_schools/public_health/research/research_centers/sc_rural_health_research_center/documents/ruralregisterednurses.pdf

Pribulick, M., Williams, I.C. & Fahs, P.S. (2010). Strategies to reduce barriers to recruitment and participation. *Online Journal of Rural Nursing & Health Care*, *10*(1), 22–33. https://link.gale.com/apps/doc/A230151147/AONE?u=anon~11b894e6&sid=googleScholar&xid=81139bc9

Project ECHO®. (2020). https://echo.unm.edu/

Sciacca, K., & Reveille, B. (2016). Evaluation of nurse practitioners enrolled in fellowship and residency programs: Methods and trends. *The Journal for Nurse Practitioners*, *12*(6), e275–e280. https://doi.org/10.1016/j.nurpra.2016.02.011

Skillman, S. M., Doescher, M. P., & Rosenblatt, R. A. (2009). *Threats to the future supply of rural registered nurses* [Policy brief]. WWAMI Rural Health Research Center. http://depts.washington.edu/uwrhrc/uploads/Rural_RNs_PB_2009.pdf

Statista Research. (2014). *Nurses in the United States in rural and urban areas as of 2014*. https://www.statista.com/statistics/328883/nurses-in-rural-and-urban-us-areas/

U.S. Department of Health and Human Services Health Resources and Services Administration (2014). *National Center for Health Workforce Analysis: Distribution of U.S. health care providers residing in rural and urban areas*. https://bhw.hrsa.gov/sites/default/files/bureau-health-workforce/data-research/nchwa-fact-sheet.pdf

US Healthcare. (2015). *America's nursing shortage: It's real, and it's back*. https://www.prnewswire.com/news-releases/americas-nursing-shortage-its-real-and-its-back-300121591.html

Williams, M. A. (2012). Rural professional isolation: an integrative review. *Journal of Rural Nursing and Health Care*, *12*(2), 3–10. http://rnojournal.binghamton.edu/index.php/RNO/article/view/51/211

Winters, C. A., Thomlinson, E. H., O'Lynn, C., Lee, H. J., McDonagh, M. K., Edge, D. S., & Reimer, M. A. (2013). Exploring rural nursing theory across borders. In Winters, C. A. (Ed.), *Rural nursing: Concepts, theory, and practice* (4th ed., pp. 35–47). Springer Publishing Company.

The World Bank. (2018). *Rural population (5 of total population)*. https://data.worldbank.org/indicator/SP.RUR.TOTL.ZS

Wros, P., Mathews, L. R., & Voss, H. (2015). An academic-practice model to improve the health of underserved neighborhoods. *Family Community Health*, *38*(2), 195–203. https://doi.org/10.1097/FCH.0000000000000065

Zhang, X., Tai, D. T., Pforsich, H., and Lin, V. W. (2018). United States registered nurse workforce report card and shortage forecast: A revisit. *American Journal of Medical Quality*, *33*(3), 229–236. https://doi.org/10.1177/10628606177383

CHAPTER 27

Transcultural Service-Learning: Preparing Nurses to Meet the Needs of Rural Indigenous Communities

Julie H. Alexander-Ruff

DISCUSSION TOPICS

- What are the benefits to nursing education that result from placing students in a cultural immersion service learning (CISL) experience as part of their undergraduate formative education?
- Should all nursing students participate in a CISL experience as a strategy to increase the exposure of student nurses to rural vulnerable communities?
- Do students gain a better understanding of social determinants of health (SDoH) and their impact on vulnerable and rural populations through CISL experiences?
- Do student nurses retain the knowledge skills and attributes attained during a 1-week CISL experience to facilitate their healthcare practices in rural communities?

INTRODUCTION

The focus of this chapter is cultural immersion service learning (CISL). Information will show how the inclusion of a CISL experience within a required undergraduate nursing course facilitated prelicensure nursing students' understanding of culturally conscious care and why the practice of cultural consciousness is an essential element of nursing practice toward the reduction of healthcare disparities seen among rural communities.

BACKGROUND

The greatest concentration of people in the United States live in large urban areas or suburban communities located next to metropolitan cities; yet the United States still has many rurally isolated communities. These isolated communities, typically in the western

United States, are often several hours drive from hospitals, other health services, retail stores, restaurants, and entertainment venues; thus restricting access to healthcare, goods, and services. Of the 500-plus American Indian (AI) reservations, the 50 largest reservations are in the most geographically remote areas of the western United States. The location of these communities contributes to challenges AIs regularly face. A lack of educational and employment opportunities, access to nutritional foods and healthcare are daily challenges that directly impact the health and well-being of Native peoples who reside on or near remote western reservations. Racial and cultural inequality compounds the issues of access associated with rurality contributing to further disparity and vulnerability. Rural AI reservation communities experience some of the most disparate health challenges of any other racial or ethnic group in the United States (Indian Health Service [IHS], 2019).

AIs comprise 2% of the national population yet AIs suffer disproportionately from all preventable health diseases or conditions including, but not limited to, unintentional injuries, suicide, cardiovascular diseases, and diabetes. Approximately 30% of AIs residing in reservation communities do not have access to electricity or clean running water. About 40% do not have Internet access leaving them cut off from health information and alerts thereby directly affecting AIs' ability to participate in self-care (Tribal Health Department, 2020).

AI communities are in regions of the country described as food desserts. Food deserts are commonplace in communities of color across the nation. Literally speaking access to fresh and healthy food is scare. Distance to a supermarket is often extreme, food prices are commonly higher than prices in urban centers, and food that is higher in calories and can be easily stored for longer periods of time are common. Knowing this information helps to explain in part unhealthy dietary choices which contribute to diseases rural vulnerable populations uniformly experience, such as obesity, diabetes, and cardiac disease. As a result, the average life span of AIs living on or near reservations is as much as 20 years less than nonnatives (IHS, 2019). Such a large disparity has implications that go beyond the individual.

Within AI communities, it is the elders of the community who carry the wisdom of the tribe, which is passed on orally to subsequent generations. Early and premature death disrupts the flow of culture from one generation to the next resulting in the loss of cultural knowledge, language, and meaning. Those with cultural and historical knowledge and those who carry the traditions of faith, spirituality, traditional healing practices, and language die from preventable health conditions disproportionately, thereby impacting the stability and continuity of an entire culture.

The United States remains the only developed country to not adopt a basic level of healthcare for all its citizens as called for in the United Nations (1948), Universal Declaration of Human Rights. Yet, American Indian and Alaska Natives (AI/AN) who have a tribal affiliation with a federally recognized tribe may access their healthcare free of charge through the IHS. The IHS is a federally funded program, which came about as part of treaty agreements in 1787 in exchange for lands and natural resources. This agreement is based on Article I, Section 8 of the U.S. Constitution. It is important to note that the IHS is consistently underfunded. Data from 2017 show a difference in funding per person on healthcare as $4,078 for AIs and $8,109 for Medicaid (Government Accountability Office, 2018). This discordance in healthcare spending has a direct correlation with the quality of preventative health services available to AI patients, appropriate levels of clinic and hospital staffing in IHS facilities, and increased mortality and morbidity of AI/AN patients. Equally important is a recognition of those individuals who identify as AI/AN but who do not have a federally recognized tribal affiliation, do not qualify for IHS services, and are more likely to be underinsured or uninsured. Additionally, adding to healthcare disparity, IHS services are divided by tribe such that a tribal member who belongs to one tribe but resides on or near a reservation associated with a different tribe must receive their healthcare from their own tribal reservation's IHS facility that is likely to be located many hundreds of miles from their home.

Rural nursing practices, especially in rural areas within the western United States, will typically include the care of AI/AN peoples who reside on or near rurally isolated reservation communities. Effective nursing practice with AI/AN peoples requires more than the knowledge and skills developed from generic evidence-based practice models. Effective practice also requires cultural consciousness in the mindful application of evidence-based practice. CISL is a pedagogy developed to facilitate such cultural consciousness. In CISL experiences, nursing faculty accompany student nurses to a specific rural community, where students work alongside community members learning about the community's culture, values, traditions, and healthcare needs. In-person learning affords a level of understanding that is not attainable through videos, assigned readings, or simulations.

The profession of nursing has historically been and continues to be a provider of service and an advocate for quality care, seeking to promote community and individual health. Bartels (1998) reminds us that the expectations for humanistic learning in nursing education include the delivery of service within a community context. In the last two decades, sweeping healthcare reform in the United States has moved from large institutional care to a focus on community health, that is, health delivered within the community context (IHS, 2019). This model is of significance for nurses working within rural communities.

CULTURAL IMMERSION SERVICE LEARNING AND HEALTH EQUITY

Health disparities are complex, multifaceted, have multivariate causes, and are a threat to individual and community health and well-being in rural communities. One of the many causes of health disparities is cultural hegemony—an incongruence of beliefs among people of different cultures, which favors one set of cultural values over another. According to the Centers for Disease Control and Prevention (2014), "Health disparities negatively affect groups of people who have systematically experienced greater social or economic obstacles to health, the social determinants of health which are historically linked to discrimination or exclusion" (p. 1). This incongruence is often tacitly held and conveyed by the beliefs of the dominant group. Nurses' understanding of "place," how rural reservation-dwelling AIs experience "place" and the impact of "place" on health, is fundamental to the social determinants of health (Office of Disease Prevention and Health Promotion, 2020). Yet, there is a disconnect between the essential understandings that nurses need to practice and the education delivered to nursing students. This incongruence is captured by Moss (2016), a member of the Lakota Nation. "As Americans, we are presented with few opportunities to learn in depth about our Indigenous people ... when presented, it is always from the dominant cultures' point of view" (p. 8). Developing health system partnerships allows student nurses to develop the skills necessary to better understand the way people of diverse cultures access and understand healthcare.

CISL is a reciprocal service-learning model that immerses students for several days or weeks into communities that are culturally dissimilar to their home community. As students share their developing nursing skills with the community, the community participants share their beliefs, values, and culture with the students. Students engage in this reciprocal process through activities that foster reflection and critical thinking about healthcare equity, and for many, it creates a disequilibrium of their current belief systems (Alexander-Ruff & Kinion, 2018).

The reciprocal activities that the student and the community participants engage in facilitates the emergence of integrative care practices, such as evidence-based best practice models synthesized with folk care models as explained in Leininger's Sunrise Enabler Model (Leininger, 1988). The nursing students bring to the community their developing understandings of professional care practices. As the community participants and clients share their folk understandings of care, the students, already disoriented by the immersion into a novel community context, question the folk care practices of the community, but also begin to question the professional practices that they have been taught. This questioning and critical reflection facilitates the development of integrative care practices.

Cultural Care Theory describes how clinicians and researchers develop and integrate knowledge of healthcare and culture to provide culturally congruent nursing care that facilitates the health of people (Leininger, 2006). This happens in four phases (McFarland & Wehbe-Alamah, 2019). First, there is a developing awareness and sensitivity to cultural care differences and similarities. Second, the healthcare provider develops an in-depth understanding of the integration of culture with evidence-based best practices resulting in culturally congruent care. Third, practitioners creatively apply their integrated knowledge of culturally congruent care to a specific individualized context or case. Finally, successful applications of integrated knowledge of culturally congruent care are implemented at the systems level to improve health outcomes for diverse populations.

The CISL model exposes nursing students to information that they would not be able to otherwise access, helping them to better understand the folk care practices and beliefs held within the community as well as the AI Elders' perspectives on the health challenges experienced by the people and their community. Such opportunities increase the student's self-efficacy and sense of belonging, which in turn facilitates the transition of the nursing student into a competent and confident nurse (Jeffreys, 2016). Additionally, a CISL experience provides nursing students from culturally homogeneous communities with access to patients from diverse backgrounds through service-learning immersion experiences.

THE CULTURAL IMMERSION SERVICE LEARNING EXPERIENCE

For nursing students attending a program in a rural, racially homogenous setting, opportunities to care for a patient who is racially or culturally different from themselves are limited. In fact, it is entirely possible for a student nurse, studying in a homogenous community, to graduate without ever caring for a patient from a culture different from their own. Community setting is important because culture informs perceptions of health risks, attitudes toward health professionals and institutions, as well as behaviors and health-related practices among individuals, agencies, and communities (Crosby et al., 2012).

The community surrounding this university has 111,876 residents with good access to healthcare, education, and social services, and an above average median household income and educational level (U. S. Census Bureau, 2018). Children in this area are largely healthy and disease free; they are rarely hospitalized, and if hospitalized, only for short periods of time. The community surrounding the university was different from many of the rural and geographically isolated communities within the state in many areas including pediatric healthcare. On the other hand, the tribal representative described the healthcare needs of the children on the reservation as profound, especially as compared to non-Indian children and stated "health care is often reactionary rather than preventative" (Personal conversation with K.S., Director of the Health Promotion and Disease Prevention Program for the Northern Plains Indian Reservation, September 18, 2010).

The CISL experience began in 2011 as an instructor-initiated partnership between the College of Nursing at a land-grant university and a Northern Plains Indian tribal community. The university–tribal community partnership aligns with the university's pediatric nursing course objectives and fosters professional development in a cross-cultural setting. Nursing students gain an understanding of the culture of two AI tribes; historical trauma and its impact on health, lifestyle, well-being, social justice, and the complex link between poverty and health while working collaboratively to meet an identified need of a host community in a cross-cultural setting.

Nursing Care of Children and Their Families is a 5-credit course focusing on the health promotion, disease prevention, illness management, and nursing care of children within the family context. Students spend a minimum of 135 clock hours at various supervised clinical sites; 60 hours of which includes the CISL experience within a Northern Plains tribal community. The CISL experience is intended to facilitate learners' initial inquiry into identifying health inequalities between AI communities and dominant-culture communities in the state and region. This approach to health promotion, maintenance, and restoration is designed in part to deconstruct technical processes of health and illness to demonstrate the social impact of healthcare on considerations of living circumstances and the public policy decisions that shape these circumstances. Discussions of basic human rights to health are intertwined with more traditional pediatric nursing care topics such as childhood obesity and diabetes, environmental air quality and asthma, and so on.

Description of Cultural Immersion Service Learning Experiential Activities

Each academic year up to 32 junior nursing students travel in groups of eight with their instructor to a rural, and geographically isolated, Northern Plains Indian Reservation where the students live, learn, and work for 1 week. Students are lodged together in a multiroom house provided by the tribal council and are responsible for preparing their own meals. Student travel expenses are supported by a university-affiliated grant. Taking students outside of the classroom and traditional clinical or practicum environment and extending the student learning experience beyond the local campus community provide the students with a challenge to consider the complexities of health inequalities, including rurality, cultural awareness in healthcare delivery, and the impact health inequities have on AI children and families.

Preexperience Activities

At the beginning of the semester students are provided with the clinical objectives, cultural expectations, logistic concerns, and other information specific to the CISL experience. In the weeks leading up to the CISL experience, students and the instructor work together to develop mutually agreed upon written expectations regarding behavior, attitude, and conduct standards for the CISL experience. The agreements are used to express needs for privacy, private time, prayer, dress preferences (modesty), special dietary needs, and any other student concerns.

Prior to departure, students are oriented to the experience by the tribal host and other guest speakers with experience in AI history and culture. Tribal health officials provide a listing of healthcare education topics they deem most important, and students prepare to teach classroom lessons, including the development of teaching materials, on each of these healthcare topics. Additionally, the students research the needs of the children in this community including healthcare issues related to rurality, wellness, and preventative healthcare.

ON-SITE ACTIVITIES

Students travel 480 miles by vehicle from the home campus to the Reservation on Sunday and return to the campus on the following Saturday. Upon arrival at the reservation, students receive their clinical assignments, and a community orientation from the tribal health director or member of his staff. Nursing students are immersed in the tribal cultures for 12 to 14 hours per day providing care to children in six tribal school health clinics and participating in cultural events. Throughout the school day, nursing students provide healthcare for children in prekindergarten through the 12th grade by performing health screenings, physical exams, healthcare education, and tending to minor injuries and acute illness as needed during the school day. In the evenings, nursing students participate in cultural events offered by the tribe, including discussions with elders, beading, arrow making, archery, horseback riding, and meal sharing. On Friday evening, students are honored with traditional dancing exhibitions in which children and community hosts teach the nursing students traditional dances and prepare a shared meal. Students then return to their home campus community on Saturday.

Each day a clinical reflective postconference is held with all nursing students and the instructor in a neutral setting, away from children, their families, and members of the community. This relaxed informal atmosphere allows students to reflect on the children and families they have seen, and their context, as well as the social and cultural framework impacting the nursing students' care, their feelings, experiences, and possible misconceptions. The daily group reflection is nonconfrontational, not graded, and seeks to leverage the whole group to help each individual student in processing their day. Late evenings are reserved for student study, individual reflection, and rest.

POSTEXPERIENCE ACTIVITIES

Students complete a pre- and postexperience reflective writing exercise with results often reflecting a significant increase in the ability to integrate cultural awareness and clinical nursing skills. For example, one student wrote:

> *Poverty contributes to poor health status, such as not being able to afford a toothbrush, leading to dental decay, leading to infection which can spread to the entire body if not corrected. Yes, I knew these things beforehand, but seeing it actually play out makes a person realize what this culture is facing on a daily basis.*

EVALUATION OF THE CULTURAL IMMERSION SERVICE LEARNING EXPERIENCE

To date, three research evaluations of this CISL experience have been completed. The first study qualitatively explored how the CISL experience facilitated cultural consciousness among nursing students during and immediately following their participation. The second study quantitatively evaluated whether there was any change in nursing students' racial attitudes immediately following the CISL using a modified version of the White Racial Attitude Scale (Helm & Parham, 1996). The third study quantitatively compared the transcultural self-efficacy scores of Bachelor of Science in Nursing (BSN) graduates who participated in the CISL experience to the transcultural self-efficacy scores of BSN graduates who shared the same curriculum but did not participate in the CISL experience.

Study 1: Evidence for Cultural Immersion Service Learning Facilitating Cultural Consciousness

METHODS

An intrinsic single case study design examined undergraduate student nurse perceptions of cultural consciousness following the CISL experience. Qualitative data was collected from two cohorts of junior-level nursing students ($n = 30$) which included (a) instructor and preceptor observations of students during the CISL experience, (b) initial student reflections during and immediately following participation in the CISL experience, and (c) follow-up student reflections written approximately 2 to 3 weeks following participation in the CISL experience. The participants were predominantly Caucasian (90%), women (93%), and under 30 years of age (70%).

Both sets of student reflections were analyzed using discourse analysis. The reflection data derived from the discourse analysis and instructor and preceptor observation data were analyzed using the constant-comparative method (Strauss, 1994). The themes, subthemes, and comparisons were synthesized to develop a grounded theory that encompassed the data. The grounded theory was then verified by going through all the data seeking contradictions to the grounded theory.

FINDINGS

Twenty-nine of the 30 students stated their goal for the CISL experience as skill development. The one exception was a student who only listed cultural engagement as a goal. One student provided evidence of cultural consciousness in her clinical observation reflections. Several weeks later in their end of course reflections, evidence of cultural consciousness was demonstrated by 19 additional students in statements linking concrete nursing skills, such as head-to-toe assessments, to the culture of the Northern Plains Indian tribes.

The process of nursing students becoming culturally conscious seemed to begin with the stark comparison of the reservation community with the community in which the university campus is situated and recognized disparity as complex and concrete. This, in turn, facilitated the recognition of privilege. Twenty-four of the students responded to this recognition with reflections indicating being overwhelmed and uncertain. Many of these students sought to restore the disequilibrium of the disparities by projecting their tacit assumptions, but before the end of the week about half of those initially projecting their assumptions began to reestablish psychological equilibrium by suspending judgment. Eight students responded to the disequilibrium created by the recognition of privilege by initially suspending judgment. Actions resulting from suspending judgment were discussed in themes about paying attention more deeply, reframing the situation, forming connections, and cultural respect.

In the clinical observation reflections, 28 of the 30 students described their experience in terms denoting themes of helping or making a difference by embracing the culture, forming connections, and paying closer attention. Six students discussed a need for increased responsibility for the quality of their help directly addressing the disparity in healthcare access.

Looking across time, most students formed an initial set of expectations based upon class discussions about what to expect colored by tacit assumptions formed by middle-class, dominant cultural experiences. The reality of the situations they encountered in the 1-week CISL experience did not match these expectations.

Recognition of Privilege. The concept of privilege emerged repeatedly as an idea in the classroom, but that idea seemed to acquire increased meaning for the students during the CISL experience. For example, one student wrote, "I worked hard to go to school and to pay for college etc. however I realize that I have been given opportunities for health and education that these children will never have." Recognizing privilege was also described through a comparison of the students' community and the reservation community. One student who was attending a clinical rotation at a private pediatric dentist's office in her home community stated "I found that overall, the children whose teeth we cared for today truly had very good oral health in comparison to the children on the reservation… It made me grateful for the resources we have available in our community."

Seeing Disparity With Clarity. The recognition of disparity and experiencing its impacts improved nursing students understanding about what healthcare disparity means and its complexity in concrete ways. For example, one student wrote, "I learned that adequate access to care is crucial; especially in rural areas ... There is a huge chance that care will not be provided in time." She continued to write, "Poverty impacts so many aspects of the health and wellbeing of children in physical, psychosocial and emotional forms ... I learned that vulnerable populations need more time and focused care." In addition to comments about healthcare access, 18 students wrote in their clinical reflections about adequacy of resources. For example, "Through this experience you see that these children are vulnerable in so many ways and experience health disparity as a result of their situations. It was a very eye-opening experience to see the lack of resources available to this population." In another example, Ivy's statement provided an apt conclusion regarding this theme. "If you do not have access to care then health declines; this was very difficult to see."

Responses to Disequilibrium. There were two types of responses to restore the disequilibrium that the nursing students experienced—suspending judgment or projecting their tacit assumptions.

Suspending Judgment. Nancy wrote in her end of course reflection, "One of the biggest things I learned is that if you don't understand the culture your patients are from, there is a tendency to be judgmental." In practice, such lifestyles may not necessarily be attainable for all patient populations because of existing disparities. For example, as one student explained in her end of course reflection, "It doesn't matter how many toothbrushes or toothpaste tubes we give children, if they don't have running water at home, there is no point."

Projecting Tacit Assumptions. Cultural norms and perceptions vary widely across cultures what is perceived by one group of individuals as acceptable may be the exact opposite for another group. Yvonne's clinical reflection showed that she was questioning her assumptions and understanding of a different perspective. She wrote:

It is so important to never make any assumptions about your patients. The conversation we had about cutting of hair really demonstrated this. I did not know that sometimes AIs cut their hair when a loved one passes away. This really showed me how easy it would be to assume this child cut her hair due to lice or simply to change their hairstyle. I would be mortified if I told someone their "haircut looked great, and I love getting my haircut" only to find out they did so because someone passed away. So, in the future, I will remind myself how easy assumptions are to make.

Actions Resulting From the Suspension of Judgment

Students who initially suspended judgment worked in the following ways to overcome feelings of disequilibrium.

Respecting and Embracing Culture. Learning about a culture or community is interpreted by community members at the Northern Plains Indian Reservation as a form of respect. Orla demonstrated her understanding of respecting and embracing culture in her clinical reflection writing:

> I have learned that in locations such as [the Northern Plains Indian Reservation], it is much harder to recruit nurses and other medical staff that are truly passionate about the population and the culture. Some health care providers who are placed on the reservation do not have the time invested in the community, I believe they do not demonstrate the appropriate care [cultural competence] about providing the absolute best care to those in need.

Another student wrote, "I learned to appreciate the culture of the population the involvement of extended family, complimentary therapies (sweat lodges), etc. My cultural awareness for this population greatly increased, and by showing cultural sensitivity, I feel as though my care improved." On the other hand, the desire to embrace the culture was mixed with degrees of uncertainty as expressed in student reflections such as "I fear that I might say something silly because I may not know enough about a particular culture."

Forming Connections. Nursing students described an essential element of their work in terms of establishing a rapport or forming a connection with their patients. This was exemplified in statements such as: "I was fairly proud of the fact that by carefully questioning the teenage girl complaining of dehydration, I was able to ascertain she was suffering from anxiety, depression and was possibly suicidal." Another student wrote:

> While also assessing the child's psychosocial situation in a conversational manner, I established a therapeutic relationship and elicited a wealth of information. Based on the information I gathered from the student I was able to tailor patient education to her areas of need and curiosity about appropriate oral care, "good" versus "bad medicines," and allowed her to auscultate her own heart sounds with my stethoscope.

Paying Deeper Attention. Four nursing students' reflections included the themes of gathering information and paying deeper attention. Nancy expressed the need to pay deeper attention by asking questions. She wrote, "I think it is also important to ask questions, to validate a child's need for help, even when the reason they approach you with is not a real issue, sometimes they need attention and to have someone listen to them."

Susan reflected on nonverbal cues as part of gathering information and paying deeper attention and wrote, "I will always try to be aware of my patients' cues." Paying deeper attention also meant looking critically at the context of the situation. Mary wrote, "I will remember that things are often more complicated or involved with other issues than they may initially seem."

Student Perceptions of Their Impact. Most students (29 of 30) expressed seeking to make a difference as an explicitly stated goal in their clinical reflections. Overall, the students who participated in this study perceived that their CISL experience provided help and in providing help their sense of increased responsibility seemed to evolve.

Feeling Increased Responsibility. Increased responsibility speaks to an acknowledgment that all of us have a responsibility in ensuring that all individuals receive high-quality care. Valerie expressed this well in her previsit writing, "I respond superficially, and have not reached a point where I am knowledgeable of other cultures." Several weeks after completing the CISL experience, she wrote:

> *Vulnerable populations, such as children and economically deprived individuals as well as communities are dependent on others to care for them. This power inequality makes this population especially vulnerable to neglect and abuse. It is important as nurses to provide care to these individuals in a way that provides choice and enables the individual to care for his or herself as much as possible.*

Her end-of-course reflection expressed increased responsibility along with help and respect.

This sense of increased responsibility was expressed by Quinn more pragmatically in writing, "I realized how important our assessments were to these kids that may be the only time they get seen for their health for the whole year."

Cultural Consciousness. Of the 30 participants, 20 demonstrated evidence of cultural consciousness in their end of course reflections. One student wrote "I observed the importance of culturally sensitive care and how a community's culture can both augment and impede the development of a community health program." This was echoed by Yvonne who wrote, "From this experience I will implement practices that allow me to slow down and look at the whole person instead of just checking things off of a list." Susan confirmed these thoughts when she stated, "Cultural understanding enables a nurse to be self-aware and deliver sensitive and specific care."

Conclusions of the Qualitative Evaluation of Cultural Immersion Service Learning

In spite of gender, ethnicity, and differences in chronological age and life experience, the 30 students who participated in the CISL experience expressed various examples of important issues facing AIs who reside in or near rural reservation communities, and the complexities of life situations in their rural communities, which directly and indirectly affect health and well-being. Many students initially struggled with their emotions when confronting the disparity of citizens within the same state in which they study and learn. They described feelings of uncertainty and being overwhelmed, moving toward new and enhanced skill development including flexibility, organization, teamwork, cultural respect, idealistic hope for the future and for change, inspiration for career enhancement, and finally cultural consciousness.

Several students expressed confirmation that concepts such as privilege and cultural awareness must be learned in situ. Yet, preparation for such an experience is key, including selected readings, exercises, and presentations. One student's final reflection summed up the experiences of the group best when she wrote, "Who knew that a bunch of sweet kiddos who live within a day's drive from me would teach me some of the hardest and most valuable lessons during my college career?"

Study 2: Evidence for the Cultural Immersion Service Learning Experience Changing Attitudes Regarding Race

METHODS
Thirty-two nursing students completed a modified version of the White Racial Identity Attitude Scale (WRIAS; Helm & Carter, 1990a) during the first week of the course and

again during the last week of the class, approximately 3 weeks after the students' CISL experience. The WRIAS was modified for use within an AI community. The original WRIAS instrument was a 50-item, 5-point Likert scale designed to assess attitudes along a continuum of five stages of White racial identity development within an African American community (Helm & Carter, 1990b). Modifications included changing the word *Black* to AI throughout the instrument and reducing the number of questions from 50 to 25 by removing items that did not apply within an AI context. Content validity was established by three expert reviewers prior to administering the modified scale. Cronbach's alpha was 0.795 on the modified instrument indicating internal reliability. A *t* test was performed to compare pre- and posttest student scores on the modified WRIAS.

RESULTS

Similar to the results in the first evaluation study, 24 of the 32 students who participated in the CISL experience demonstrated cultural consciousness in their written reflections at the end of the semester. Quantitatively, postexperience scores on the modified WRIAS (Helm & Carter, 1990b) were statistically significant ($t = 7.906$, degrees of freedom [df] 31, $p < .0001$). Twenty-five of the 32 participants demonstrated more than a 10-point difference between their pretest WRIAS score and posttest score. Furthermore, the effect size of the CISL intervention was calculated at 1.902. Typically, an effect size of 0.8, even with a small sample, is considered a worthwhile process to replicate.

Study 3: Evidence for the Cultural Immersion Service Learning Experience Impacting BSN Graduates' Transcultural Self-Efficacy

METHODS

This study used a quasi-experimental design to determine whether a difference existed in transcultural self-efficacy of BSN graduates among five campuses. One campus conducted a mandatory CISL experience during the graduates' junior year and the four other campuses did not offer such an experience. Participants in this study were 53 graduates from each of five campuses of a racially homogenous university. All graduates mastered the same curriculum objectives including meeting cultural competency standards; however, individual instructors determined the instructional activities. On one campus, an instructor embedded a CISL experience into the pediatrics course taken by nursing students during the second semester of their junior year.

After receiving Institutional Review Board exemption approval, 94 BSN graduates were sent an email containing the link to a survey 30 days prior to graduation. Two rounds of follow-up requests were made, one 15 days prior to graduation and the other 20 days following graduation. Completed surveys were reviewed for outliers and completeness, and then placed into SPSS for analysis. Descriptive statistics calculations as well as an analysis of variance (ANOVA) were performed comparing the total score and subtest scores by campus.

Fifty-five BSN graduates responded to the Transcultural Self-Efficacy tool (TSET) (Jeffreys, 2016). Two of the responses received were incomplete. The sample size for this study was 53 (56.4%). Of those completing the survey, 48 were women (91%) and 52 identified as Caucasian (98%). The remaining person was AI. All participants were less than 40 years of age, with most students (72%) being less than 25 years old. Of the students responding, 18 (34%) students were from the campus participating in the CISL experience. Seventeen (32%) students responded from the nursing college's only urban campus. The remaining 18 (34%) students were distributed across the remaining three campuses.

As a result, 18 participants (34%) received the intervention, and 35 (66%) did not receive the intervention.

RESULTS

The results demonstrated that transcultural self-efficacy was significantly greater in those graduates who participated in the CISL experience compared to graduates from the other four campuses ($F = 7.26$, df 4,48, $p < .0001$); yet, no difference in transcultural self-efficacy was found among graduates of the four campuses not offering the CISL experience. Furthermore, in analyzing the subtest scores, a significant difference between the graduates participating in the CISL experience and those who had not participated. Table 27.1 provides the mean scores and SD of scores by campus. Table 27.2 shows the analysis of variance results and effect size by subtest scores.

As shown in Table 27.1, the graduates at the campus requiring the CISL experience self-reported a higher and more narrow range in transcultural self-efficacy scores overall and in each subtest area than graduates on other campuses. Furthermore, the self-reports of transcultural self-efficacy from all the other campuses were similar regarding the total score means as well as the score means of each subscale.

Table 27.2 shows that there was a significant difference ($p < .0001$) between the graduates at the campus requiring the CISL experience and all other campuses regarding total scores as well as a significant difference in each of the subtest scores. Furthermore, the effect size of transcultural self-efficacy for graduates participating in the CISL experience is moderate to high. Effect size is important when considering the practicality of implementation in terms of cost versus benefits. The total score effect size of 0.83 for graduates participating in the CISL experience indicates the probability that an individual graduate at the campus requiring the CISL experience at the 50th percentile would be 79th percentile at any of the four other campuses regarding transcultural self-efficacy.

TABLE 27.1 Mean and SD of Scores by Campus

Campus	Total Score Mean (SD)	Cognitive Subscore	Practical Subscore	Affective Subscore
1	7.64 (1.31)	7.84 (1.73)	6.95 (1.76)	8.35 (1.46)
CISL	9.23 (0.80)	9.40 (0.74)	9.18 (1.14)	9.08 (1.80)
3	7.67 (1.09)	7.93 (1.14)	7.93 (1.15)	7.83 (1.03)
4	7.14 (1.33)	7.09 (1.80)	7.09 (1.93)	7.29 (1.85)
5	7.32 (1.07)	7.37 (1.43)	7.37 (1.44)	7.78 (2.04)
Combined	8.11 (1.35)	8.26 (1.55)	8.26 (1.73)	8.37 (1.47)

SD, standard deviation.

TABLE 27.2 Analysis of Variance Results and Effect Size by Subtest Domain

	Degrees of Freedom Between/within/total	F-Ratio	p Value	Effect Size
Cognitive	4/48/52	5.215	.001	.74
Practical	4/48/52	7.775	<.0001	.53
Affective	4/48/52	5.173	.002	.48
Total	4/48/52	7.264	<.0001	.83

A Tukey Honestly Significant Difference post hoc test was performed to compare the differences transcultural self-efficacy scores among each of the campuses. The transcultural self-efficacy scores were significantly different among the campus requiring the CISL experience and three other campuses ($p < .011$, .026, and .013, respectively). Yet, no significant difference was found between the self-efficacy scores of graduates from campus 3 and the campus requiring the CISL experience. Furthermore, there was no significant difference found among any of the campuses that did not offer the CISL experience.

This study demonstrated that a CISL experience embedded within a nursing education curriculum seems to have facilitated the transcultural self-efficacy of BSN graduates to the extent of improving transcultural self-efficacy scores almost a full *SD* (.83) in comparison with other BSN graduates who were educated within the same curriculum but did not have the CISL experience. Such findings are particularly important when nurses are educated in communities that are racially and ethnically homogeneous because the patient populations encountered during clinical experiences within such communities reflect the diversity of the community.

CONCLUSION

AIs living in rural communities experience a heavier burden of health disparities than any other racial or ethnic group in the United States (IHS, 2019). One approach toward alleviating such health disparity is to prepare nurses who can provide transcultural nursing care (Leininger, 1988). Culturally congruent healthcare practices facilitate improved nursing care outcomes. The American Association of Colleges of Nursing (2008) includes practice in a multicultural environment and the skills *needed to* provide culturally competent care as essential elements of nursing education in its standards for the preparation of professional nurses. Yet, the Robert Woods Johnson Foundation (2014) reported that the majority of the approximately 17,000 nursing students in the United States are educated based on the models of nursing education that have remained unchanged for decades.

Institutionalism prevails within our nursing preparation programs. CISL experiences will require more than just instructor support, it requires the support of college administrators to provide the resources for change, and instructional colleagues to adjust their course schedules to allow students taking concurrent courses to participate in an immersion experience. Nonetheless, immersing students in communities with different beliefs and cultures to hone their clinical skills provides the students a reason to question their own beliefs and tacit biases, as well as to develop authentic relationships, which facilitate a student's ability to adopt social change perspectives, and thus enables students to see themselves as change agents. Without transcultural self-efficacy, without nurses seeing themselves as change agents, healthcare inequities that affect disproportionately rural and vulnerable communities will continue unabated.

Evaluation studies demonstrate a connection between a 1-week CISL experience and improved cultural consciousness, greater understanding and tolerance in racial attitudes, and enhanced transcultural self-efficacy among BSN graduates. Such CISL experiences may serve to shape the learner and the professional nurse they will become. Transcultural nursing knowledge and skills are required to provide culturally congruent care to patients and the patients' families living in rural and geographically isolated communities. Culturally congruent nursing care is directly associated with improved health outcomes for diverse peoples (Leininger, 2006).

REFERENCES

Alexander-Ruff, J. H., & Kinion, E. (2018). Engaging nursing students in a rural Native American community to facilitate cultural consciousness. *Journal of Community Health Nursing*, 35(4), 196–206. doi: 10.1080/07370016.2018.1516423

American Association Of Colleges Of Nursing. (2008). *The essentials of baccalaureate education for professional nursing practice*. Author.

Bartels, J. E. (1998). Humanistic learning in the context of service: The liberal arts in nursing education. In J. S. Norbeck, C. Connolly, & J. Koerner (Eds.), *Caring and community: Concepts and models for service learning in nursing* (pp. 7–18). American Association for Higher Education.

Centers for Disease Control and Prevention. (2014). *Definitions for social determinants of health*. http://www.cdc.gov/nchhstp/socialdetermininants/definitions.html

Crosby, R. A., Wendel, M. L., Vanderpool, R. C., & Casey, B. R. (Eds.). (2012). *Rural populations and health: Determinants, disparities, and solutions*. Jossey-Bass.

Government Accountability Office. (2018). *Indian health service: Spending levels of the HIS compared to three other federal healthcare programs*. https://www.gao.gov/assets/700/695871.pdf

Helms, J. E., & Carter, R. T. (1990a). Development of the White Racial Identity Attitude Scale. In J. E. Helms (Ed.), *Black and White racial identity attitudes: Theory, research, and practice* (pp. 67–80). Greenwood Press.

Helms, J. E., & Carter, R. T. (1990b). Relationships of White and Black racial identity attitudes and demographic similarity to counselor preferences. *Journal of Counseling Psychology*, 38, 446–457.

Indian Health Service. (2019). *Disparities factsheet 2000–2013. U.S. Health and Human Services* https://www.ihs.gov/newsroom/factsheets/disparities/

Jeffreys, M. R. (2016). *The cultural competence education resource toolkit* (3d ed.). Springer Publishing Company.

Leininger, M. M. (1988). *Transcultural nursing: Concepts, theories, and practices*. Wiley & Sons.

Leininger, M. M. (2006). Culture care diversity and universality theory and evolution of the ethnonursing method. In M. M. Leininger & M. R. McFarland (Eds.), *Culture care diversity and universality: A worldwide nursing theory* (2nd ed., pp. 1–41). Jones & Bartlett.

McFarland, M. R., & Wehbe-Alamah, H. B. (2019). Leininger's theory of culture care diversity and universality: An overview with a historical retrospective and a view toward the future. *Journal of Transcultural Nursing*, 30(6), 540–557. doi:10.1177/1043659619867134.

Moss, M. P. (2016). *American Indian health and nursing*. University of Oklahoma Press.

Office of Disease Prevention and Health Promotion. (2020). *Health people 2030*. https://www.healthy-people.gov/

Robert Woods Johnson Foundation. (2014). *Charting nursing's future*. Robert Woods Johnson Foundation.

Strauss, A. L. (1994). *Qualitative analysis for social scientists*. Cambridge University.

Tribal Health Department. (2020). *Community health assessment*. Same as author.

United Nations. (1948). *The universal declaration of human rights*. United Nations. https://www.un.org/en/universal-declaration-human-rights/

U.S. Census Bureau (2018). *American Community Survey 5-year estimates*. http://censusreporter.org/profiles/04000US30-montana/

SECTION V

Vulnerable Populations

Section V focuses on nursing care of vulnerable populations. This section includes three new chapters and one chapter updated from the previous edition. Authors of the new chapters focus on the healthcare needs of migrant and seasonal farmworkers (Chapter 28), American Indian perspectives on palliative and end-of-life care (Chapter 29), and neonates in opioid withdrawal and the rise of neonatal abstinence syndrome (Chapter 30). The remaining chapter updates strategies needed to conduct research with a vulnerable population (Chapter 31).

CHAPTER 28

Risks to Safety and Health for Migrant and Seasonal Farmworkers

SALLY MOYCE

DISCUSSION TOPICS

- Migrant and seasonal farmworkers (MSFWs) face risks to health due to their migratory lifestyle, their socio-economic position, and a potential lack of legal authorization to live in the United States. Brainstorm potential ways nurses may work with social workers, outreach workers, and other health personnel to meet the needs of this population.
- While MSFWs face health risks due to occupational exposures, many poor health conditions result from places where the workers live. Discuss potential hazards that may be present in farmworker homes that could threaten health. Provide potential solutions to help mitigate these risks.
- Nurses working in migrant health centers know that services should be provided at a single visit, so as not to lose the patient to follow up. Propose roles for other health professionals who should be included in the patient's care to provide wrap-around services in a single visit.
- How might nurses work with Migrant Head Start or the school system to provide essential screening, immunization, and health promotion activities for children who move with their parents or are exposed to agricultural hazards.

INTRODUCTION

In 2020, an estimated 272 million people worldwide were immigrants, and two-thirds of those left their country of origin for employment opportunities in other countries (McAuliffe et al., 2019). The largest driver of labor migration is economic disparity in one's country of origin and the search for work in a host country. In the United States, an estimated 2.4 million persons are migrant and seasonal farmworkers (MSFWs). International migration is an important part of global social and economic development. Immigrant workers contribute to the economies of their home countries via remittances, or money sent back to home countries, which totaled $689 billion in 2018 (McAuliffe et al., 2019). They also develop new skills that are potentially used upon their return. In addition, migrants provide needed labor and skills to the host countries. However, migration is a complex issue that presents challenges in ensuring equal protection of migrant workers, particularly in relation to occupational health. This chapter discusses the occupational safety and health of MSFWs, a group of immigrant laborers who have shouldered higher occupational health risks than the native-born population and who require specialized nursing skills to meet their needs.

MIGRANT AND SEASONAL WORKERS

Definitions

The term migrant is used in many contexts, often to refer to a person from another country who works in agriculture. However, healthcare reimbursement mechanisms require a standardized definition when providing care to this special population. Therefore, an understanding of the federal definitions of terms is important. A migrant farmworker is someone who leaves their permanent residence for work in the agricultural sector. This person often follows the crops as they harvest, moving from south to north as temperatures and seasons change. A seasonal farmworker, in contrast, does not leave their home to work in agriculture. This individual is employed in agriculture only seasonally, or when the harvest requires. They may have other sources of income. While most farmworkers in the United States are immigrant laborers – mostly from Mexico and South America – immigration from a foreign country is not a requirement to meet these definitions. The definition of agricultural work is broad – persons may be employed in harvesting fruits or vegetables, working in canneries or meat/fish packing plants, or in nurseries, dairies, or ranches.

Funded by the U.S. Department of Labor, the National Agricultural Workers Survey (NAWS) is an important source of information about this group. Findings from the survey revealed that only 16% of respondents were actual migrant workers. Most were seasonal and almost 85% reported they did not have full-time employment (Hernandez & Gabbard, 2019). Some international migrant farmworkers come to the United States on guest worker visas, called H2A visas. These visas require that a worker is sponsored by an agricultural employer and last only as long as the work lasts. The NAWS found that approximately one half of the workers surveyed lacked any legal authorization to live and work in the United States, and the lack of documentation put them at risk for occupational exploitation and negative health outcomes.

Health and Safety Risks in the Occupational Setting

The work of MSFWs has been labeled as 3-D—dirty, dangerous, and degrading (Quandt et al., 2013). These jobs lack the protections other positions may have and result in lower pay, longer working hours, and poor conditions for migrant workers. Agriculture is the most dangerous occupation in the United States and has a fatality rate of 22.8 fatalities per 100,000 workers, compared to an overall fatality rate of 3.4 fatalities per 100,000 workers in all other industries (Bureau of Labor Statistics, 2016). MSFWs experience occupational morbidities at rates that are higher than other occupations, as well, and are at risk for musculoskeletal injuries, lacerations, falls, accidents with farm animals or heavy machinery, exposure to pesticides and chemicals, and adverse weather.

The higher rates of occupational morbidity and mortality among MSFWs may be attributed to a variety of factors, including inherent risks in the jobs themselves and the lack of training and protection for immigrant workers. Some of the additional risks shouldered by the immigrant workforce are inherent in the jobs themselves, such as exposures to hazardous environmental conditions. Other risks are due to the workers' position in society, including their socio-economic status, and barriers to accessing healthcare. These are discussed in the next section.

WORKPLACE HAZARDS

Despite regulations in many occupational settings, safety standards in places where immigrant workers are employed are not always followed (Moyce & Schenker, 2018). For example, while personal protective equipment (PPE) is required, it may be up to the worker to provide their own equipment or the costs of the equipment are deducted from the worker's paycheck (Quandt et al., 2006). Additionally, safety trainings may not be offered in the worker's native language or, due to a migratory lifestyle, the worker may miss the trainings at the beginning of the season (Liebman et al., 2016). However, due to the dangerous nature of the work, safety trainings and adherence to state and federal regulations are essential to protecting health.

EXTREME WEATHER

Agricultural work exposes workers to temperature extremes and weather events including hail, freezing fog, and lightning strikes. Work often starts before dawn, when temperatures are low, and continues into the late afternoon, when summer temperatures exceed safe working conditions recommended by the National Institute of Occupational Safety and Health (NIOSH). Agricultural workers in the United States die from heat-related illness at a rate that is 20 times that of all other occupations (Centers for Disease Control and Prevention, 2013). Workers employed in fishing experience the opposite exposure, and frequent contact with ice cold water leads to hypothermia (Garcia & De Castro, 2016).

EXPOSURE TO HAZARDOUS CHEMICALS

Employed in jobs that are dangerous entail coming into contact with hazardous chemicals, and immigrant workers have high rates of chemical exposures. For example, migrants who work in agriculture are exposed to pesticides and herbicides daily. In the United States, 2.1 billion pounds of pesticides are applied each year, although injury data related to pesticides are only reported by 12 states to NIOSH. NIOSH estimates injury rates of 18.6/100,000 workers (Calvert, 2016). An estimated 88% of pesticide-related injuries and illnesses go unreported (Prado et al., 2017). Pesticides are designed to be toxic and potent, and MSFWs are repeatedly exposed to these chemicals in the application of pesticides and when harvesting pesticide-treated crops. Workers and families who live near agricultural fields are also at risk due to pesticide drift. Additionally, workers may inadvertently bring pesticide residue into their homes on their clothes and boots. Pesticide exposure has been linked to a variety of health concerns, including respiratory illness, dermatological conditions, cancer, and reproductive disorders (García-García et al., 2016; Gomes et al., 1999).

PHYSICAL DEMANDS

The agricultural sector has high rates of musculoskeletal injury. Farmers and ranchers risk injury from large animals, crush injuries from machines, falls, and repetitive motion injuries (Liebman et al., 2016). In one study, researchers found tractor injuries to be more dangerous and fatal than high-speed motorcycle accidents (Eraybar et al., 2019). Tractors create back injury due to the constant vibrating motion and the need to turn and look over one's shoulder when towing something (Cardenas et al., 2018).

WORKPLACE ABUSE

The immigrant worker experiences more abuse on the job than a native-born worker. Those employed in day labor – an work arrangement that lasts for a short period of time without a formal contract – experience wage theft and threats of termination from employment on a regular basis (Haro et al., 2020). These jobs rarely provide protective measures from potential exposures, and due to the lack of a formal contract, limit the ability of the worker to advocate on their own behalf (Fuentes et al., 2016). Other abuses at the workplace include verbal abuse, discrimination, and sexual assault (Fava et al., 2020; Villegas, 2019).

Labor trafficking is relatively high in developed nations, including the United States. An estimated 14.2 million persons worldwide are trafficked into jobs in the manufacturing, agricultural, construction, or domestic work sectors (International Labor Organization, 2017; Weiss, 2015). While sex trafficking often gets more attention in the media and research, labor trafficking is higher in the United States and often involves children (Koegler et al., 2019). Persons who are trafficked may receive little to no wages for long and arduous work without the ability to leave their employment situation. The individual's passport may have been confiscated, and the person is forced to work under threats to their personal safety or the safety of their family (Logan et al., 2009). Trafficked workers experience trauma that leads to depression, anxiety, post-traumatic stress disorder, and substance abuse (Hopper et al., 2018).

Social and Economic Hazards

POVERTY

Manual farmwork has been deemed *unskilled* labor, despite the actual skill required to pick, clean, and pack produce. This deskilling of the work results in low wages. MSFWs often earn wages that are below the federal poverty level and live in poverty. According to the NAWS, the average annual income for an MSFW was about $18,000. Thirty-three percent of those surveyed had family incomes below the federal poverty level (Hernandez & Gabbard, 2019). Despite earning relatively little, MSFWs send money home – either to their home countries or to their homes in the United States – to support their families. Some workers have housing provided by their employer, but most must pay for their own housing. Their low incomes lead many to share housing, which means they live in overcrowded settings. Many pay for transportation to and from work, PPE, and in some cases, water at the worksite (Villarejo, 2003).

Poverty contributes to a host of health problems, one of them being food insecurity. Even though they contribute to the food supply in the United States, MSFWs are often food insecure. A lack of nutritious food results in many chronic illnesses, including obesity, cardiovascular disease, and diabetes (Smith & Cuesta, 2018). Other health concerns related to poverty arise when workers live in crowded, substandard housing; when they lack access to running water or refrigeration; and when they do not have money for transportation to access health or social services.

LANGUAGE AND CULTURAL BARRIERS

MSFWs often do not speak the primary language of the host country and may not understand important safety trainings at the worksite. Perhaps due to this language barrier, workers who have lower levels of education or limited language proficiency also suffer more occupational injuries than those with higher levels of education or better language skills. Safety warnings and signs are often posted in the host language and are ineffective in protecting a worker who cannot read what they say (Liebman et al., 2016; Moyce & Schenker, 2018).

Language barriers limit access to resources for MSFWs. Some states offer workers' compensation benefits to anyone employed in agriculture, regardless of legal authorization to work status, and if a worker is injured on the job but does not know that he has compensation, he may lose wages until he recovers. Worse, and far too often, a worker may continue to work through an injury so as not to lose wages.

Cultural differences between MSFWs and their host communities can lead to several adverse health outcomes. Culturally inappropriate care leads to delaying needed medical care or not following medical advice. MSFWs are at risk for low-quality care and more expensive care due to misunderstandings about where to access care. The cultural divide between a farmworker patient and a provider may lead to isolation, feelings of stress, and exacerbated illness (Kim-Godwin & Bechtel, 2004).

HEALTH INSURANCE AND ACCESS TO CARE

Employers of seasonal or temporary workers often do not offer health insurance. Immigrant workers may not be authorized to work in the United States, and while the Affordable Care Act (ACA) extended health insurance benefits to many individuals, it did not include coverage for undocumented persons. One of the most significant barriers to accessing healthcare is a lack of health insurance or the economic means to pay for medical care (Hoffman & Paradise, 2008). If a worker is injured on the job or loses a job, there is no safety net available to help with medical costs, which can create a significant financial burden (Sano et al., 2011). Language barriers can provide an additional barrier, as MSFWs who do not speak English may not understand how to apply for insurance or may be unclear about what health insurance is or the terms associated with it. Additionally, if a worker is undocumented, he may be anxious about filling out paperwork or may think he does not have the necessary documentation to apply for insurance (Olukotun et al., 2019).

Other barriers to accessing care include not knowing where to go for services or how the services in the host country are offered. MSFWs often live on the farms where they are employed or live in rural areas close to agricultural fields. These isolated areas have a limited supply of healthcare providers, and a lack of transportation makes it difficult for MSFWs to get to appointments (Preibisch & Otero, 2014). Often, workdays are long with inflexible hours and include weekend hours, which limit a worker's ability to schedule an appointment. MSFWs are rarely given paid time off, which means attending to a health concern results in lost wages. Cultural differences and attitudes about health and language barriers make communicating with providers difficult, as well (Ahmed et al., 2016; Edward & Biddle, 2017; Luque et al., 2018).

AUTHORIZATION TO WORK

Workers who do not have documentation or legal authorization to work are more than twice as likely to experience wage violations compared to workers who have legal documentation (Bernhardt et al., 2009). Undocumented workers are often afraid to complain about unjust working conditions, stolen wages, or safety violations for fear of being deported and a lack of legal options available to those without legal status. In addition, workers who are in the country illegally are excluded from legal protections designed to keep workers safe (Flynn et al., 2015). They are also unable to access various services, including health insurance, workers' compensation, and driver's licenses (Flynn et al., 2015). Unauthorized workers experience high levels of stress related to their immigration status.

In the United States, workers who are hired under work visas (H-2 visas) are guaranteed certain occupational protections, including contracted wages, workers' compensation benefits, and the legal right to live in the United States. However, these visas are directly tied to the work and are sponsored by the employer, and if the worker loses the job, they lose the legal authority to live in the United States. Therefore, workers are reluctant to complain about unsafe conditions for fear of losing the right to live in the United States. This creates an incentive for the worker to continue working, even in dangerous conditions (Liebman et al., 2013; Moyce & Schenker, 2018).

Other Factors

CHILDREN

There are an estimated one million migrant children in the United States. Children of MSFWs may move with their parents, which means they lack regular access to school or a pediatrician. Children who are constantly on the move often miss important vaccinations or well-child checks. Alternatively, if the parents do not have the child's medical records, the child may be over-immunized. Children whose parents are unauthorized to work in the United States often miss medical appointments due to a parent's fear of accessing health services. If children do not move with their parents, they are likely to live in poverty near agricultural worksites. Living near agricultural fields put children at risk for pesticide drift, and pesticide exposure has been linked to delayed development among children (Eskenazi et al., 2014).

Children who grow up in agricultural settings are at risk for injuries on the farms. Parents who are unable to afford childcare bring their children to work with them where they are exposed to pesticides, heat stress, organic dusts, and zoonotic diseases. Children who are employed in farmwork often enter at a young age and are too small for PPE and are at increased risk for injuries because they are too young to understand safety trainings or to read warning signs (Arcury et al., 2019).

FEMALE GENDER

Women in farmwork experience sexual harassment and assault. They often delay using the toilet due to fears of being sexually assaulted in the bathrooms (Moyce et al., 2017). Women who migrate because of their partner's employment find themselves in a double role of being a family caregiver while also needing to earn money in the local economy. If a family has children, the woman traditionally shoulders the childcare responsibilities. Her work is secondary to her role in the home, and in order to work, she must find adequate and affordable childcare. This can present a challenge and limit the type of work a woman can obtain, and many women settle for lower-paying, hourly work rather than a full-time job to manage their childcare responsibilities (Bonizzoni, 2014).

If a woman experiences intimate partner violence, her health is at risk, but particularly if she is an immigrant. A woman may not have a source of community support outside of her home. Reporting her husband or partner to the authorities means losing the only social structure she has. If she is undocumented or without legal authorization to live in the host country, she is at even greater risk because she is unlikely to leave her partner or seek help due to her own fears of deportation and retribution (Rai & Choi, 2018). Women who feel a strong sense of family obligation or a religious requirement to stay in a marriage may experience cultural dissonance with social service agencies or nurses who encourage her to leave an abusive situation (Ghafournia, 2017).

RURAL LOCATIONS

The rural location of farmwork puts MSFWs at risk for poor health outcomes. Rural communities are not always accepting outsiders/newcomers (Long & Weinert, 1989; also See Chapter 2) , nor are they accustomed to persons of diverse backgrounds and may not have the health infrastructure established to provide services in a culturally and linguistically appropriate manner (Jensen, 2006). Providers who speak languages other than English are rare in rural healthcare facilities, and immigrant workers do not trust that interpreters – often accessed over the phone – are conveying their messages correctly (Greder & Reina, 2019). Discrimination is higher among immigrants in rural settings compared to urban settings and may discourage workers from seeking health services (Greder & Reina, 2019; Jensen, 2006; Sangaramoorthy & Guevara, 2017).

In rural communities, services are often unavailable, inadequate, or at a greater distance than in urban settings, and public transportation may not exist. Immigrant workers who do not know how to drive or who cannot afford a car are often isolated from services or clinics. Women who work in the home caring for the family but who do not drive experience isolation, depression, and limitations on their ability to buy groceries or take a sick child to a clinic (Sano et al., 2011; Schmalzbauer, 2014). Rural communities also lack an ethnic enclave for immigrants to help with integration or cultural mediation (Raffaelli et al., 2012).

NURSING CARE FOR MIGRANT AND SEASONAL FARMWORKERS

The above health risks to this vulnerable population require a specialized skillset among nurses and healthcare providers. The health concerns are similar to those found in other at-risk populations, but MSFWs are at an increased disadvantage due to mobility, language and cultural barriers, lack of familiarity with local health resources, and limited health insurance coverage. The migratory lifestyle creates a particular set of challenges for MSFWs, especially if they need to manage a chronic health condition.

Role of the Nurse

The nurse may be the only connection an MSFW has with the health system, and if the nurse has a limited amount of time to interact with a patient, confronting the host of health issues may seem overwhelming. Nurses may focus on prevention techniques aimed at educating and protecting workers from injuries and illnesses. Nurses can do medication reconciliation to make sure patients understand their prescribed medications and have a long-term supply if a patient migrates. Nurses may also address the social determinants of health and ensure that the patient has adequate food, housing, transportation, or PPE. Nurses are instrumental in providing referral services and connecting patients to necessary care.

Some nurses practice in a mobile environment inside a specially equipped motorhome. These mobile clinics have all the supplies and equipment of a regular exam room and can be driven to migrant camps or towns where MSFWs live. Nurses can provide essential health screenings, education, and immunizations. These mobile clinics also have the advantage that they can operate after work hours or on days when workers are resting.

Nurses can also be advocates for MSFW patients in other clinical settings as well. Providing medical appointments during alternative hours, after work, can help patients access services. Ensuring that a patient has transportation to and from appointments increases the likelihood that a patient will attend a scheduled visit. Nurses may arrange for translation or interpreting services if they know a patient does not speak English. Nurses can also advocate for providing wrap-around services, designed to meet all the patient's needs in one place, or to *wrap around* the patient to fully support him. Bundling appointments with the provider, a social worker, the diabetes educator, and a health insurance specialist make it easier to meet the patient's needs rather than scheduling separate appointments for each service. Clinics that have on-site pharmacies can offer medications to MSFWs, often at reduced costs, which can improve medication compliance.

The nurse may need to navigate cultural and language barriers with the patient, as well. Working with an interpreter is a learned skill and requires practice. Nurses should avoid using a family member as an interpreter. When a family member is asked to interpret, messages can be missed or not communicated due to a lack of understanding medical terminology. Asking a child to interpret for an adult puts an unfair burden on the child, especially if grave news needs to be delivered. When at all possible, a medical interpreter should be provided. These trained professionals can often be accessed over the telephone. When speaking to a patient through an interpreter, the nurse must remember that the patient is the center of the visit. The interpreter, if in person, should be positioned behind the patient, and the nurse should speak directly to the patient, not to the interpreter. Avoid side conversations with the interpreter, as they may be misconstrued as conversations about the patient. The nurse should speak slowly and in short segments, allowing time for the interpreter to translate messages. These appointments may take longer than other appointments and should not be rushed.

Working with Victims of Trafficking

Nurses may unknowingly care for a victim of human trafficking, as trafficked persons may have reason to visit a healthcare provider while in employment bondage. Nurses who are aware of the potential for human trafficking can screen for signs of abuse and can connect individuals with resources. A nurse should be alert to a potential trafficking situation when a person accompanying a patient refuses to allow the patient to be examined alone. If possible, a nurse can ask questions to assess the patient's safety, including questions about the patient's ability to act independently, carry identification, or leave their current employment (Polaris Project, 2011) (See Table 28.1).

Careful documentation about the suspected abuse and collaboration with a social worker to assist the patient to safety is important. Nurses can also contact the National Human Trafficking Resource Center for advice (Coppola & Cantwell, 2016).

IMPROVING ACCESS TO CARE FOR MSFWS

To provide consistent services to MSFWs as they move around the country, some primary care clinics are part of the Migrants Clinicians Network. Federal funding for providers who serve MSFWs is available through the Bureau of Primary Health Care from the Health Resources and Services Administration (HRSA). The Migrant Clinicians Network provides support to providers through trainings, workforce development, and advocacy efforts.

TABLE 28.1 Questions to Ask a Suspected Victim of Trafficking

Is it safe for you to talk to me right now?

Is there anything I can do to make you feel safer?

When you are working, are you able to leave if you choose?

Are you able to use the bathroom independently when you want?

Do you have consistent access to food? Are you ever forced to go without food?

How are you paid? Are you paid the full amount you are owed?

Are there locks on the windows and doors where you live or work or sleep?

Are you allowed to communicate with your family or friends?

Do you have control over your own personal documents?

Have you been threatened or harmed in any way by your employer? Has your family?

Another federally funded program is the Migrant Health Program from the National Center for Farmworker Health, Inc. This organization offers grant funding to health centers who care for MSFWs. Many of these clinics provide health services on a sliding-scale fee or without cost to those who qualify. This network of community clinics allows providers to communicate in anticipation of an MSFW patient's arrival and to coordinate care when the patient moves to a new site.

A specialized education program targeting young children of MSFWs is the Migrant Head Start Program. Funded by the U.S. Department of Health and Human Services (2020), these programs provide early childhood development programs to children from infancy to 5 years of age. Services are offered in education, transportation, nutrition, emotion, and family development.

CONCLUSION

Despite their importance to the nation's agricultural sector, MSFWs are an invisible population. The mobile lifestyle, occupational hazards, and unique socio-cultural position of MSFWs create a host of potential risks for poor health. Nurses working with this vulnerable population can provide quality care in a culturally and linguistically sensitive manner. Understanding the health risks may inform questions the nurse asks in a clinical setting. A comprehensive occupational evaluation or an awareness of the potential for pesticide exposure, for example, may help identify the source of non-specific health symptoms. Nurses who work with migrant populations can ensure patients have adequate medications and referrals to services in the patient's next destination. Additionally, creative service delivery options may offer healthcare options to a population who may otherwise go without adequate care.

REFERENCES

Ahmed, S., Shommu, N. S., Rumana, N., Barron, G. R., Wicklum, S., & Turin, T. C. (2016). Barriers to access of primary healthcare by immigrant populations in Canada: A literature review. *Journal of Immigrant and Minority Health, 18*(6), 1522–1540. https://doi.org/10.1007/s10903-015-0276-z

Arcury, T. A., Arnold, T. J., Mora, D. C., Sandberg, J. C., Daniel, S. S., Wiggins, M. F., & Quandt, S. A. (2019). "Be careful!" Perceptions of work-safety culture among hired Latinx child farmworkers in North Carolina. *American Journal of Industrial Medicine, 62*(12), 1091–1102. https://doi.org/10.1002/ajim.23045

Bernhardt, A., Milkman, R., Theodore, N., Heckathorn, D. D., Auer, M., DeFilippis, J., González, A. L., Narro, V., & Perelshteyn, J. (2009). *Broken laws, unprotected workers: Violations of employment and labor laws in America's cities*. University of California, Los Angeles. http://escholarship.org/uc/item/1vn389nh.pdf

Bonizzoni, P. (2014). Immigrant working mothers reconciling work and childcare: The experience of Latin American and Eastern European women in Milan. *Social Politics, 21*(2), 194–217. https://doi.org/10.1093/sp/jxu008

Bureau of Labor Statistics. (2016). *Foreign-born workers: Labor force characteristics—2015*. U.S. Department of Labor. http://www.census.gov/content/dam/Census/library/working-papers/2015/demo/POP-twps0103.pdf

Calvert, G. M. (2016). Acute occupational pesticide-related illness and injury—United States, 2007–2011. *MMWR. Morbidity and Mortality Weekly Report, 63*, 11–16. https://doi.org/10.15585/mmwr.mm6355a3

Cardenas, V. M., Cen, R., Clemens, M. M., Conner, J. L., Victory, J. L., Stallones, L., & Delongchamp, R. R. (2018). Morbidity and mortality from farm tractor and other agricultural machinery-related injuries in Arkansas. *Journal of Agricultural Safety and Health, 24*(4), 213–225. https://doi.org/10.13031/jash.12828

Centers for Disease Control and Prevention. (2013). *Preventing heat-related illness or death of outdoor workers*. U.S. Department of Health and Human Services, Public Health Service, Centers for Disease Control and Prevention, National Institute for Occupational Safety and Health. https://doi.org/10.26616/NIOSHPUB2013143

Coppola, J. S., & Cantwell, R. (2016). Health professional role in identifying and assessing victims of human labor trafficking. *The Journal for Nurse Practitioners, 12*(5), e193–e200. https://doi.org/10.1016/j.nurpra.2016.01.004

Edward, J., & Biddle, D. J. (2017). Using geographic information systems (GIS) to examine barriers to healthcare access for Hispanic and Latino immigrants in the US south. *Journal of Racial and Ethnic Health Disparities, 4*(2), 297–307. https://doi.org/10.1007/s40615-016-0229-9

Eraybar, S., Atmaca, S., Nennicioglu, Y., Torun, G., Aydin, O., Varisli, B., Sandal, N., Buyukyilmaz, T., Seyit, M., & Yildirim, H. (2019). Comparison of fatal injuries resulting from tractor and high speed motorcycle accidents in Turkey: A multicenter study. *Emergency Medicine International, 2019*. https://doi.org/10.1155/2019/9471407

Eskenazi, B., Kogut, K., Huen, K., Harley, K. G., Bouchard, M., Bradman, A., Boyd-Barr, D., Johnson, C., & Holland, N. (2014). Organophosphate pesticide exposure, PON1, and neurodevelopment in school-age children from the CHAMACOS study. *Environmental Research, 134*, 149–157. https://doi.org/10.1016/j.envres.2014.07.001

Fava, N. M., Sanchez, M., Wuyke, G., Diez-Morel, S., Vazquez, V., Ravelo, G. J., Villalba, K., & Rojas, P. (2020). Associations between sexual trauma and sexual relationship power among Latina immigrant farmworkers: The moderating role of gender norms. *Journal of Traumatic Stress, 33*, 1093–1101. https://doi.org/10.1002/jts.22561

Flynn, M. A., Eggerth, D. E., & Jacobson, C. J. (2015). Undocumented status as a social determinant of occupational safety and health: The workers' perspective. *American Journal of Industrial Medicine, 58*(11), 1127–1137. https://doi.org/10.1002/ajim.22531

Fuentes, C. M. D., Pantoja, L. M., Tarver, M., Geschwind, S. A., & Lara, M. (2016). Latino immigrant day laborer perceptions of occupational safety and health information preferences. *American Journal of Industrial Medicine, 59*(6), 476–485. https://doi.org/10.1002/ajim.22575

Garcia, G. M., & De Castro, B. (2016). Working conditions, occupational injuries, and health among Filipino fish processing workers in Dutch Harbor, Alaska. *Workplace Health & Safety, 65*(5), 219–226. https://doi.org/10.1177/2165079916665396

García-García, C. R., Parrón, T., Requena, M., Alarcón, R., Tsatsakis, A. M., & Hernández, A. F. (2016). Occupational pesticide exposure and adverse health effects at the clinical, hematological and biochemical level. *Life Sciences, 145*, 274–283. https://doi.org/10.1016/j.lfs.2015.10.013

Ghafournia, N. (2017). Muslim women and domestic violence: Developing a framework for social work practice. *Journal of Religion & Spirituality in Social Work: Social Thought, 36*(1–2), 146–163. https://doi.org/10.1080/15426432.2017.1313150

Gomes, J., Lloyd, O. L., & Revitt, D. M. (1999). The influence of personal protection, environmental hygiene and exposure to pesticides on the health of immigrant farm workers in a desert country. *International Archives of Occupational and Environmental Health*, 72(1), 40–45. https://doi.org/10.1007/s004200050332

Greder, K., & Reina, A. S. (2019). Procuring health: Experiences of Mexican immigrant women in rural midwestern communities. *Qualitative Health Research*, 29(9), 1334–1344. https://doi.org/10.1177/1049732318816676

Haro, A. Y., Kuhn, R., Rodriguez, M. A., Theodore, N., Melendez, E., & Valenzuela, A. (2020). Beyond occupational hazards: Abuse of day laborers and health. *Journal of Immigrant and Minority Health*, 22(6), 1172–1183. https://doi.org/10.1007/s10903-020-01094-3

Hernandez, T., & Gabbard, S. (2019). *Findings from the National Agricultural Workers Survey (NAWS) 2015–2016. A demographic and employment profile of United States farmworkers* (No. 13). JBS International. https://www.dol.gov/sites/dolgov/files/ETA/naws/pdfs/NAWS_Research_Report_13.pdf

Hoffman, C., & Paradise, J. (2008). Health insurance and access to health care in the United States. *Annals of the New York Academy of Sciences*, 1136(1), 149–160. https://doi.org/10.1196/annals.1425.007

Hopper, E. K., Azar, N., Bhattacharyya, S., Malebranche, D. A., & Brennan, K. E. (2018). STARS experiential group intervention: A complex trauma treatment approach for survivors of human trafficking. *Journal of Evidence-Informed Social Work*, 15(2), 215–241. https://doi.org/10.1080/23761407.2018.1455616

International Labor Organization. (2017). *Global estimates of modern slavery: Forced labour and forced marriage*. http://www.ilo.org/global/topics/forced-labour/lang--en/index.htm

Jensen, L. (2006). *New immigrant settlements in rural America: Problems, prospects, and policies* (Vol. 1). Carsey Institute. https://scholars.unh.edu/cgi/viewcontent.cgi?article=1016&context=carsey

Kim-Godwin, Y. S., & Bechtel, G. A. (2004). Stress among migrant and seasonal farmworkers in rural southeast North Carolina. *The Journal of Rural Health*, 20(3), 271–278. https://doi.org/10.1111/j.1748-0361.2004.tb00039.x

Koegler, E., Mohl, A., Preble, K., & Teti, M. (2019). Reports and victims of sex and labor trafficking in a major Midwest metropolitan area, 2008–2017. *Public Health Reports*, 134(4), 432–440. https://doi.org/10.1177/0033354919854479

Liebman, A. K., Juarez-Carrillo, P. M., Reyes, I. A. C., & Keifer, M. C. (2016). Immigrant dairy workers' perceptions of health and safety on the farm in America's Heartland. *American Journal of Industrial Medicine*, 59(3), 227–235. https://doi.org/10.1002/ajim.22538

Liebman, A. K., Wiggins, M. F., Fraser, C., Levin, J., Sidebottom, J., & Arcury, T. A. (2013). Occupational health policy and immigrant workers in the agriculture, forestry, and fishing sector. *American Journal of Industrial Medicine*, 56(8), 975–984. https://doi.org/10.1002/ajim.22190

Logan, T. K., Walker, R., & Hunt, G. (2009). Understanding human trafficking in the United States. *Trauma, Violence, & Abuse*, 10(1), 3–30. https://doi.org/10.1177/1524838008327262

Long, K. A., & Weinert, C. (1989). Rural nursing: Developing the theory base. *Scholarly Inquiry for Nursing Practice: An International Journal*, 3(2), 113–127.

Luque, J. S., Soulen, G., Davila, C. B., & Cartmell, K. (2018). Access to health care for uninsured Latina immigrants in South Carolina. *BMC Health Services Research*, 18(1), 310. https://doi.org/10.1186/s12913-018-3138-2

McAuliffe, M., James, Khadria, B., & International Organization for Migration. (2019). *World migration report 2020*. https://publications.iom.int/system/files/pdf/wmr_2020.pdf

Moyce, S. C., & Schenker, M. (2018). Migrant workers and their occupational health and safety. *Annual Review of Public Health*, 39, 351–365. https://doi.org/10.1146/annurev-publhealth-040617-013714

Moyce, S., Mitchell, D., Armitage, T., Tancredi, D., Joseph, J., & Schenker, M. (2017). Heat strain, volume depletion and kidney function in California agricultural workers. *Occupational & Environmental Medicine*, 74(6), 402–409. https://doi.org/10.1136/oemed-2016-103848

Olukotun, O., Mkandawire-Valhmu, L., & Kako, P. (2019). Navigating complex realities: Barriers to health care access for undocumented African immigrant women in the United States. *Health Care for Women International*, 42(2), 145–164. https://doi.org/10.1080/07399332.2019.1640703

Polaris Project. (2011). *Human trafficking assessment for domestic workers*. National Human Trafficking Resource Center. https://humantraffickinghotline.org/sites/default/files/Assessment%20Tool%20for%20Domestic%20Workers.pdf

Prado, J. B., Mulay, P. R., Kasner, E. J., Bojes, H. K., & Calvert, G. M. (2017). Acute pesticide-related illness among farmworkers: Barriers to reporting to public health authorities. *Journal of Agromedicine*, 22(4), 395–405. https://doi.org/10.1080/1059924X.2017.1353936

Preibisch, K., & Otero, G. (2014). Does citizenship status matter in Canadian agriculture? Workplace health and safety for migrant and immigrant laborers. *Rural Sociology*, 79(2), 174–199. https://doi.org/10.1111/ruso.12043

Quandt, S. A., Arcury-Quandt, A. E., Lawlor, E. J., Carrillo, L., Marín, A. J., Grzywacz, J. G., & Arcury, T. A. (2013). 3-D jobs and health disparities: The health implications of Latino chicken catchers' working conditions. *American Journal of Industrial Medicine*, 56(2), 206–215. https://doi.org/10.1002/ajim.22072

Quandt, S. A., Grzywacz, J. G., Marín, A., Carrillo, L., Coates, M. L., Burke, B., & Arcury, T. A. (2006). Illnesses and injuries reported by Latino poultry workers in western North Carolina. *American Journal of Industrial Medicine*, 49(5), 343–351. https://doi.org/10.1002/ajim.20299

Raffaelli, M., Tran, S. P., Wiley, A. R., Galarza-Heras, M., & Lazarevic, V. (2012). Risk and resilience in rural communities: The experiences of immigrant Latina mothers. *Family Relations*, 61(4), 559–570. https://doi.org/10.1111/j.1741-3729.2012.00717.x

Rai, A., & Choi, Y. J. (2018). Socio-cultural risk factors impacting domestic violence among South Asian immigrant women: A scoping review. *Aggression and Violent Behavior*, 38, 76–85. https://doi.org/10.1016/j.avb.2017.12.001

Sangaramoorthy, T., & Guevara, E. M. (2017). Immigrant health in rural Maryland: A qualitative study of major barriers to health care access. *Journal of Immigrant and Minority Health*, 19(4), 939–946. https://doi.org/10.1007/s10903-016-0417-z

Sano, Y., Garasky, S., Greder, K. A., Cook, C. C., & Browder, D. E. (2011). Understanding food insecurity among Latino immigrant families in rural America. *Journal of Family and Economic Issues*, 32(1), 111–123. https://doi.org/10.1007/s10834-010-9219-y

Schmalzbauer, L. (2014). *The last best place?: Gender, family, and migration in the New West*. Stanford University Press.

Smith, J., & Cuesta, G. (2018). Hunger in the fields: Food insecurity and food access among farmworker families in Migrant and Seasonal Head Start. *Journal of Latinos and Education*, 9(3), 1–12. https://doi.org/10.1080/15348431.2018.1500291

United States Department of Health and Human Services Office of Head Start. (2020). *Head start services*. https://www.acf.hhs.gov/ohs/about/head-start

Villarejo, D. (2003). The health of US hired farm workers. *Annual Review of Public Health*, 24(1), 175–193.

Villegas, P. E. (2019). "I made myself small like a cat and ran away": Workplace sexual harassment, precarious immigration status and legal violence. *Journal of Gender Studies*, 28(6), 674–686. https://doi.org/10.1080/09589236.2019.1604326

Weiss, M. S. (2015). Human trafficking and forced labor: A primer. *ABA Journal of Labor & Employment Law*, 31(1), 1.

CHAPTER 29

American Indian Perspectives on Palliative and End-of-Life Care

YOSHIKO Y. COLCLOUGH AND MARY J. ISAACSON

DISCUSSION TOPICS

- Discuss how to engage with American Indian (AI) communities in a culturally respectful manner using community-based participatory principles.
- Describe opportunities for development of palliative and end-of-life (EOL) care with AI communities.
- Identify challenges for implementing and sustaining palliative and EOL care in tribal communities.

INTRODUCTION

In the United States, there are 574 federally recognized tribes across 35 states (National Congress of American Indians, 2020). According to the 2010 U.S. Census, about 5.2 million (1.6%) reported their race as American Indian/Alaska Native (AI/AN) and 2.9 million (0.9%) reported AI/AN as their only race (U.S. Census Bureau, 2012). Fifty-four percent of AIs/ANs live in rural regions, with 68% residing in or close to their tribal reservation (Rural Health Information Hub, 2018a).

In the following, two nurse scientists briefly review healthcare services for AI/AN people, define hospice and palliative care, and describe their individual approaches to understanding end-of-life (EOL) and palliative care in two AI tribal communities. They conclude with lessons learned and implications for rural nursing practice, research, and education.

INDIAN HEALTH SERVICE

Provision of healthcare services is a "federal promise" granted to federally recognized AI/AN tribes through treaties with the federal government (National Indian Health Board, 2015, p. 1). The Indian Health Service (IHS) is the federally designated healthcare provider (HCP) for AIs/ANs from federally recognized tribes. Funding for IHS is appropriated from Congress through discretionary dollars and since its inception lacks sufficient funding to meet the basic healthcare needs of tribal communities (NCAI, 2016; Warne & Frizzell, 2014).

HOSPICE AND PALLIATIVE CARE

Palliative care seeks to enhance quality of life for patients with serious illness through the delivery of specialized medical care and can be used along with aggressive treatment (Center to Advance Palliative Care, n.d.). Hospice incorporates the same principles of palliative care; however, patients have a life expectancy of less than 6 months and are not seeking curative therapy (National Institute on Aging, 2017). Despite the benefits and supportive rules, use of hospice by the AI/AN population is significantly lower than Whites (0.4%/82.5%, respectively) (National Hospice and Palliative Care Organization, 2019). Due to the serious hospice use disparity for AI/AN populations, the National Institute of Nursing Research began soliciting for proposals in 2019 seeking *Strategies to Provide Culturally Tailored Palliative and EOL Care for Seriously Ill AI and AN Individuals*. Currently, the most common strategy to provide palliative and EOL care for AI/AN patients is to train HCPs to be culturally competent and sensitive. This is not sufficient. It is essential that prior to training HCPs, we must first understand the tribal communities' perspectives specific to death and dying. Then we must collaborate with these communities to culturally tailor palliative and EOL programs to these perspectives. This chapter describes two nurse scientists' (Y.C. & M.I.) individual approaches to understanding EOL and palliative care in two AI tribal communities.

BLACKFEET COMMUNITY HOSPICE PROJECT

This section describes opportunity, engagement, and challenges that the first author (Y.C.) experienced when beginning the hospice project as an academic partner of the Blackfeet Nation. First, an application of community-based participatory research (CBPR) is explained. An overview of the Blackfeet Nation, Y.C.'s academic transformation, and progress of the hospice project follow.

Community-Based Participatory Research

After 1 year of struggling and stagnating in seeking a minority-population partner to work on EOL care issues, a turning point arrived. The Montana Consortium for Community-Based Research in Health conducted two CBPR workshops in 2006. CBPR requires community involvement in every step of the research process to lead to direct benefits to the community and scientific discovery that benefits all (Wallerstein et al., 2017). Bringing together researchers and communities, establishes trust, shares power, fosters co-learning, enhances strengths and resources, builds capacity, and examines and addresses community-identified needs and health problems (Christopher et al., 2011; Israel et al., 2012; Wallerstein et al., 2017).

The two workshops were held separately to avoid any perceived coercion: one for community partners and the other for academic partners. Following the workshops, Consortium leaders introduced individuals with common interests, connecting Y.C. and the Director of Nursing (DON) at the IHS Blackfeet Community Hospital. Y.C. learned over time that there had been several earlier attempts to introduce hospice to the Blackfeet community; however, these efforts were not successful as they did not reach out to the public in a meaningful way. The DON requested that project development moves at a slow pace to ensure the success of the project and that an "open door" policy be created for project membership to enhance community involvement. All project development meetings and presentations of the study findings were held on the reservation with community members and healthcare workers participating.

Overview of the Blackfeet Nation

Montana is home to seven Indian reservations and one state-recognized nation (Montana. Gov, n.d.[a]). The Blackfeet Indian Reservation was established with a treaty in 1855. It is 1.5 million acres – one of the 10 largest reservations in the United States. It is located in a frontier setting in northwest Montana and bordered on the north by Canada and on the west by Glacier National Park. While it is home to the 17,321 member Blackfeet Nation, about 7,000 live on or near the reservation (Blackfeet Nation, 2020; Montana.Gov, n.d.[b]).

The Blackfeet shares similarities with the general AI/AN population. Their relational worldview values harmony and balance. Disease is not only a physical or psychologic ailment; rather, it is considered an imbalance among self, family, spiritual forces, community, other animals/creatures, and the environment (Bastien & Chief, 2004; Cohen, 2003/2006; Kahn-John, 2021). Many AIs are soft-spoken, observant, and use nonverbal communication styles with limited direct eye contact. Humor enhances their relationships and relieves tension. The oral tradition is a powerful method of transmitting traditional knowledge, values, beliefs, and ethical teaching to the next generation through stories, symbols, metaphors, and songs (Bastien & Chief, 2004; Cohen, 2003/2006). Thus, older adults are respected for their wisdom.

The family is central with AIs/ANs. Family includes extended kinships, where persons are considered family even if they are not related by blood. Families provide the foundation for a collective ideology through balance, harmony, and commitment to tribal life (Cohen, 2003/2006; Kahn-John, 2021). Spirituality is another key concept (Cohen, 2003/2006). Activities such as powwow, smudging, and prayers are ways of expressing spirituality. These activities honor and communicate with all beings and the creator to restore individual/collective balance, harmony, and healings (Colclough, 2017; Fitzgerald & Fitzgerald, 2006).

However, for the Blackfeet and other AI/AN tribes, their traditional worldviews have been gravely impacted by Euro-American contact. This contact has led to widespread abuses, such as loss of land, family, and identity resulting in historical trauma. Historical trauma or generational trauma is cumulative emotional and psychologic wounding emanating from massive group trauma (Brave Heart, 2003). It occurs across generations and explains AI/AN challenges with healthcare disparities, loss of identity, and their lack of trust toward IHS and Euro-Americans (Brave Heart et al., 2011).

Academic Transformation

The partnership with the Blackfeet initiated Y.C.'s academic transformation. The most intense challenges occurred in the first 2 to 3 years of the partnership, which Y.C. describes in three themes. These themes are (a) a psychologic-behavioral cycle, (b) a challenge of physical and psychologic distance, and (c) the process of initial transformation – attitude change from intrapersonal to interpersonal (Colclough, 2011).

First, Y.C.'s inexperience in CBPR along with her Type-A personality heightened her anxiety with facing uncertain circumstances and caused an internal vicious cycle. This cycle included extensive work to do her best, personal reflection of her individual work as unwilling paternalism, and deep concern that this individual work could be interpreted as exploitation. Since academic pressure of productivity threatened her, she hoped several factors would work in her favor to quickly establish trusting relationships. These factors included an Asian appearance similar to AIs, being a nurse, the most trusted professional, a communication style of less explicit and sensitive to nonverbal expression, and previous residency in the community. However, at her first meeting, tribal members were very inquisitive as to her reasons for being there. Y.C. was an outsider within the Blackfeet Community; thus, three to four meetings were necessary for tribal members to trust and share traditional knowledge with her.

Second, the challenges of physical (300 miles one way) and psychologic distance were eased by monthly interactions and additional personal visits with the community. Moreover, an invitation to the AI regional conference by the director of tribal health and the use of humor by community members buoyed her spirits. Finally, academic personal growth occurred when Y.C. realized the meaning of community involvement by changing her attitude from intrapersonal to interpersonal. Y.C. learned that asking for the community members' input and feedback was crucial, and that she needed to understand individual team member's priorities. Distance, once felt as an unavoidable obstacle, turned out to symbolize the remoteness of the community, which reflected its strength, endurance, and perseverance. Over time, the team matured along with progression of the project.

Development of the Blackfeet Community Hospice Project

With mentorships and financial support through internal and external grants, the infrastructure of the team was established. Project development began with an assessment study on EOL experiences from 58 tribal members who were affected by cancer (i.e., patients, family, and HCPs) to identify key values, describe contributing factors in EOL care, and develop a culturally appropriate intervention. Key findings were similar to previous studies (Avis et al., 2009; Caxaj et al., 2017; Centers for Medicare & Medicaid Services, 2017; Duggleby et al., 2015; Gebauer et al., 2016; Guadagnolo et al., 2014; Isaacson & Lynch, 2018). The assessment revealed that EOL experiences for ill family members were characterized as a struggle due to a lack of knowledge (e.g., unfamiliar word of hospice by both HCPs and community people and no or a misunderstanding of hospice) and feelings of conflict and ambivalence toward the Westernized practices (Colclough & Brown, 2014a). Moreover, it confirmed that a taboo perception on talking about death and dying prevailed on the reservation.

For those who knew about the Medicare hospice benefit, a choice of "do not resuscitate" and a requirement of a 6-month prognosis were additional barriers from the perspective of Blackfeet traditional values and beliefs for hospice use. Despite the Blackfeet Community's historical mistrust of White authority, study participants stated that they trust their physicians to give them direction regarding their care (Colclough & Brown, 2014b). They were not aware of autonomous/informed decision-making in healthcare, which implies a complicated and vacillating trust/mistrust relationship.

A period of project stagnation occurred when the team encountered difficulty achieving consensus among tribal stakeholders to make the project a priority. To affirm the team's commitment and validity of the project, the team conducted interviews with 10 older adults, who indicated support for continuation of the project. In 2017, the modified Duke EOL Care Survey (Johnson et al., 2009) was conducted with 92 survey participants.

The findings indicated a shift of taboo perception on the topic of death; 76% of the respondents noted feeling comfortable talking about death (Colclough & Brown, 2019b).

In October 2018, the community held a public workshop to increase awareness of the EOL care options. The workshop significantly increased the participants' (28 out of 30) EOL knowledge with positive evaluations noted (Colclough & Brown, 2019b). Organizing regular workshops to be held in new locations was supported in order to expand the project and to help overcome the taboo perception of hospice. In 2020, the project was placed on hold due to the COVID-19 pandemic restrictions.

SOUTH DAKOTA AI PERSPECTIVES ON PALLIATIVE AND END-OF-LIFE CARE

This section shares the second author's (M.I.) experience working as a collaborative partner with one specific South Dakota tribe. It begins with an overview of health disparities experienced by AIs in South Dakota, reviews the current palliative care climate in South Dakota, illustrates the process of CBPR with this tribal community in defining their unique understanding of palliative and EOL care, and concludes with a discussion on the development of an Elder-led advance care planning program.

American Indians in South Dakota

AIs comprise 9% of South Dakota's population (U.S. Census Bureau, 2019), yet suffer health disparities at a significantly higher rate than their White counterparts. Specifically, South Dakota AI women experience breast cancer at higher rates, are diagnosed at later stages, and have rising rates of late-stage breast cancer (South Dakota Department of Health, 2019). South Dakota AIs also have higher incidence and mortality rates from colorectal and lung cancer (SD DOH, 2019). In addition, AIs residing in the Northern Plains have greater prevalence of diabetes and heart disease (Blevins, 2017). Even with these higher morbidity and mortality rates, South Dakota AIs have limited or no access to palliative and EOL care (Isaacson et al., 2015).

As stated previously, IHS is the principal provider of healthcare to AIs. However, access to these services is challenging for South Dakota AIs related to the state's vast geographical landscape (Isaacson et al., 2016). For example, AI reservations and trust land comprise 12% of South Dakota's 77,116 square miles (U.S. Department of Justice, n.d.) and are located in predominantly rural or frontier (< 6 people/square mile) counties (Rural Health Information Hub, 2018b; U.S. Department of Agriculture, n.d.). The rurality of South Dakota's reservations, along with poor road conditions, unreliable transportation, and the inability to afford gas, compounds the host of issues associated with access to primary care services, let alone specialty services such as palliative care.

Palliative Care and South Dakota Reservations

The Center to Advance Palliative Care's (2019) most recent report gives South Dakota an "A" rating for hospital-based palliative care. This achievement is based on the state's nine hospitals with over 50 beds; eight report having a palliative care program. However, what this report does not recognize is that these hospitals are in predominantly urban and/or metro counties. In facilities with fewer than 50 beds, 40% report offering some types of palliative care, yet IHS does not provide palliative care (Isaacson et al., 2015).

South Dakota's AI population would benefit from palliative care services. In addition, there is a limited published research on palliative care programs for AIs. Existing evidence emphasizes that prior to developing palliative and EOL care programs for AIs it is essential to: (1) enhance HCPs communication practices with AIs, (2) improve HCP cultural awareness and sensitivity, (3) receive guidance and input from the AI community specific to the program, and (4) reduce barriers of insurance coverage and mistrust in the IHS system (Isaacson, 2018; Isaacson & Lynch, 2018; Isaacson et al., 2015).

Developing Collaborative Relationships

Establishing trust is critical in the development of collaborative relationships with tribal communities. M.I.'s relationship with this community began in 2008 and is grounded in CBPR principles and practices. CBPR recognizes that together the researcher and community identify questions, prepare plans, create and implement interventions, and assess the outcomes postintervention (Minkler & Wallerstein, 2008). Within this framework, all members' contributions are valued and the researcher's commitment to the community is longstanding (Israel et al., 2008). M.I. and this community's interest in palliative care began in 2012, when a palliative medicine physician asked this profound question, "Why do so many AI families travel from the west to the east side of the state to receive palliative care services?" (J. Bennett, personal communication, September 15, 2012).

UNDERSTANDING THE NARRATIVE

M.I. is a certified hospice/palliative nurse and a nurse scientist. M.I. initiated a conversation with the tribal health administrator and learned of the many challenges AI families experience when caring for their seriously ill-loved ones at home. Home health, home hospice, and outpatient palliative care services do not exist; symptom management is typically provided as an inpatient. Moreover, there is limited understanding by AI patients and families specific to hospice and palliative care services; thus, they are unable to advocate or request these specialized services.

If seriously ill AI patients are receiving inpatient care off the reservation and wish to return to their home community, they are often denied admission to the hospital by IHS. Reasons cited by IHS for denial are a lack of expertise in symptom management or a lack of inpatient EOL beds.

AI PERSPECTIVES ON HOSPICE AND PALLIATIVE CARE

To garner AI perspectives regarding hospice and palliative care, including cultural considerations, M.I. conducted Talking Circles with tribal older adults and tribal health educators over a period of 5 months. Talking Circles (i.e., focus groups) provide a culturally appropriate platform for AIs to share thoughts/ideas regarding a specific topic (Isaacson et al., 2018). M.I. shared the guiding principles of hospice and palliative care; participants indicated that hospice and palliative care are culturally acceptable and congruent with their tribal lifeways (Isaacson, 2018). Participants identified that while some tribal communities avoid discussions about dying, death is "part of the circle of life" (Isaacson, 2018, p. 162). Many indicated that providing these services would be beneficial to this community; but prior to implementing such a program, IHS personnel must have cultural awareness training. In addition, participants strongly advocated for development of a community education program specific to living wills, last wills, and advance directives.

ADVANCE DIRECTIVES—"CARE FOR OUR OLDER ADULTS"

In 2015, three AI older adults who had participated in the previously discussed Talking Circles led the development and implementation of an older-adult -driven advance directive education program. The older adults edited an existing advance directive brochure by adding culturally appropriate designs and including terms in the Native language. M.I. provided training to the older adults in the differences in palliative and hospice care, and how to discuss living wills, last wills, and advance directives. Information specific to these topics was obtained from the CaringInfo Web site (NHPCO, 2020). Once the older adults felt comfortable delivering the education, they traveled to 11 older-adult meal locations, covering over 1,000 miles and meeting/discussing advance directives to 270 participants (Isaacson, 2017). This community-based participatory project highlights the importance of community ownership; where the older adults identified the urgent need, defined how to address the need, designed the intervention, and determined how best to deliver the intervention. M.I.'s role was to facilitate meetings, support the older adults, and provide guidance and direction specific to palliative and EOL care.

The results of this project led to the development, submission, and funding of a National Cancer Institute grant to develop a culturally congruent palliative care model for AIs in Western South Dakota. Community Advisory Board meetings with three of the reservations are underway. However, due to the COVID-19 pandemic, tribal health/review boards have requested that the research team employ video or teleconferencing to conduct Talking Circles and interviews instead of the traditional methods of data collection (i.e., face to face).

APPLICATION AND IMPLICATION OF RURAL NURSING THEORY

Table 29.1 provides a snapshot view of how the theoretical statements within Rural Nursing Theory apply to the Blackfeet and Lakota. It is evident that the theoretical statements have limited applicability to these tribal communities. The two authors concur with the recommendation made by Lee and Winters (2018) regarding the need to explore the applicability of Rural Nursing Theory with other populations and cultures, for example, AI/AN.

Implications for Rural Nursing Practice, Research, and Education

It is essential that HCPs, who are not members of the tribal community, practice with an understanding of cultural humility. Prior to caring for tribal members, HCPs should attend cultural awareness education specific to the tribal community. This education provides a beginning foundation in learning about traditional lifeways, appropriate greetings, and respectful practices.

Individuals who wish to conduct research with tribal communities need to identify and contact a gatekeeper with access to the tribal community. CBPR is a helpful methodology to employ. The two authors use of CBPR with their respective tribal communities helped them learn: (1) the importance of establishing, maintaining, and strengthening trusting relationships among all members; (2) respecting the community and culture's way of doing business; (3) understanding community members' priorities may differ from the researcher; (4) listening to the community members' voices; and (5) investing the time needed for sustainability and future projects.

TABLE 29.1 Application of Rural Nursing Theory with Two AI Tribal Communities

Rural Concepts	Theoretical Statements	Blackfeet	Lakota
Health beliefs, work beliefs, and *health-seeking behavior* in which *isolation* and *distance* assist in understanding	• Health as being able to do what they want to do; it is a way of life and a state of mind; there is a goal of maintaining balance in all aspects of life. • For older residents and those with ties to extractive industries, health in a functional manner – to work, to be productive, and to do usual tasks	• Health is a state of harmony and balance among self, family, spiritual forces, community, other animals/creatures, and environment. Disease is not only a physical or psychologic ailment	• The definition of health is dependent upon if the individual is more traditional or contemporary in their views. Yet, whether traditional or contemporary, being in balance with nature, with your community, and with yourself is necessary for health. The Medicine Wheel guides this understanding of balance within the physical, mental, spiritual, and emotional realms. Balance is more than a state of mind. • Elders are highly revered by the Lakota. They provide guidance and wisdom to the younger generations. For those residing on the reservation, access to industry is limited.
Self-reliance and *independence*	• Rural residents make decision to seek care for illness, sickness, or injury depending on their self-assessment of the severity of their present health condition and of the resources needed and available. • Rural residents with infants and children experiencing illness, sickness, or injury will seek care more quickly than for themselves	• Access to healthcare should be privilege since the federal government "promised" it to AIs/ANs. Hold feelings of conflict and ambivalence toward the Westernized practices while relying upon their physician to make healthcare decisions. Concept of informed decision in healthcare is rarely held	• Tribal healers or helpers receive their ability as a gift from the Creator. Decisions regarding when to seek care have evolved. IHS provides the Western medicine for illness; there is a limited access to preventive healthcare services. Many Lakota will use a combination of the Western and traditional medicine for illness. • Lakota with children may also combine traditional and the Western medicine for their families

(continued)

TABLE 29.1 Application of Rural Nursing Theory with Two AI Tribal Communities (*continued*)

Rural Concepts	Theoretical Statements	Blackfeet	Lakota
Lack of anonymity Insider/outsider	• HCPs must deal with a lack of anonymity and much greater role diffusion than providers in urban or suburban settings	• A distinction between insider/ outsider will be maintained until trust and residency are established	• Primary care providers working for South Dakota IHS facilities often are locum tenens, thus it is difficult for patients to become comfortable and familiar with their primary care provider. A lack of anonymity is more likely to occur with those working as CHRs. However, as a collectivistic society and with broader definitions of family, this concept is less likely to be identified by CHRs.

AI, American Indian; AN, Alaska Native; CHR, community health representative; HCP, healthcare provider; IHS, Indian Health Service

Nurse educators working in states with tribal communities should incorporate education modules regarding AI/AN tribes in their curricula. This education should include, but not be limited to, such topics as colonization, boarding schools, forced assimilation, and historical trauma (Montana State University, n.d.). Moreover, with the high serious illness rates experienced by tribal communities, nursing students would benefit from receiving education on primary palliative and EOL care.

CONCLUSION

The Western medicine concepts of palliative and EOL care offer great potential for improving quality of life for AIs, yet prior to implementation must be culturally adapted to tribal communities. This cultural adaptation must be done in partnership with the tribes. CBPR is a useful methodology for guiding partnership development between non-Native researchers and tribal communities, ensuring the community and the researchers work collaboratively in the development of culturally tailored interventions. As nonnative nurse researchers, the authors' collaborative work with these two tribal communities demonstrates the importance of listening and understanding the communities' needs and wishes.

REFERENCES

Avis, F. P., Whitford, L., & Horn, K. (2009, May 8). Reducing cancer disparities for American Indians in the rural intermountain west. *Governor's Conference for Partnership Aging*, Browning, MT.

Bastien, B., & Chief, D. M. (2004). *Blackfoot ways of knowing: The worldview of the Siksikaitsitapi*. University of Calgary Press. https://doi.org/10.2307/j.ctv6gqrdz

Blackfeet Nation. (2020, May 11). https://blackfeetnation.com/

Blevins, B. (2017, September 6). *Addressing American Indian health disparities: Q & A with Dr. Don Warne.* The Rural Monitor. https://www.ruralhealthinfo.org/rural-monitor/don-warne/

Brave Heart, M., Chase, J., Elkins, J., & Altschul, D. B. (2011). Historical trauma among indigenous peoples of the Americas: Concepts, research, and clinical considerations. *Journal of Psychoactive Drugs,* 43(4), 282–290. https://doi.org/10.1080/02791072.2011.628913

Brave Heart, M. Y. (2003, January-March). The historical trauma response among natives and its relationship with substance abuse: A Lakota illustration. *Journal of Psychoactive Drugs,* 35(1), 7–13. https://doi.org/10.1080/02791072.2003.10399988

Caxaj, C. S., Schill, K., & Janke, R. (2017). Priorities and challenges for a palliative approach to care for rural indigenous populations: A scoping review. *Health & Social Care in the Community,* 26(3), e329–e336. https://doi.org/10.1111/hsc.12469

Center to Advance Palliative Care. (n.d.). *About palliative care.* https://www.capc.org/about/palliative-care/

Center to Advance Palliative Care. (2019, September). *South Dakota: Palliative care in your state.* America's Care of Serious Illness: A State-by-State Report Card on Access to Palliative Care in Our Nation's Hospitals. https://reportcard.capc.org/state/south-dakota/

Centers for Medicare & Medicaid Services. (2017). *LTSS Research: Hospice in Indian country literature review.* https://www.cms.gov/Outreach-and-Education/American-Indian-Alaska-Native/AIAN/LTSS-TA-Center/pdf/ltss-research-hospice-in-indian-country-5-9-2017.pdf

Christopher, S., Saha, R., Lachapelle, P., Jennings, D., Colclough, Y., Cooper, C., Cummins, C., Eggers, M. J., FourStar, K., Harris, K., Kuntz, S. W., LaFromboise, V., LaVeaux, D., McDonald, T., Bird, J. R., Rink, E., & Webster, L. (2011). Applying indigenous community-based participatory research principles to partnership development in health disparities research. *Family & Community Health,* 34(3), 246–255. https://doi.org/10.1097/FCH.0b013e318219606f

Cohen, K. (2003/2006). *Honoring the medicine.* Ballantine Books.

Colclough, Y. Y. (2011). *Forging a culturally-based collaborative research partnership within an American-Indian community.* Montana State University.

Colclough, Y. Y. (2017). Native American death taboo: Implications for health care providers. *American Journal of Hospice and Palliative Medicine,* 34(6), 584–591. https://doi.org/10.1177/1049909116638839

Colclough, Y. Y., & Brown, G. M. (2014a). American Indians' experiences of life-threatening illness and end of life. *Journal of Hospice and Palliative Nursing,* 16(7), 404–413. https://doi.org/10.1097/NJH.0000000000000086

Colclough, Y. Y., & Brown, G. M. (2014b). End-of-life treatment decision making: American Indians' perspective. *American Journal of Hospice & Palliative Medicine,* 31(5), 503–512. https://doi.org/10.1177/1049909113489592

Colclough, Y., & Brown, G. M. (2019a). *Development of the Blackfeet community hospice project: Pilot workshop* [Research]. Montana State University.

Colclough, Y. Y., & Brown, G. M. (2019b). Moving toward openness: Blackfeet Indians' perception changes regarding talking about end of life. *American Journal of Hospice & Palliative Medicine,* 36(4), 282–289. https://doi.org/10.1177/1049909118818255

Duggleby, W., Kuchera, S., MacLeod, R., Holyoke, P., Scott, T., Holtslander, L., Letendre, A., Moeke-Maxwell, T., Burhansstipanov, L., & Chambers, T. (2015). Indigenous people's experiences at the end of life. *Palliative & Supportive Care,* 13(6), 1721–1733. https://doi.org/http://dx.doi.org/10.1017/S147895151500070X

Fitzgerald, M. O., & Fitzgerald, J. (Eds.). (2006). *Indian spirit* (2nd ed.). World Wisdom, Inc.

Gebauer, S., Knox Morley, S., Haozous, E. A., Finlay, E., Camarata, C., Fahy, B., FitzGerald, E., Harlow, K., & Marr, L. (2016). Palliative care for American Indians and Alaska Natives: A review of the literature. *Journal of Palliative Medicine,* 19(12), 1331–1340. https://doi.org/10.1089/jpm.2016.0201

Guadagnolo, B. A., Huo, J., Buchholz, T. A., & Petereit, D. G. (2014, Autumn). Disparities in hospice utilization among American Indian medicare beneficiaries dying of cancer. *Ethnicity & Disease,* 24(4), 393–398.

Isaacson, M., Hulme, P., Cowan, J., Kerkvliet, J. L., & Minton, M. (2016). *Implementation of Survivorship care plans at three health system-based cancer centers in a rural state.* [Research Report]. South Dakota State University, Office of Nursing Research.

Isaacson. M. J. (2017). Wakanki ewastepikte: An advance directive education project with American Indian elders. *Journal of Hospice and Palliative Nursing*, 19(6), 580–587. https://doi.org/10.1097/NJH.0000000000000392.

Isaacson, M. J. (2018). Addressing the palliative and end-of-life care needs with Native American elders. *International Journal of Palliative Nursing*, 24(4), 160–168. https://doi.org/10.12968/ijpn.2018.24.4.160

Isaacson, M. J., Bott-Knutson, R. C., Fishback, M. B., Varnum, A., & Brandenburger, S. (2018). Native elder and youth perspectives on mental well-being, the value of the horse, and navigating two worlds. *Online Journal of Rural Nursing and Health Care*, 18(2), 265–302. http://dx.doi.org/10.14574/ojrnhc.v18i2.542

Isaacson, M. J., & Lynch, A. R. (2018). Culturally relevant palliative and end-of-life care for U.S. Indigenous populations: An integrative review. *Journal of Transcultural Nursing*, 29(2), 180–191. https://doi.org/10.1177/1043659617720980

Isaacson, M., Karel, B., Varilek, B. M., Steenstra, W. J., Tanis-Heyenga, J. P., & Wagner, A. J. (2015). Insights from health care professionals regarding palliative care options on South Dakota reservations. *Journal of Transcultural Nursing*, 26(5), 473–479. https://doi.org/10.1177/1043659614527623

Israel, B. A., Eng, E., Schulz, A. J., & Parker, E. A. (2012). *Methods for community-based participatory research for health* (2nd ed.). Jossey-Bass.

Israel, B. A., Schulz, A. J., Parker, E. A., Allen, A. J., & Guzman, R. (2008). Critical issues in developing and following CBPR principles. In M. Minkler & N. Wallerstein (Eds.), *Community-based participatory research for health* (2nd ed., pp. 48–66). Jossey-Bass.

Johnson, K. S., Kuchibhatla, M., & Tulsky, J. A. (2009). Racial differences in self-reported exposure to information about hospice Ccare. *Journal of Palliative Medicine*, 12(10), 921–927. https://doi.org/10.1089/jpm.2009.0066

Kahn-John, M. (2021). Navajos (Dine). In J. N. Giger & L. G. Haddad (Eds.), *Transcultural nursing: Assessment and intervention* (8th ed., pp. 241–261). Elsvier.

Lee, H. J., & Winters, C. A. (2018). Rural nursing theory: Past, present, and future. In C. A. Winters & H. J. Lee (Eds.), *Rural nursing: Concepts, theory, and practice* (5th ed.). Springer Publishing Company.

Minkler, M., & Wallerstein, N. (2008). Introduction to community-based participatory research: New issues and emphases. In M. Minkler & N. Wallerstein (Eds.), *Community-based participatory research for health* (2nd ed., pp. 5–23). Jossey-Bass.

Montana.Gov. (n.d.[a]). *Montana governor's office of Indian affairs*. https://tribalnations.mt.gov/tribalnations

Montana.Gov. (n.d.[b]). *Montana governor's office of Indian affairs*. https://tribalnations.mt.gov/blackfeet

Montana State University. (n.d.). *Indian education for all in Montana for one MUS*. http://www.montana.edu/iefa/

National Congress of American Indians. (2016). *Health care: Reducing disparities in the federal health care budget*. NCAI Fiscal Year 2016 Budget Request. http://www.ncai.org/policy-issues/tribal-governance/budget-and-approprations/07_FY2016_Health_NCAI_Budget.pdf

National Congress of American Indians. (2020, February). *Tribal nations and the United States: An introduction*. http://www.ncai.org/tribalnations/introduction/Indian_Country_101_Updated_February_2019.pdf

National Hospice and Palliative Care Organization. (2019, July 2). *NHPCO facts and figures, 2018 edition*. https://39k5cm1a9u1968hg74aj3x51-wpengine.netdna-ssl.com/wp-content/uploads/2019/07/2018_NHPCO_Facts_Figures.pdf

National Hospice and Palliative Care Organization. (2020). *Patients and caregivers*. https://www.nhpco.org/patients-and-caregivers/

National Indian Health Board. (2015, March). *The legal foundations for delivery of health care to American Indians and Alaska Natives*. https://www.nihb.org/docs/05202015/Foundations%20of%20Indian%20Health%20Care%20(March%202015).pdf

National Institute on Aging. (2017, May 17). *What are palliative care and hospice care?* https://www.nia.nih.gov/health/what-are-palliative-care-and-hospice-care

Rural Health Information Hub. (2018a, November 28). *Rural tribal health*. https://www.ruralhealthinfo.org/topics/rural-tribal-health

Rural Health Information Hub. (2018b, June 7). *Health and healthcare in frontier areas*. https://www.rural-healthinfo.org/topics/frontier

South Dakota Department of Health. (2019, March). *South Dakota American Indian cancer disparities data report*. https://getscreened.sd.gov/documents/AmericanIndianCancerDisparitiesReport.pdf

United States Census Bureau. (2012. January). *The American Indian and Alaska Native population: 2010*. https://www.census.gov/library/publications/2012/dec/c2010br-10.html

United States Census Bureau. (2019, July 1). *QuickFacts South Dakota*. https://www.census.gov/quickfacts/SD

United States Department of Agriculture. (n.d.). *South Dakota*. https://www.ers.usda.gov/webdocs/DataFiles/53180/25596_SD.pdf?v=0

United States Department of Justice. (n.d.). *Indian country*. The United States Attorney's Office District of SD. https://www.justice.gov/usao-sd/indian-country

Wallerstein, N., Duran, B., Oetzel, J., & Minkler, M. (2017). *Community-based participatoryresearch for health: Advancing social and health equity* (3rd ed.). Jossey-Bass.

Warne, D., & Frizzell, L. B. (2014). American Indian health policy: Historical trends and contemporary issues. *American Journal of Public Health*, 104(S3), S263–S267. https://doi.org/12.2015/AJPH.2013.301682

CHAPTER 30

An Evidence-Based Policy and Educational Program for Neonates Experiencing Opioid Withdrawal

Amy Olson, Stacy M. Stellflug, and Sandra W. Kuntz

DISCUSSION TOPICS

- What limitations to implementing an evidence-based project exist in rural locations? What are ways to prepare for these limitations prior to implementation?
- What differences exist between rural and urban healthcare systems that should be considered when designing and implementing an evidence-based project?
- How can the results of this project be applied to other rural locations? How should the project be adjusted?

INTRODUCTION

Neonatal abstinence syndrome (NAS) is an emergent issue due to the increase in prenatal maternal opioid use. The term NAS is used to describe a neonate experiencing withdrawal symptoms, ranging from feeding difficulties to seizures, as a result of exposure to maternal opioid use (Haycraft, 2018). In the United States between 2000 and 2012, the incidence of NAS diagnosis increased from 1.2 to 5.8 per 1,000 hospital births, affecting over 21,000 neonates (Patrick et al., 2012, 2015). The fourfold increase cost an estimated $316 million nationally in 2012 (Corr & Hollenbeak, 2017). According to the Montana Office of Epidemiology and Scientific Support, the rate of NAS in Montana neonates increased from 0.8 to 9.0 per 1,000 hospital births between 2000 and 2013 (Montana Department of Public Health and Human Services [MTDPHHS] Montana Hospital Discharge Data System, 2013). The rates of NAS in Montana have increased dramatically, even when compared to the increase on a national level.

BACKGROUND

Treatment for NAS primarily depends on the severity of withdrawal symptoms and often can be assessed and treated on the postpartum unit. However, some cases necessitate admission to an NICU. NICUs provide highly specialized treatment for neonates, including high-risk intravenous medications, cardiac monitoring, and respiratory support. Having a neonate admitted to an NICU is a "psychological crisis that might cause many emotional problems for parents" (Hosseini et al., 2019, p. 272).

Montana is the fourth largest state in the union, with seven people per square mile, and ranks 48th out of the 50 states for population density (United States Census Bureau, 2010). Within Montana, there are 69 hospitals of which 48 are considered critical access hospitals (CAH) (Health Resources & Services Administration, 2018). CAH designation applies to hospitals located in rural communities, more than 35 road miles from another hospital with less than 25 acute care beds (Montana Hospital Association, 2016). CAHs often do not have NICUs with nurses trained in caring for neonates needing extra support. Nurses and providers in a CAH need to have the skills, tools, and confidence to identify, monitor, and treat a neonate with withdrawal symptoms. Although neonates suffering from withdrawal often can remain on a postpartum unit, rural healthcare providers must be able to recognize when a neonate needs a higher level of care than is available at the CAH. The care team can be guided on treatment management and level of severity by using a validated, reliable scale to monitor withdrawal symptoms.

Current evidence recommends all nursery units develop a policy to address management of neonates at risk of NAS (Jansson, 2018). The policy should include a scoring system and management protocols, supportive care measures, skin care, and breastfeeding recommendations (Jansson, 2018). A standardized NAS hospital policy with a consistent NAS scoring system is associated with lower length of pharmacologic treatment, length of stay, and neonates discharged on medications for NAS (Patrick et al., 2016). Although a standardized policy suggests improved outcomes in neonates diagnosed with NAS, Romisher et al. (2018) suggested the need for NAS-specific education programs in addition to the hospital policy. Franza (2016) discussed that educational programs for the care team resulted in increased confidence levels in caring for neonates with NAS and increased confidence in communicating with opioid-addicted parents. Education on the guidelines for using the assessment tool provides the care team with consistent and accurate scores for diagnosing NAS and treatment management (Timpson et al., 2018).

In a 2012 policy statement released by the American Academy of Pediatrics (AAP), greater than 50% of neonates exposed to opioids will develop NAS (Hudak & Tan, 2012). The report also contained recommendations for the management of NAS. The recommendations included encouraging all hospital staffs to develop a policy to standardize care for neonates diagnosed with NAS. The policy should include maternal screening of all pregnant women by interview to identify risk factors for opioid use. If the woman is positive for risk factors or suspected of opioid use, the policy should include urine and biological screening of the neonate (urine, meconium, or cord tissue) (Hudak & Tan, 2012). A large variation in patient management for these withdrawing neonates remain despite the AAP policy statement release in 2012 (Raffaeli et al., 2017). In addition to provider expertise, some of the variations among facilities include environmental and hospital factors. Environmental factors may include mother–neonate rooming-in and breastfeeding. Hospital-related factors have included assessment tools used, noise level of the nursery, policies, and protocols. The variations of environmental and hospital factors affect management of withdrawing neonates if the variation does not follow the AAP recommendations (Raffaeli et al., 2017).

The remainder of this chapter will describe a Doctor of Nursing Practice professional project completed in 2019 at a CAH hospital in Montana. The purpose of the project was to assess the change in team member confidence when providing care for neonates suspected of substance withdrawal at a CAH in Montana by: (a) developing and implementing a policy on care and treatment of a drug-dependent newborn; (b) educating the team providing care to these neonates on the use of NAS scoring tools; and (c) evaluating the education and improved confidence levels of the healthcare team.

REVIEW OF EXTANT LITERATURE

Neonatal Abstinence Scoring Tools

The most used assessment tool for identifying, diagnosing, and managing NAS in neonates is the Finnegan Neonatal Abstinence Scoring Tool (FNAST). The FNAST was originally developed in 1975 to provide a quantitative evaluation of the clinical status of a neonate withdrawing. The tool assisted in the standardization of assessment and treatment in these neonates (Finnegan et al., 1975). The signs and symptoms of NAS are broken into three categories: (a) central nervous system disturbances, (b) metabolic, vasomotor, and respiratory disturbances, and (c) gastrointestinal disturbances. Each category has four to nine assessment items to score (Finnegan et al., 1975). Although this tool has been widely used, there is a limited evidence of the reliability and validity. Retskin and Wright (2014) evaluated the FNAST for interobserver reliability in a cross-sectional study. The median total score resulted in an interclass correlation coefficient (ICC) of 0.996 indicating excellent reliability between observers (Retskin & Wright, 2014). However, the individual scores on the 21-item FNAST had much less interobserver reliability (ICC of 0.694) (Retskin & Wright, 2014) indicating a concern about whether clinical decisions of pharmacologic treatment are made based off the reliability of these scores. Some of the items are subjective, such as excessive irritability or poor feeding leading to discrepancies in scoring. Therefore, education of the observer/assessor and utilizing more than one rater to account for interrater variability are important components to improve consistency (Retskin & Wright, 2014; Timpson et al., 2018). Although the FNAST is a widely used NAS-scoring tool, other tools have been developed, such as the Lipitz Withdrawal Scale (LWS) and the Maternal Opioid Treatment: Human Experimental Research NAS Scale (MNS). All the tools have been compared to the FNAST with limited guidance on which tool is superior (Fox et al., 2016; Jones et al., 2016; Newman, 2014).

Recently, a new NAS scoring tool developed by Grossman et al. (2017) is gaining popularity. The Eat, Sleep, Console (ESC) Model was developed by Grossman as an alternative to the FNAST for neonates diagnosed with NAS. The ESC Model considered three parameters: "the neonate's ability to eat, to sleep, and to be consoled" (p. e3). If the neonate met these parameters, then no pharmacologic intervention was initiated or increased. Reliability and validity have not been established for the ESC Model. The results of the research study conducted by Grossman et al. (2017) included a reduction of average length of stay for neonates from 22.4 to 5.9 days, a decrease in morphine use in methadone-exposed neonates from 98% to 14% and a $30,000 reduction in NICU costs. No adverse events occurred while using this functional assessment approach (Grossman et al., 2017). Grossman et al. (2018) published a follow-up research article of smaller scale indicating similar results: decrease in morphine use when using ESC versus FNAST.

Treatment and Management

The initial treatment of neonates identified with NAS should be supportive and nonpharmacologic. Nonpharmacologic interventions include parental presence and breastfeeding. Multiple primary research studies and systematic reviews have identified positive associations between shorter length of inpatient stay and decreased need for pharmacologic therapy in neonates receiving nonpharmacologic interventions (Abrahams et al., 2007, 2010; Crook & Brandon, 2017; Dryden et al., 2009; Grossman et al., 2017; Holmes et al., 2016; Howard et al., 2017; Hudak & Tan, 2012; Hünseler et al., 2013; Isemann et al., 2011; MacMillan et al., 2018; Newman et al., 2015; O'Connor et al., 2013; Pritham et al., 2012; Saiki et al., 2010; Short et al., 2016; Wachman et al., 2018; Welle-Strand et al., 2013).

Although pharmacologic intervention is not the first-line treatment for a neonate exhibiting signs of withdrawal, it can be an important part of the short-term treatment plan to control symptoms. There have been several research studies comparing morphine, methadone, and buprenorphine in the treatment of NAS symptoms. Some findings have been contradictory in identifying which medication is superior for use in neonates withdrawing from opioids (Brown et al., 2015; Hall et al., 2016, 2018; Kraft et al., 2017; Young et al., 2015). Ultimately, systematic reviews and clinical guidelines have supported the use of all three medications (Jansson, 2018; Wachman et al., 2018).

Confidence Levels of Care Team

There has been limited research on confidence levels of the care team treating a neonate with NAS. The results of three quality improvement projects implementing an educational intervention and policy suggest an improvement in nurse knowledge and confidence caring for and assessing neonates withdrawing from opioids (Cook et al., 2017; Franza, 2016; Timpson et al., 2018). Other research addressing nurses' experience, knowledge, and attitudes while caring for this population identified frustration, stress, and gaps in education for the healthcare team (Fraser et al., 2006; Lucas & Knobel, 2012; Maguire et al., 2012; Murphy-Oikonen et al., 2010).

METHODS

The purpose of this project was to improve confidence in the team providing care for neonates suspected of substance withdrawal at a CAH in Montana by: (a) developing and implementing a policy on care and treatment of a drug-dependent newborn; (b) educating the team providing care to these neonates on the use of NAS-scoring tools; and (c) evaluating the education and improved confidence levels of the healthcare team. This chapter includes an overview of the design, setting, population, protection of human subjects, procedures for implementation and data collection, and how the data were analyzed.

Design Overview

The quality improvement project was nonexperimental. An evidence-based policy and education program were implemented on the hospital unit. A pretest/posttest design was used to evaluate change in nursing knowledge on NAS-scoring tools. A survey was administered prior to and following the education program to evaluate confidence in caring for neonates diagnosed with NAS. The data were analyzed using a two-tailed paired samples t test to compare the means represented at two different times, pretest versus posttest, for the confidence survey and knowledge test. The average mean difference in scores, *standard deviation (SD)* of the divergence, *standard error (SE)* of the difference, and confidence levels were calculated based on the *t* test.

Setting/Sample and Population

The setting for this quality improvement project was a CAH in rural Montana. The hospital had 25-inpatient beds with inpatient services covering medical, surgical, and OB patients. Within the inpatient OB department, there was a labor and delivery unit, postpartum unit, and nursery. The staff included 10 nurses, 2 obstetricians, and 5 pediatric providers. The hospital averaged 180 births per year. The incidence of NAS on this unit had not previously been established due to unclear diagnostic criteria with providers coding and discrepancy on NAS-withdrawal symptoms relating to healthcare team education on the topic, however, in a 6-month timeframe in 2018, at least two were noted (A. Sorenson, personal communication, February 25, 2018). The obstetricians did not provide newborn care so for the sake of this project; the two obstetricians were omitted from the project; the remaining 15 healthcare team members (including providers and nurses) were invited to participate in this project.

Procedures/Measures

The evidence-based policy was developed through careful review of the literature and other facilities' policies regarding NAS. The policy included symptoms of neonatal withdrawal, nonpharmacologic and pharmacologic treatment options, blood tests to consider, special considerations and patient teaching. The policy underwent thorough evaluation by the OB manager on the unit and pediatric providers. Pharmacologic treatment options needed to be cleared by hospital administration and pharmacy. The staff made the final decision on whether the FNAST or ESC method was to be used and included in the policy.

With permission, a test was adapted from a similar quality improvement project completed by Jeanne Franza to evaluate the care team knowledge of NAS and FNAST before and after the education program was implemented. Franza (2016) completed the project at the Midstate Medical Center in Meriden, Connecticut. "Content validity was verified by three experts" (Franza, 2016, p. e6). The pre- and posttests were identical with 13 questions.

A confidence survey was administered before and after the education program to evaluate the confidence level of each healthcare team member on caring for infants diagnosed with NAS and the confidence in using NAS-scoring tools. This confidence survey was adapted, with permission, from a similar quality improvement project performed by Christy Cook, Shannon Dahms, and Sonja Meiers. Cook et al. (2017) implemented the quality improvement project at a rural Midwest hospital assessing nurses' knowledge and confidence in caring for neonates with NAS. The pre- and postsurveys were identical with 15 survey questions. The participants rated their confidence on a scale from 1 to 4 (not confident to very confident).

The education program was adapted, with permission, from Franza (2016) who assisted by providing valuable knowledge on changes to be made to the PowerPoint presentation used in the education program. Although she used an educational DVD during implementation of her quality improvement project, she did not feel this portion of the educational program added to the overall knowledge of NAS and NAS-scoring tools (J. Franza, personal communication, September 6, 2018).

Following the administration of the consent, confidence survey, and pretest, the educational program was organized by this author and delivered in a conference room on the unit. The educational program, consisting of a PowerPoint presentation, was reviewed in detail with the healthcare professionals providing care to neonates suspected of substance withdrawal. The educational training was offered on two dates identified by the OB manager and was presented to the staff as a mandatory training. Immediately following the educational training, the post-test and confidence survey were administered.

RESULTS

The purpose of the project was to determine the effect of education on the care of neonates suspected of substance withdrawal at a CAH in Montana on healthcare provider knowledge and confidence. Secondarily, an NAS evidence-based policy was developed and implemented on the unit. The results are shown in Table 30.1.

Demographic information was collected on all staff agreeing to participate in the project. Eleven total participants, including nine nurses (81.8%; eight full-time nursing staff and one travel nurse) and two pediatric providers (MD) (18.2%), attended the educational training and completed both surveys. All attendants were female, and age was not assessed. The total average year of experience was 10 years (range 1.5 to 26 years, median 6 years) with a total average years of experience at this facility of 3.4 years (range 0.2 to 9 years, median 3.5 years). The physician-specific total average experience was less than 3 years. Of the two physicians participating in the project, both provided pediatric care; however, only one physician with 2 years experience trained specifically as a pediatrician; the other physician trained as a family practice physician.

Sample size for the project was 11. Surveys completed preeducation had a mean knowledge score of 67.8% (Table 30.2). The *SD* was 18% with a range of 30.7% to 100%. The knowledge survey was distributed immediately following the education session, and participants returned the survey prior to leaving the conference room. Posteducation,

TABLE 30.1 Demographic Data of Participants in NAS Education Program Measuring Healthcare Provider Knowledge and Confidence

Roles	Nurses	9	81.8%
	Pediatric providers (MD)	2	18.2%
Sex	Female	11	100%
	Male	0	0%
Experience in role	Mean/Median [Range]	10/6 [1.5–26]	
	Less than 5 years	5	45.5%
	5–10 years	1	9.1%
	10–15 years	2	18.2%
	Greater than 15 years	3	27.3%
Experience in role on current unit	Mean/Median [Range]	3.4 / 3.5 [0.2–9]	
	Less than 5 years	8	72.7%
	5–10 years	3	27.3%
	10–15 years	0	0%
	Greater than 15 years	0	0%

TABLE 30.2 Mean, *SD*, and Range of Scores for Pre- and Postintervention on Knowledge

	Sample Size (*n*)	Mean Score (% Correct)	SD	Range of Scores (% correct)
Preintervention KNOWLEDGE	11	67.8%	18%	30.7%–100%
Postintervention KNOWLEDGE	11	92.3%	8.6%	76.9%–100%

SD, standard deviation.

TABLE 30.3 Paired Samples *t* test Examining Effect of NAS Education Program on Healthcare Provider Knowledge

	Mean	SD	SE Mean	95% Confidence Interval of the Difference		*t*	df	Sig. (2-tailed)
				Lower	Upper			
Preintervention to Postintervention	0.25	0.16	0.04	0.15	0.34	2.18	12	0.0001

NAS, neonatal abstinence syndrome; SD, standard deviation; SE, standard error.

participants answered 92.3% of the questions correctly. The *SD* was 8.6% with a range of 76.9% to 100%.

A paired samples *t* test was conducted to assess the effect of the NAS education program and the implementation of an NAS evidence-based policy on healthcare provider knowledge of neonates suspected of substance withdrawal as compared to no education/policy (Table 30.3). There was a significant improvement in the scores for knowledge prior to the education session ($M = 0.68$, $SD = 0.18$) when compared to knowledge after the education session ($M = 0.92$, $SD = 0.09$); $t(12) = 2.18$, $p = .0001$, an alpha of 0.05 was set a priori. The results suggest implementation of an NAS educational program including education regarding the implementation of a corresponding evidence-based policy has a statistically significant effect on provider and nurse knowledge about NAS. Specifically, the results suggest NAS education improved provider/nurse knowledge.

The confidence survey was completed prior to the education session. All 11 participants completed the 15-question confidence survey (Table 30.4). Preintervention, the mean confidence score was 2.36 on a four-point scale indicating a result between somewhat confidence and quite confident. The *SD* was 0.45 with a range of 1.47 to 3.27. The confidence survey was distributed with the knowledge survey immediately following the education session. Participants were required to complete the postintervention confidence survey prior to leaving the conference room. Postintervention, the mean confidence score was 3.01 on a four-point scale indicating a result between quite confident and highly confident. The *SD* was 0.34 with a range in scores from 2 to 3.47.

A paired samples *t* test was conducted to assess whether the implementation of a NAS evidence-based policy and an NAS education program improves healthcare provider confidence in caring for neonates suspected of substance withdrawal as compared to no education/policy (Table 30.5). There was a statistically significant improvement in the scores for confidence prior to the education session ($M = 2.36$, $SD = 0.45$) when compared to confidence after the education session ($M = 3.01$, $SD = 0.34$); $t(12) = 2.14$, $p < .0001$, $\alpha = 0.05$.

TABLE 30.4 Mean, SD, and Range of Scores for Pre- and Postintervention on Confidence

	Sample Size (n)	Mean Score	SD	Range of Scores
Preintervention CONFIDENCE	11	2.36	0.45	1.47–3.27
Postintervention CONFIDENCE	11	3.01	0.34	2-3–47

SD, standard deviation.

TABLE 30.5 Paired Samples *t* test Examining Effect of NAS Education Program on Healthcare Provider Confidence

	Mean	SD	SE Mean	95% Confidence Interval of the Difference		*t*	df	Sig. (2-tailed)
				Lower	Upper			
Preintervention to Postintervention	0.65	0.2	0.05	0.54	0.76	2.14	12	<0.0001

NAS, neonatal abstinence syndrome; SD, standard deviation; SE, standard error.

DISCUSSION

The opioid use among pregnant women has increased, which has led to a rise in the rate of NAS. Neonates with NAS are delivered at rural and urban locations throughout the country. The rural CAH often lacks the resources (policy development and education updates) to prepare healthcare team members for safe care of neonates that present with NAS. The goal of the project was to provide resources and education to better prepare healthcare team members to care for this population.

The project was a quality improvement project and was thus nonexperimental. The AAP policy statement released in 2012 encouraged all hospitals to develop a policy to standardize care for neonates diagnosed with NAS (Hudak & Tan, 2012). In following recommendations by the AAP, an evidence-based policy was developed for the unit. The policy included information and guidance on the treatment of NAS, including nonpharmacologic treatment options, pharmacologic, education, and follow-up care. Morphine was chosen as the pharmacologic treatment to include in the policy as staff are most comfortable with morphine. Literature supports morphine, methadone, or buprenorphine as the pharmacologic treatment method (Jansson, 2018; Wachman et al., 2018). The ESC Model was selected by the unit as the preferred scoring tool despite the units' previous use of FNAST. The choice of the ESC Model was made based on the ease of use and decreased risk of interobserver variability when compared to the FNAST.

Romisher et al. (2018) suggested the need for NAS-specific education programs in addition to the hospital policy. Education on the guidelines for using the assessment tool provides the care team with consistent and accurate scores for diagnosing NAS and treatment management (Timpson et al., 2018). An education program was implemented on NAS and evaluated using surveys. The results suggest implementation of an NAS educational program including education regarding the implementation of a corresponding evidence-based policy has a statistically significant effect on provider and nurse knowledge and confidence about NAS. Specifically, the results suggest NAS education improved provider/nurse knowledge and confidence in caring for neonates affected by NAS. The results were consistent with previous research on confidence levels and knowledge surrounding neonates affected by NAS (Cook et al., 2017; Franza, 2016; Fraser et al., 2006; Lucas & Knobel, 2012; Maguire et al., 2012; Murphy-Oikonen et al., 2010; Romisher et al., 2018; Timpson et al., 2018).

Limitations and Lessons Learned

There were several limitations in the project. The OB manager changed between the initial discussion of the project and the implementation, which added some confusion and resulted in last-minute changes to the project. The new OB manager wanted the staff to be educated on the ESC and FNAST scoring tools to allow a consensus to be made on which option to use. Once the method was decided, the author was able to finish the policy, which caused a delay in the policy being finalized. The delay may have altered the results of the surveys, specifically the survey question on confidence in using the policy on the unit since the policy was not finalized prior to the staff taking the posteducation survey.

Most of the correspondence between the author and the facility staff were done from a distance. Since the preparation for the project was completed from a distance, the project implementation date had to be decided in advance to make travel arrangements. Multiple staff members contracted the flu the week of implementation. All the education documents were provided to the staff who were unable to attend, but surveys were not collected, decreasing the population size for the project. Ideally, future projects would occur at a facility within a comfortable travel distance for the author, which would allow for increased flexibility with scheduling project implementation. Additionally, if the author were employed within the facility, she would have a better sense of changes in staffing, including management changes within the unit to avoid last-minute changes to the project.

Implications for Rural Healthcare

The implications for practice became clear within 6 months of project implementation. The OB manager stated, "We have implemented the NAS policy with the ESC Model and have used it on two separate occasions. Both times that we used it, it was fantastic and so easy to use" (A. Davis, personal communication, August 20, 2019). Within 6 months, two neonates with NAS remained on the postpartum unit of the CAH with their parents and were successfully discharged home. The unit was able to avoid adverse outcomes associated with an NICU transfer, including emotional issues for the parents and cost.

The results of this project support the potential benefits for other rural hospitals to enhance the providers' skills and confidence of caring for neonates suspected of opioid withdrawal. Avoiding NICU transfer of the neonate provides the opportunity for early bonding for the parents.

CONCLUSION

The inquiry question for this project was to providers caring for neonates suspected of drug withdrawal: Does implementation of an NAS evidence-based policy and an NAS education program improve healthcare provider knowledge, confidence, and perceived ability to care for neonates suspected of substance withdrawal as compared to no policy/education? The results strongly suggest the answer to the original question is yes. The results along with the unit feedback indicated the project had statistical and clinical significance.

REFERENCES

Abrahams, R. R., Kelly, S. A., Payne, S., Thiessen, P. N., Mackintosh, J., & Janssen, P. A. (2007). Rooming-in compared with standard care for newborns of mothers using methadone or heroin. *Canadian Family Physician, 53*(10), 1722–1730.

Abrahams, R. R., MacKay-Dunn, M. H., Nevmerjitskaia, V., MacRae, G. S., Payne, S. P., & Hodgson, Z. G. (2010). An evaluation of rooming-in among substance-exposed newborns in British Columbia. *Journal of Obstetrics and Gynaecology Canada, 32*(9), 866–871.

Brown, M. S., Hayes, M. J., & Thornton, L. M. (2015). Methadone versus morphine for treatment of neonatal abstinence syndrome: A prospective randomized clinical trial. *Journal of Perinatology, 35*(4), 278–283. doi:10.1038/jp.2014.194

Cook, C. L., Dahms, S. K., & Meiers, S. J. (2017). Enhancing care for infants with neonatal abstinence syndrome: An evidence-based practice approach in a rural midwestern region. *Worldviews on Evidence-Based Nursing, 14*(5), 422–423. doi:10.1111/wvn.12217

Corr, T. E., & Hollenbeak, C. S. (2017). The economic burden of neonatal abstinence syndrome in the United States. *Addiction, 112*, 1590–1599. doi:10.1111/add.13842

Crook, K., & Brandon, D. (2017). Prenatal breastfeeding education: impact on infants with neonatal abstinence syndrome. *Advances in Neonatal Care, 17*(4), 299–305. doi:10.1097/ANC.0000000000000392

Dryden, C., Young, D., Hepburn, M., & Mactier, H. (2009). Maternal methadone use in pregnancy: Factors associated with the development of neonatal abstinence syndrome and implications for healthcare resources. *International Journal of Obstetrics & Gynaecology, 116*(5), 665–671. doi:10.1111/j.1471-0528.2008.02073

Finnegan, L. P., Connaughton, J. F., Kron, R. E., & Emich, J. P. (1975). Neonatal abstinence syndrome: Assessment and management. *Addictive Diseases, 2*, 141–158.

Fox, K., Kavanagh, P., & Fielder, A. (2016). A comparison of two neonatal withdrawal scales: A retrospective case note audit. *Journal of Neonatal Nursing, 22*(6), 284–291. doi:10.1016/j.jnn.2016.06.002

Franza, J. (2016). Nursing care of newborn infants with neonatal abstinence syndrome: Increasing knowledge through education. *Advances in Neonatal Care*, E6. doi:10.1097/ANC.0000000000000298

Fraser, J. A., Barnes, M., Biggs, H. C., & Kain, V. J. (2006). Caring, chaos and the vulnerable family: Experiences in caring for newborns of drug-dependent parents. *International Journal of Nursing Studies, 44*(8), 1363–1370. doi:10.1016/j.ijnurstu.2006.06.004

Grossman, M. R., Berkwitt, A. K., Osborn, R. R., Xu, Y., Esserman, D. A., Shapiro, E. D., & Bizzarro, M. J. (2017). An initiative to improve the quality of care of infants with neonatal abstinence syndrome. *Pediatrics, 139*(6), e1–e9. doi:10.1542/peds.2016-3360

Grossman, M. R., Lipshaw, M. J., Osborn, R. R., & Berkwitt, A. K. (2018). A novel approach to assessing infants with neonatal abstinence syndrome. *Hospital Pediatrics, 8*(1), 1–6. doi:10.1542/hpeds.2017-0128.

Hall, E. S., Isemann, B. T., Wexelblatt, S. L., Meinzen-Derr, J., Wiles, J. R., Harvey, S., & Akinbi, H. T. (2016). A cohort comparison of buprenorphine versus methadone treatment for neonatal abstinence syndrome. *Journal of Pediatrics, 170*, 39–44. doi:10.1016/j.jpeds.2015.11.039

Hall, E. S., Rice, W. R., Folger, A. T., & Wexelblatt, S. L. (2018). Comparison of neonatal abstinence syndrome treatment with sublingual buprenorphine versus conventional opioids. *American Journal of Perinatology, 35*(4), 405–412. doi:10.1055/s-0037-1608634

Haycraft, A. L. (2018). Pregnancy and the opioid epidemic. *Journal of Psychosocial Nursing and Mental Health Services, 56*(3), 19–23. doi:10.3928/02793695-20180219-03.

Health Resources & Services Administration. (2018). Data. https://data.hrsa.gov/

Holmes, A. V., Atwood, E. C., Whalen, B., Beliveau, J., Jarvis, J. D., Matulis, J. C., & Ralston, S. L. (2016). Rooming-in to treat neonatal abstinence syndrome: Improved family-centered care at lower cost. *Pediatrics, 137*(6), e20152929. doi:10.1542/peds.2015-2929

Hosseini, S. N., Ghodousi, A., Sadeghi, N., & Abbasi, S. (2019). Comparing neonatal intensive care unit nursing support in mothers with newborn abstinence syndrome (NAS) and mothers of healthy neonates. *International Journal of Medical Toxicology and Forensic Medicine, 9*(4), 271–278. https://doi.org/10.32598/ijmtfm.v9i4.26184

Howard, M. B., Schiff, D. M., Penwill, N., Si, W., Rai, A., Wolfgang, T., Moses, J. M., & Wachman, E. M. (2017). Impact of parental presence at infants' bedside on neonatal abstinence syndrome. *Hospital Pediatrics, 7*(2), 63–69. doi:10.1542/hpeds.2016-0147

Hudak, M. L., & Tan, R. C. (2012). Clinical report: Neonatal drug withdrawal. *Pediatrics, 129*(2), e540–e560. doi:10.1542/peds.2011-3212.

Hünseler, C., Brückle, M., Roth, B., & Kribs, A. (2013). Neonatal opiate withdrawal and rooming-in: A retrospective analysis of a single center experience. *Klinische Pädiatrie NLM, 225*(5), 247–251. doi: 10.1055/s-0033-1347190

Isemann, B., Meinzen-Derr, J., & Akinbi, H. (2011). Maternal and neonatal factors impacting response to methadone therapy in infants treated for neonatal abstinence syndrome. *Journal of Perinatology, 31*(1), 25–29. doi:10.1038/jp.2010.66

Jansson, L. M. (2018). *Neonatal abstinence syndrome.* UpToDate. www.uptodate.com.

Jones, H., Seashore, C., Johnson, E., Horton, E., O'Grady, K, Andringa, K., Grossman, M. R., Whalen, B., & Holmes, A. (2016). Psychometric assessment of the neonatal abstinence scoring system and the MOTHER NAS scale. *American Journal on Addictions, 25*(5), 370–373. doi:10.1111/ajad.12388.

Kraft, W. K., Adeniyi-Jones, S. C., Chervoneva, I., Greenspan, J. S., Abatemarco, D., Kaltenbach, K., & Ehrlich, M. E. (2017). Buprenorphine for the treatment of the neonatal abstinence syndrome. *New England Journal of Medicine, 376*(24), 2341–2348. doi:10.1056/NEJMoa1614835

Lucas, K., & Knobel, R. B. (2012). Implementing practice guidelines and education to improve care of infants with neonatal abstinence syndrome. *Advances in Neonatal Care, 12*(1), 40–45. doi:10.1097/ANC.0b013e318241bd73

MacMillan, K. D., Rendon, C. P., Verma, K., Riblet, N., Washer, D. B., & Holmes, A. V. (2018). Association of rooming-in with outcomes for neonatal abstinence syndrome: A systematic review and meta-analysis. *JAMA Pediatrics, 172*(4), 345–351. doi:10.1001/jamapediatrics.2017.5195

Maguire, D., Webb, M., Passmore, D., & Cline, G. (2012). NICU nurses' lived experience: Caring for infants with neonatal abstinence syndrome. *Advances in Neonatal Care, 12*(5), 281-285. doi: 10.1097/ANC.0b013e3182677bc1

Montana Department of Public Health and Human Services (MTDPHHS) Montana Hospital Discharge Data System (MHDDS). (2013). *Neonatal abstinence syndrome in Montana newborns, 200-2013 [Data file].* dphhs.mt.gov

Montana Hospital Association. (2016). *Critical access hospital.* https://mtha.org/critical-access-hospital/

Murphy-Oikonen, J., Brownlee, K., Montelpare, W., & Gerlach, K. (2010). The experiences of NICU nurses in caring for infants with neonatal abstinence syndrome. *Neonatal Network, 29*(5), 307-313.

Newman, A., Davies, G. A., Dow, K., Holmes, B., Macdonald, J., McKnight, S., & Newton, L. (2015). Rooming-in care for infants of opioid-dependent mothers: Implementation and evaluation at a tertiary care hospital. *Canadian Family Physician, 61*(12), e555–e561.

Newman, K. M. (2014). The right tool at the right time: Examining the evidence surrounding measurement of neonatal abstinence syndrome. *Advances in Neonatal Care, 14*(3), 181–186. doi:10.1097/ANC.000000000000095.

Patrick, S., Schumacher, R., Horbar, J., Buus-Frank, M., Edwards, E., Morrow, K., Ferrelli, K. R., Picarillo, A. P., Gupta, M., & Soll, R. (2016). Improving care for neonatal abstinence syndrome. *Pediatrics, 137*(5), 1324–1332. doi:10.1377/hlthaff.2015.1496.

Patrick, S. W., Davis, M. M., Lehmann, C. U., & Cooper, W. O. (2015). Increasing incidence and geographic distribution of neonatal abstinence syndrome: United States 2009) to 2012. *Journal of Perinatology, 35*, 650–655. doi:10.1038/jp.2015.36

Patrick, S. W., Schumacher, R. E., Benneyworth, B. D., Krans, E. E., McAllister, J. M., & Davis, M. M. (2012). Neonatal abstinence syndrome and associated health care expenditures: United States, 2000–2009. *Journal of American Medical Association, 307*(18), 1934–1940. doi:10.1001/jama.2012.3951

Pritham, U. A., Paul, J. A., & Hayes, M. J. (2012). Opioid dependency in pregnancy and length of stay for neonatal abstinence syndrome. *Journal of Obstetric, Gynecologic & Neonatal Nursing, 41*(2), 180–190. doi:10.1111/j.1552-6909.2011.01330.x

O'Connor, A. B., Collett, A., Alto, W. A., & O'Brien, L. M. (2013). Breastfeeding rates and the relationship between breastfeeding and neonatal abstinence syndrome in women maintained on buprenorphine during pregnancy. *Journal of Midwifery & Women's Health, 58*(4), 383–388. doi:10.1111/jmwh.12009

Raffaeli, G., Cavallaro, G., Allegaert, K., Wildschut, E.D., Fumagalli, M., Agosti, M.,… Mosca, F. (2017). Neonatal abstinence syndrome: Update on diagnostic and therapeutic strategies. *Pharmacotherapy*, *37*(7), 814–823. doi:10.1002/phar.1954.

Retskin, C. M., & Wright, M. E. (2014). Interobserver reliability of the Finnegan Neonatal Abstinence Scoring Tool in an acute care setting. *Journal of Obstetric, Gynecologic & Neonatal Nursing*, *43*(1), S61. doi:10.1111/1552-6909.12345.

Romisher, R., Hill, D., & Cong, X. (2018). Neonatal abstinence syndrome: Exploring nurses' attitudes, knowledge, and practice. *Advances in Neonatal Care*, *0*, 1–9. doi:10.1097/ANC.0000000000000462.

Saiki, T., Lee, S., Hannam, S., & Greenough, A. (2010). Neonatal abstinence syndrome: Postnatal ward versus neonatal unit management. *European Journal of Pediatrics*, *169*(1), 95–98. doi:10.1007/s00431-009-0994-0

Short, V. L., Gannon, M., & Abatemarco, D. J. (2016). The association between breastfeeding and length of hospital stay among infants diagnosed with neonatal abstinence syndrome: a population-based study of in-hospital births. *Breastfeeding Medicine*, *11*, 343–349. doi:10.1089/bfm.2016.0084

Timpson, W., Killoran, C., Maranda, L., Picarillo, A., & Bloch-Salisbury, E. (2018). A quality improvement initiative to increase scoring consistency and accuracy of the Finnegan tool: Challenges in obtaining reliable assessments of drug withdrawal in neonatal abstinence syndrome. *Advances in Neonatal Care*, *18*(1), 70–78. doi:10.1097/ANC.0000000000000441.

United States Census Bureau. (2010). *Montana quick facts*. www.census.gov.

Wachman, E. M., Schiff, D. M., & Silverstein, M. (2018). Neonatal abstinence syndrome: Advances in diagnosis and treatment. *Journal of the American Medical Association*, *319*(13), 1362–1374. doi:10.1001/jama.2018.2640.

Welle-Strand, G. K., Skurtveit, S., Jansson, L. M., Bakstad, B., Bjarkø, L., & Ravndal, E. (2013). Breastfeeding reduces the need for withdrawal treatment in opioid-exposed infants. *Acta Paediatrica*, *102*(11), 1060–1066. doi:10.1111/apa.12378

Young, M. E., Hager, S. J., & Spurlock, D. (2015) Retrospective chart review comparing morphine and methadone in neonates treated for neonatal abstinence syndrome. *American Journal of Health-System Pharmacy*, *72*(23 Suppl. 3), S162–S167. doi:10.2146/sp150025

CHAPTER 31

The Rural Participatory Research Model

Sandra W. Kuntz, Tanis Hernandez,
and Charlene A. Winters

DISCUSSION TOPICS

- You are a university nurse researcher. How would you apply the Rural Participatory Research Model (RPRM) for a study you will lead in a distant rural community?
- Describe strategies to engage rural community members in research from onset to completion of a project.
- Explain the notion of "erosion of trust" that can occur following a technologic disaster.

INTRODUCTION

Partnerships between community members and academic investigators are integral to the success of human studies in rural communities. Research to explore the holistic impact of a rural, slow-motion, technologic environmental disaster relies on questions raised and examined by community members living with the direct or indirect social, emotional, physical, or economic effects of exposure. In October 2005, clinicians from the Center for Asbestos Related Disease (CARD) contacted Montana State University (MSU) nurse researchers and queried the possibility of collaborating with MSU on a specific project. The CARD clinic is devoted to healthcare, outreach, and research to benefit all people impacted by exposure to Libby amphibole asbestos (LAA) (CARD, 2020). The CARD clinicians were looking for a partner to help analyze a data set that included results from the St. George's Respiratory Questionnaire (SGRQ) survey linked to clinical data from 1,200 CARD clients. The SGRQ is "an index deigned to measure and quantify health-related health status in patients with chronic airflow limitation ... [the SGRQ] has been shown to correlate well with established measures of symptom level, disease activity and disability" (Jones et al., 1992, p. 1321).

The initial partnership resulted in the joint submission of a grant to the Health Resources and Services Administration (HRSA) Office of Rural Health Policy [R04RH07544]. The funding supported Study 1, a comprehensive understanding of the biopsychosocial health status of persons exposed to LAA and the human response to chronic illness resulting from asbestos exposure. The study utilized a community-based participatory research (CBPR) approach and analysis of the CARD clinic existing client data. Results of this study are reported in the *International Scholarly Research Network* (Weinert et al., 2011), *Journal of Environmental and Public Health* (Winters et al., 2011), and *BMJ Open* (Winters et al., 2012).

Next, the CARD/MSU team developed Study 2 in response to the National Institutes of Health (NIH) Public Trust Initiative to explore ways to improve the communication and interaction between the researchers and the public. The funded proposal, *Exploring Research Communication and Engagement in a Rural Community: The Libby Partnership Initiative,* included the following three aims and specifically called for the development of a rural CBPR model as a part of the grant deliverables.

- Determine the research milieu in Libby, Montana, by conducting a focused community assessment to include:
  - History of research in the community
  - Infrastructure (services and resources) available to support the communication and translation of research in the community
  - Libby residents' awareness, knowledge, and acceptance of research
  - Libby residents' preferred method of communication about research
- Design, implement, and evaluate strategies for communicating research opportunities and results to Libby residents to
  - Be used by researchers to facilitate research communication in Libby, Montana
  - Increase community residents' awareness, knowledge, and acceptance of research
  - Enhance the existing local research infrastructure for communication of research to community members.
- Develop the foundation for a rural CBPR model that fosters community involvement in research and guides researchers working in rural communities.

Finally, Study 3 contributed further insight toward the development of the model described in the third aim of Study 2. An MSU master's in nursing student and Libby community member, Natasha Nicole Blata-Pennock, worked with the CARD/MSU team to conduct a study entitled *Communication and Information Exchange in Libby, Montana: A Secondary Data Analysis of Community Advisory Group Meeting Summaries.* This retrospective, qualitative study was launched based on the following problem statement:

Effective communication is an essential component to the success of community-based activities. Although the Libby Community Advisory Group (CAG) was developed [by the Environmental Protection Agency (EPA)] as a forum for two way communication and information exchange between the community and agencies involved in the (Libby) clean-up efforts, little is known about preferred modes of communication and the community's acceptance and resistance to biomedical and behavioral research (Blata-Pennock, 2010, p. 10).

The study of existing EPA documents identified "concerns, perceptions, and preferences of rural Libby residents related to research communication and other issues critical to the population's health and well-being" (p. 10). The qualitative analysis of themes utilized Rural Nursing Theory (Long & Weinert, 1989; Winters & Lee, 2018), Covello's Risk Communication Model (Covello & Allen, 1988), and increased awareness of communication preferences related to research in a rural community.

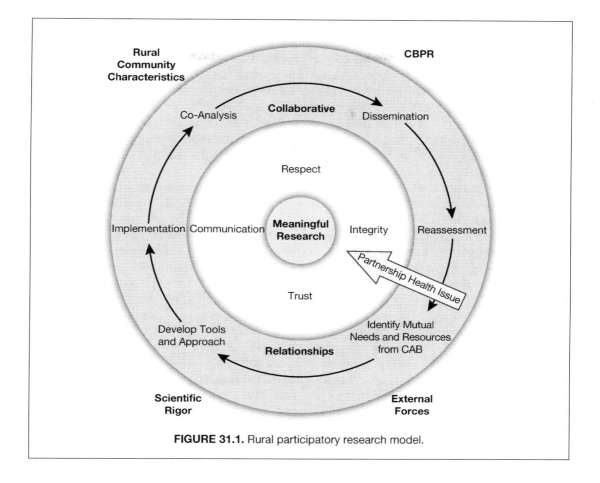

FIGURE 31.1. Rural participatory research model.

The purpose of this chapter is to report on the development of the community-generated Rural Participatory Research Model (RPRM) that emerged from results of the three studies conducted in Libby, Montana between 2006 and 2010. The RPRM (Figure 31.1) was developed to help guide researchers working with rural communities experiencing the ongoing effects of an environmental disaster.

BACKGROUND

Libby, Montana is considered rural (population 2,663) (U.S. Census Bureau, 2018); the surrounding county is designated frontier with a population of 19,980 and 5.4 people/square mile (U.S. Census Bureau, 2019). From the 1920s until 1990, vermiculite ore contaminated with amphibole asbestos was mined, processed, and distributed from Libby to more than 200 processing facilities across the United States accounting for 80% of the world's supply (U.S. Environmental Protection Agency, 2017). Vermiculite is a natural-occurring fibrous mineral widely used in industry and construction (U.S. EPA, 2003). Contaminated vermiculite was also widely disbursed in south Lincoln County as it was available by the truck load, free of charge, and used as a soil conditioner in gardens, as insulation for homes and business, and as foundations for school running tracks and driveways.

In 1999, a media exposé revealed possible community-wide amphibole asbestos exposure. Amphibole asbestos is a toxic mineral associated with lung cancer, mesothelioma, and nonmalignant lung and pleural disorders, including asbestosis, pleural plaques, pleural thickening, and pleural effusions (Amandus et al., 1987a, b). In 2000 and 2001, medical screening of more than 6,668 current and former Libby residents revealed pleural abnormalities in 18% of participants and interstitial abnormalities in less than 1%. By comparison, the rate of pleural abnormalities in non–asbestos-exposed populations in the United States ranged from 0.2% to 2.3% (Agency for Toxic Substances and Disease Registry, 2003). In an analysis of death records, asbestosis mortality in Libby was found to be 40 to 80 times higher than expected and lung cancer mortality 1.2 to 1.3 times higher than expected when compared to Montana and the United States, respectively (ATSDR, 2002).

The extent of community-wide asbestos contamination warranted EPA designation as a Superfund site in 2002. Seven years later, the first public health emergency in U.S. history was declared in Libby under the Comprehensive Environmental Response, Compensation, and Liability Act (CERCLA), also known as the Superfund Law, due to the high rates of morbidity and mortality (U.S. Department of Health & Human Services, 2009). At that point in time, generations of individuals had been exposed over a 70-year span of time. Since respiratory compromise can take 10 to 40 years to materialize following asbestos exposure, it was clear that the community needed a long-term healthcare response as the disaster was continuing to unfold. The CARD clinic, a nonprofit community-based clinic in Libby, continues to this day to screen people for asbestos-related diseases (ARDs) and lung cancer. From July 1, 2011, through May 31, 2020, CARD screened 7,020 people; 2,680 were diagnosed with ARD. CARD also provides ongoing healthcare for those diagnosed as well as outreach and education to a regional audience.

METHODS

Development of the RPRM (see Figure 31.1) evolved over time as the CARD/MSU team addressed research questions posed by community members, CARD clinicians, and MSU nurse researchers. Study 1 provided entry to the community and the initial opportunity to work with the CARD clinic personnel. All three studies in this analysis used a CBPR approach and created an opportunity to work continuously with the CARD clinicians. To assure community engagement and voice, a community advisory board (CAB) was formed at the beginning of the first study to provide input to the investigators at every stage of the research. The research design and methods used for each study varied based on the project goals and specific aims.

For Study 1 (Winters et al., 2008), a descriptive cross-sectional study design was used by the team to explore the (1) respiratory health status and respiratory health-related quality of life (HRQOL) of a cohort of persons exposed to LAA (Winters et al., 2012); (2) the psychosocial health status (depression, stress, and acceptance of illness) and differences in psychosocial health based on age, gender, residence, exposure pathway, insurance status, and access to care (Weinert et al., 2011); and (3) the perceived satisfaction with access and financial aspects of care among the CARD clinic's local and distant clients (Winters et al., 2011).

For Study 2, case study research methods (Yin, 2009) were applied to the study aims. The embedded single-case design followed three principles of data collection. First, multiple sources of both quantitative and qualitative evidence were collected (archival records, direct observation, and community member surveys) and analyzed to begin building the case during the first year of the project. Second, a case study database was created to organize and document the evidence. The database contributed to outcome reliability, project evaluation, and the final report. Finally, construct validity and an enhanced quality of case design was achieved as the chain of evidence was maintained. Throughout the 2-year investigation, a study protocol guided each phase of the project and provided structure for the evaluation of project inputs (e.g., research and process data), formative outputs (e.g., data analysis), and summative outcomes (e.g., final case study and foundation for the rural research model). The initial case study research protocol developed by the CARD/MSU team was enhanced and revised through community input and feedback from the CAB (Winters et al., 2014).

Study 3 (Blata-Pennock, 2010), a retrospective, descriptive, qualitative study, used content and thematic analysis of existing EPA documents to search for and identify concerns, perceptions, preferences, and research communication themes critical to the population's health and wellbeing within the Libby community. Four years of meeting summaries (2001, 2003, 2006, and 2008) from the CAG formed by the EPA were selected for analysis. Years chosen for review coincided with seminal events associated with asbestos mitigation in the community. For instance, year 2001 was the first year of CAG and the year ATSDR released the asbestos medical screening report. Year 2003 represents the year after Libby was placed on the EPA National Priorities List (NPL) as a Superfund site. Year 2006 represents a time of continued clean-up efforts by the EPA, and 2008 is the year leading up to the CAG dissolvement and the period of time shortly before the federal public health emergency was declared in Libby. A total of 53 meeting summaries were analyzed with themes sorted based on five topics: primary information exchange; communication characteristics; community awareness, knowledge, concerns, perceptions, preferences, acceptance and resistance to healthcare and clean-up; acceptance and resistance to biomedical and behavioral research; characteristics of rural residents; and evidence of rules of risk communication. Analysis of the primary information exchange topic and characteristics of rural residents/rules of risk communication proved most valuable to the RPRM model development and confirmation.

RESULTS: RURAL PARTICIPATORY RESEARCH MODEL COMPONENTS

Findings related to all three studies contributed to the development of the RPRM. The components of the model are *italicized* in this section.

Study 1

In Study 1, the direct contribution to RPRM included the importance of establishing a relationship with the community by responding to specific needs raised by CARD on behalf of community members impacted by exposure to LAA. The research questions were generated from the community and a partnership was established that respected the tenets of CBPR. Study 1 allowed the MSU team entry to the community and *an opportunity to build trust, establish mutual respect, observe and exhibit integrity, and create effective methods of communicating with the CARD clinicians and community members.* For instance, in addition to creating the CAB, the MSU/CARD team planned special evening events and participated in community-based research rallies to better inform and connect with community members. At the center of the RPRM, *meaningful research* is surrounded by basic principles of partnership and *collaborative relationships – mutual trust, respect, integrity, and communication.*

For Study 1, the research team first used existing clinical data of 329 clients (chest radiographs, pulmonary function tests, smoking history, demographic characteristics, and SGRQ results) to examine the respiratory health status (55% had pleural abnormalities; 21% had both pleural and interstitial abnormalities; 18% had no documented lung abnormality based on chest x-ray) and HRQOL scores from the SGRQ. The SGRQ results for the Libby cohort indicated significantly lower scores for HRQOL compared to healthy people and "appreciably worse than some persons with chronic obstructive pulmonary disease" (Winters et al., 2012, p. 8).

Next, the team applied three measures (Center for Epidemiological Studies-Depression Scale [CES-D]; Perceived Stress Scale [PSS]; and Acceptance of Illness Scale [AOI]) to determine the psychosocial health status (depression, stress, and acceptance of illness) of 386 CARD clinic clients. Results indicated "participants demonstrated moderate levels of stress and acceptance of illness however more than one-third (34.5%) had depression scores indicating a clinically significant level of psychological distress" (Weinert et al., 2011, p. 9). For the CARD/MSU research team, these findings pointed to the importance of caring for not just the physical/pulmonary health of citizens exposed to LAA but the emotional health needs as well. "Psychological distress identification, prevention, and intervention strategies, including self-management skills, are needed for persons exposed to environmental and workplace contamination such as the LAA disaster." (p. 9)

The final inquiry in Study 1 addressed the perceived satisfaction with access/financial aspects of care among the CARD clinic's local and distant clients. Two of seven subscales of the Medical Outcomes, Patient Satisfaction Questionnaire (PSQ-III) were used. The 12-item Access, Availability, and Convenience subscale measured perception of availability of medical resources, waiting times, and continuity of care. The Financial Aspects of Care subscale assessed perception of difficulty in paying for medical care (Ware & Hays, 1988). The two PSQ-III subscales were administered to 426 CARD clients during regular clinic visits. The research team concluded:

> *The presence of the CARD clinic providing .... specialty care services may serve as a stopgap and somewhat of an equalizing factor for the provision of care to ... patients; however, when compared to persons with other chronic illnesses, the Libby cohort was significantly less satisfied with access and financial aspects of care. Among the Libby cohort, younger participants were less satisfied with access and financial aspects of care than older members, while exposure through a family member or household contact (versus other routes of exposure) and having a limited source of insurance .... resulted in the lowest scores on satisfaction with financial aspects of care (Winters et al., 2011, p. 6).*

In addition to a robust biopsychosocial description of a sample of CARD patients exposed to LAA, the three inquiries for Study 1 helped demonstrate the value and capability of the team to apply *scientific rigor* to community questions. At each stage of the research *(identification of needs and resources, selection of tools and approaches, implementation, co-analysis of the results, dissemination, and reassessment needs for the next project)*, community members on the CAB and clinicians of the CARD clinic provided insight and an explanation of the meaning of the findings to the researchers.

Study 2

Study 1 set the stage for the development of RPRM. Study 2 took the model to the next step by exploring "the community's history of asbestos-related research, community-based research infrastructure, and rural residents' views on and willingness to participate in research" (Winters et al., 2014, p. 214). The case study investigation involved multiple data sources and a complex data management tracking system. The results were summarized based on the four study propositions that related directly to the issues raised by community members. The case study model was grounded in theory and advanced based on context and proposition development. Data were collected from a variety of archival sources (records, media, and meeting minutes) or generated from interviews and surveys as needed. The result (discovery) led to the case results and confirmation of RPRM key components.

The first proposition addressed community history and the erosion of trust that took place over a period of at least three decades. Early studies uncovered high mortality rates among mineworkers and subsequently, family members who received secondary exposure to asbestos. When community environmental hazards are identified, decisions to remove the public from potential exposures often result in closing areas or moving people away from the hazard. However, in Libby, the EPA conducted the clean-up as citizens went about their daily lives. Communication conflicts between the public and scientific/technical experts, business, community, and political leaders and policymakers frequently resulted in skepticism, mistrust, and increased public wariness. The obstacles and stages of risk communication (Covello & Allen, 1988) provide credence to the value of reciprocal listening and consistent messaging since once *trust, respect, integrity/ authenticity, and communication* are lost, all are difficult to reclaim.

The second proposition involved the infrastructure to support communication and translation of research. A critical resource noted by community members is the CARD specialty clinic, which not only provides diagnostic and supportive care to clients but also serves as liaison and gatekeeper between the community and outside researchers. Rural Nursing Theory proved valuable in understanding the value of CARD as an internal resource to community members. *Characteristics of rural people* include "hardiness, self-sufficiency, independence, work oriented, distrusting of 'outsiders' and 'newcomers' and trustful and respectful of 'old timers' (people who have lived in the community for an extended period of time" (Long & Weinert, 1989; Winters et al., 2011, pp. 215–216). Trusted gatekeepers with insight into community characteristics, beliefs, and values are best suited to support communication and translation of research.

The third proposition identified divergent views between residents (community members) and researchers related to communication resources including the most common, effective, trusted, and preferred methods for receiving (by residents) or transmitting (by researchers) research information. Residents identified the local newspaper (72%) and the local radio station (61%) as the most common methods for learning about research. The most effective but least trusted communication source was word of mouth (50%). Conversely, when researchers were asked about the preferred methods for transmitting research information, the researchers chose scientific publications, public forums like CAG, or CARD-sponsored research rallies. This communication *dissemination* variation depicts an important cultural gap between residents and researchers, which should be investigated and resolved with the help of a community liaison.

The fourth proposition highlighted the importance of community engagement factors and confirmed agreement between residents and researchers. Residents indicated they were more likely to participate in research if the research "was worthwhile (52%); helped the community (49%); benefited their family (48%); or improved their healthcare (40%)" (Winters et al., 2011, p. 222). Researchers believed residents would be more likely to participate "if the research was perceived as having a potential to benefit participant health" (p. 223). A principal components analysis related to Propositions 3 and 4 (communication and community engagement factors) examined "empirical dimensions of attitudes towards research participation including community engagement at a designated Superfund site" (Winters et al., 2016, p. 7). Principal components showed four dimensions of community members' attitudes toward research engagement: (1) researcher communication and contributions to the community; (2) identity and affiliation of the researchers requesting participation; (3) potential personal barriers including data confidentiality, painful or invasive procedures, and effects on health insurance, and (4) research benefits for the community, oneself, or family.

Study 3

"The purpose of (the third) study was to use existing documents (CAG meeting summaries) to identify concerns, perceptions, and communication preferences of rural Libby residents related to research and other issues critical to the community's health and well-being" (Blata-Pennock, 2010, p. 48). Qualitative results from analysis of 53 CAG meeting summaries identified critical *external forces* that impacted the community from 2001 to 2008 including political and economic impacts; governmental intervention by the EPA; external research funding; health issues; mine ownership litigation; federal asbestos and healthcare legislation; and public health emergency and Superfund designations. This study identified 11 primary information exchange topics that emerged from participants of CAG and were noted in the meeting summaries.

Of the 11 most and least topics discussed during the 53 CAG meetings, the top four primary information exchange topics included first, cleanup activities in Libby ($n = 51$); second, government agency involvement in activities ($n = 50$); third, funding and finances ($n = 48$); and fourth, health issues among community members ($n = 43$). The least discussed topics included the Superfund designation ($n = 11$); the public health emergency designation ($n = 19$); the community economy ($n = 23$); and, the CAG purpose and process ($n = 24$). The qualitative themes uncovered in the Blata-Pennock (2010, p. 50) analysis provided the granular-level concerns of community members as they discussed issues critical to the community's health.

Examples of *rural community characteristics* including independence/self-reliance, hardiness/resilience, distance/isolation, and insider/outsider perceptions are captured in comments from CAG community members (Blata-Pennock, 2010, pp. 86–88).

- Independence and self-reliance: "We need to continue working hard and persistently with the tools available to us. The heavens are not going to open and rain money on us" (p. 87).
- Hardiness and resilience: "As frustrating as things are, we should recognize how far we have come ... It is important not to dwell on the negative" (p. 87).
- Distance and isolation: "Community isolation from specialty healthcare services ... [caused concern] since the only pulmonologist that worked with the community [was retirement age]" (p. 87).
- Outsider/insider: "People in Libby have trust and confidence in the CARD clinic and willing to provide information to it. They may not be as willing to share their information with an outside university" (p. 88).

Study 3 confirmed and reinforced many of the RPRM concepts, especially precepts located in the outer circle of the model: *rural community characteristics, external forces, CBPR, and scientific rigor of research.*

CONCLUSION

The rural community of Libby, Montana, was thrust into the national spotlight in the 1990s and, to this day, the population continues to deal with the sequelae and fallout of this technologic, environmental disaster. The RPRM was developed to help guide researchers working with rural communities experiencing the ongoing effects of an environmental disaster. Although not specifically designed or patterned after logic-model metrics, the CARD/MSU team recognized the critical nature of inputs (knowledge of community history, patterns, and beliefs); activities and outputs conducted based on community member insights (meaningful research grounded on mutual respect, integrity/authenticity, trust, and communication); a research plan with short-term and long-term outcomes (publishable scientific data that will lead to new knowledge and improved health outcomes for the population).

The RPRM may be used by research teams when conducting research within and with other rural communities, whether experiencing an environmental disaster or another type of event. Research in rural communities cannot be adequately conducted by the application of research models developed for urban or suburban areas but requires unique approaches emphasizing the special needs of these communities and populations. Building upon the tenets of rural nursing theory and CBPR, the RPRM is well suited for research conducted in partnership with rural residents.

REFERENCES

Agency for Toxic Substances and Disease Registry. (2002). *Mortality in Libby, Montana (1979–1998)*. https://www.atsdr.cdc.gov/hac/pha/LibbyAsbestosSite/MT_LibbyHCMortalityRev8-8-2002_508.pdf

Agency for Toxic Substances and Disease Registry. (2003). *Public health assessment*. https://www.atsdr.cdc.gov/news/libby-pha.pdf

Amandus, H. E., Althouse, R., Morgan, W. K., Sargent, E. N., & Jones, R. (1987a). The morbidity and mortality of vermiculite miners and millers exposed to tremolite-actinolite: Part III. Radiographic findings. *American Journal of Industrial Medicine*, 11(1), 27–37. https://doi.org/10.1002/ajim.4700110104

Amandus, H. E., Wheeler, R., Jankovic, J., & Tucker, J. (1987b). The morbidity and mortality of vermiculite miners and millers exposed to tremolite–actinolite: Part I. Exposure estimates. *American Journal of Industrial Medicine*, 11(1), 1–14. https://doi.org/10.1002/ajim.4700110102

Blata-Pennock, N. (2010). *Communication and information exchange in Libby, Montana: A secondary data analysis of community advisory group meeting summaries* [masters thesis, Montana State University] ScholarWorks.

Center for Asbestos Related Disease. (2020). Welcome *to CARD*. https://libbyasbestos.org/

Covello, V., & Allen, F. (1988). The EPA's seven cardinal rules of risk communication. http://www.wvdhhr.org/bphtraining/courses/cdcynergy/content/activeinformation/resources/epa_seven_cardinal_rules.pdf

Jones, P. W., Quirk, F. H., Baveystock, C. M., & Littlejohns, P. (1992). A self-complete measure of health status for chronic airflow limitation. *The St. George's Respiratory Questionnaire. American Review Respiratory Disease*, 145(6), 1321–1327. https://doi.org/10.1164/ajrccm/145.6.1321

Long, K. A., & Weinert, C. (1989). Rural nursing: Developing the theory base. *Scholarly Inquiry for Nursing Practice*, 3(2), 113–127. https://doi.org/10.1891/sinp.3.2

U.S. Census Bureau. (2018). *American community survey: Libby, Montana*. https://data.census.gov/cedsci/table?q=Libby,%20Montana&g=1600000US3043450&layer=VT_2018_160_00_PY_D1&hidePreview=false&tid=ACSDP5Y2018.DP05&cid=DP05_0001E&vintage=2018

U.S. Census Bureau. (2019). QuickFacts: Lincoln County, Montana. https://www.census.gov/quickfacts/fact/table/lincolncountymontana,US/PST045219

U.S. Department of Health & Human Services. (2009). *EPA announces public health emergency in Libby, Montana.* https://yosemite.epa.gov/opa/admpress.nsf/bd4379a92ceceeac8525735900400c27/0d16234d252 c98-f9852575d8005e63ac!opendocument

U.S. Environmental Protection Agency. (2003). *ABCs of asbestos in schools.* https://www.epa.gov/sites/ production/files/documents/abcsfinal.pdf

U.S. Environmental Protection Agency. (2017). *Libby site background.* https://cumulis.epa.gov/ supercpad/cursites/csitinfo.cfm?id=0801744

Ware, J. E. Jr., & Hays, R. D. (1988). Methods for measuring patient satisfaction with specific medical encounters. *Medical Care, 26*(4), 393–402.

Weinert, C., Hill, W. G., Winters, C. A., Kuntz, S. W., Rowse, K., Hernandez, T., Black, B., Cudney, S. (2011). Psychosocial health status of persons seeking treatment for exposure to Libby amphibole asbestos. *ISRN Nursing, 2011*, 735936. https://doi.org/10.5402/2011/735936

Winters, C. A., Hill, W. G., Kuntz, S. W., Weinert, C., Rowse, K., Hernandez, T., & Black, B. (2011). Determining satisfaction with access and financial aspects of care for persons exposed to Libby amphibole asbestos: Rural and national environmental policy implications. *Journal of Environmental and Public Health, 2011*, 789514. https://doi.org/10.1155/2011/789514

Winters, C. A., Hill, W. G., Rowse, K., Black, B., Kuntz, S. W., & Weinert, C. (2012). Descriptive analysis of the respiratory health status of persons exposed to Libby amphibole asbestos. *BMJ Open, 2*(6). https://doi.org/10.1136/bmjopen-2012-001552

Winters, C. A., Kuntz, S. W., Weinert, C., & Black, B. (2014). A case study exploring research communication and engagement in a rural community experiencing an environmental disaster. *Applied Environmental Education & Communication, 13*(4), 213–226. https://doi.org/10.1080/15330 15X.2014.970718

Winters, C. A., & Lee, H. S. (Eds.). (2018). *Rural nursing: Concepts, theory and practice* (5th ed.). Springer Publishing Company.

Winters, C. A., Moore, C. F., Kuntz, S. W., Weinert, C., Hernandez, T., & Black, B. (2016). Principal components analysis to identify influences on research communication and engagement during an environmental disaster. *BMJ Open, 6*(8), e012106. https://doi.org/10.1136/bmjopen-2016-012106

Winters, C. A., Rowse, K., Kuntz, S. W., & Weinert, C. (2008). *The Libby Project.* Health Services and Resources Administration 1P20NR07790-01.

Yin, R. (2009). *Case study research: Design and methods* (4th ed.). Sage.

Index